Pediatric Critical Care

Editors

LAUREN R. SORCE
JOY D. HOWELL

CRITICAL CARE CLINICS

www.criticalcare.theclinics.com

Consulting Editor
GREGORY S. MARTIN

April 2023 • Volume 39 • Number 2

ELSEVIER

1600 John F. Kennedy Boulevard • Suite 1800 • Philadelphia, Pennsylvania, 19103-2899

http://www.theclinics.com

CRITICAL CARE CLINICS Volume 39, Number 2
April 2023 ISSN 0749-0704, ISBN-13: 978-0-323-93875-4

Editor: Joanna Gascoine
Developmental Editor: Hannah Almira Lopez

Critical Care Clinics (ISSN: 0749-0704) is published quarterly by Elsevier Inc., 360 Park Avenue South, New York, NY 10010-1710. Months of issue are January, April, July, and October. Business and Editorial Offices: 1600 John F. Kennedy Blvd., Suite 1800, Philadelphia, PA 19103-2899. Customer Service Office: 6277 Sea Harbor Drive, Orlando, FL 32887-4800. Periodicals postage paid at New York, NY and additional mailing offices. Subscription prices are $274.00 per year for US individuals, $779 per year for US institutions, $100.00 per year for US students and residents, $305.00 per year for Canadian individuals, $976.00 per year for Canadian institutions, $348.00 per year for international individuals, $976.00 per year for international institutions, $100.00 per year for Canadian students/residents, and $150.00 per year for foreign students/residents. To receive student/resident rate, orders must be accompanied by name of affiliated institution, date of term, and the signature of program/residency coordinator on institution letterhead. Orders will be billed at individual rate until proof of status is received. Foreign air speed delivery is included in all Clinics subscription prices. All prices are subject to change without notice. POSTMASTER: Send address changes to Critical Care Clinics, Elsevier Periodicals Customer Service, 11830 Westline Industrial Drive, St. Louis, MO 63146. **Customer Service: 1-800-654-2452 (US). From outside of the US, call 1-314-447-8871. Fax: 1-314-447-8029. E-mail: journalscustomerservice-usa@elsevier.com (for print support) or journalsonlinesupport-usa@elsevier.com (for online support).**

Reprints. For copies of 100 or more of articles in this publication, please contact the Commercial Reprints Department, Elsevier Inc., 360 Park Avenue South, New York, NY 10010-1710. Tel.: 212-633-3874; Fax: 212-633-3820; E-mail: reprints@elsevier.com.

Critical Care Clinics is also published in Spanish by Editorial Inter-Medica, Junin 917, 1er A, 1113, Buenos Aires, Argentina.

Critical Care Clinics is covered in MEDLINE/PubMed (Index Medicus), EMBASE/Excerpta Medica, Current Concepts/Clinical Medicine, ISI/BIOMED, and Chemical Abstracts.

Contributors

CONSULTING EDITOR

GREGORY S. MARTIN, MD, MSC
Professor, Division of Pulmonary, Allergy, Critical Care and Sleep Medicine, Research Director, Emory Critical Care Center, Director, Emory/Georgia Tech Predictive Health Institute, Co-Director, Atlanta Center for Microsystems Engineered Point-of-Care Technologies (ACME POCT), President, Society of Critical Care Medicine, Atlanta, Georgia, USA

EDITORS

LAUREN R. SORCE, PhD, RN, CPNP-AC/PC, FCCM, FAAN
Founders Board Nurse Scientist, Associate Director Nursing Research, Ann & Robert H. Lurie Children's Hospital of Chicago, Assistant Professor, Division of Pediatric Critical Care Medicine, Northwestern University Feinberg School of Medicine, Pediatric Critical Care Nurse Practitioner, Chicago, Illinois, USA

JOY D. HOWELL, MD, FAAP, FCCM
Assistant Dean for Diversity and Student Life, Vice Chair for Diversity in Pediatrics, Professor of Clinical Pediatrics, Weill Cornell Medicine, Office of Student Diversity, Department of Pediatrics, Division of Pediatric Critical Care Medicine, New York, New York, USA

AUTHORS

HIBA ABUELHIJA, MD
Fellow in Pediatric Critical Care Medicine, Pediatric Critical Care, Hadassah University Medical Center, Hadassah Ein Kerem, Jerusalem, Israel

MANZILAT AKANDE, MD, MPH
Section of Critical Care, Department of Pediatrics, Oklahoma University Health Sciences Center, Oklahoma City, Oklahoma, USA

RYAN P. BARBARO, MD, MSC
Division of Pediatric Critical Care, University of Michigan Medical School, Susan B. Miester Child Health Evaluation and Research Center, University of Michigan, Ann Arbor, Michigan, USA

RONALD A. BRONICKI, MD, FCCM, FACC
Division of Critical Care Medicine, Department of Pediatrics, Baylor College of Medicine, Texas Children's Hospital, Houston, Texas, USA

RACHEL CHAPMAN, MD
Department of Pediatrics, Division of Neonatology, Fetal and Neonatal Institute, Children's Hospital, Department of Pediatrics, Keck School of Medicine of University of Southern California, Los Angeles, California, USA

PAUL A. CHECCHIA, MD, FCCM, FACC
Division of Critical Care Medicine, Department of Pediatrics, Baylor College of Medicine, Texas Children's Hospital, Houston, Texas, USA

THOMAS CONLON, MD
Division of Critical Care Medicine, Department of Anesthesiology and Critical Care Medicine, Children's Hospital of Philadelphia, University of Pennsylvania, Philadelphia, Pennsylvania, USA

MARTHA A.Q. CURLEY, PhD, RN, FAAN
Ruth M. Colket Endowed Chair in Pediatric Nursing, Children's Hospital of Philadelphia, Professor, Department of Family and Community Health, University of Pennsylvania School of Nursing, Professor, Department of Anesthesia and Critical Care Medicine, Perelman School of Medicine, University of Pennsylvania, Philadelphia, Pennsylvania, USA

MARY DAHMER, PhD
Division of Critical Care, Department of Pediatrics, University of Michigan, Ann Arbor, Michigan, USA

LISA DELSIGNORE, MD
Assistant Professor, Tufts University School of Medicine, Division of Pediatric Critical Care, Tufts Children's Hospital, Tufts Medical Center, Boston, Massachusetts, USA

LESLIE A. DERVAN, MD, MS
Co-Director, Neurocritical Care Program, Seattle Children's Hospital, Associate Professor, Division of Pediatric Critical Care Medicine, University of Washington, Seattle, Washington, USA

IVIE ESANGBEDO, MD
Associate Professor, Division of Pediatric Critical Care, Seattle Children's Hospital, University of Washington School of Medicine, Seattle, Washington, USA

ERICKA L. FINK, MD, MS
Department of Critical Care Medicine, UPMC Children's Hospital of Pittsburgh, Pittsburgh, Pennsylvania, USA

SARAH GINSBURG, MD
Division of Critical Care Medicine, Department of Pediatrics, The University of Texas Southwestern Medical Center, Dallas, Texas, USA

KATELIN HOSKINS, PhD, MBE, CRNP
Assistant Professor of Nursing, University of Pennsylvania School of Nursing, Philadelphia, Pennsylvania, USA

ROBERT HYSLOP, RN
Heart Institute, Children's Hospital Colorado, Aurora, Colorado, USA

SHARON Y. IRVING, PhD, CRNP, Associate Professor of Pediatric Nursing, Division of Critical Care Medicine, Cincinnati Children's Hospital Medical Center, University of Cincinnati, Cincinnati, Ohio, USA

AIMEE JENNINGS, CPNP-AC/PC, FCCM
Division of Critical Care Medicine, Advanced Practice, Seattle Children's Hospital, Seattle, Washington, USA

CHRISTINE JOYCE, MD
Department of Pediatrics, Division of Pediatric Critical Care Medicine, Weill Cornell Medicine, New York, New York, USA

OLIVER KARAM, MD, PhD
Professor, Department of Pediatrics, Yale School of Medicine, New Haven, Connecticut, USA

ELINORE J. KAUFMAN, MD, MSHP
Assistant Professor of Surgery, Division of Traumatology, Surgical Critical Care, and Emergency Surgery, Perelman School of Medicine, University of Pennsylvania, Penn Presbyterian Medical Center, Philadelphia, Pennsylvania, USA

ROXANNE KIRSCH, MD, MBE
Division of Cardiac Critical Care, Department of Critical Care Medicine, Clinical Bioethics Associate, Department of Bioethics, The Hospital for Sick Children, Toronto, Ontario, Canada

ANISHA KSHETRAPAL, MD, MSEd
Assistant Professor, Department of Pediatrics, Division of Emergency Medicine, Ann & Robert H Lurie Children's Hospital of Chicago, Chicago, Illinois, USA

JOEL K.B. LIM, MBBS, MRCPCH
Children's Intensive Care Unit, Department of Pediatric Subspecialties, KK Women's and Children's Hospital, Singapore

GRAEME MACLAREN, MBBS, MSC
Cardiothoracic Intensive Care Unit, National University Health System, Singapore

PAULA MAGEE, MD, MPH
Division of Critical Care Medicine, Department of Pediatrics, Ann & Robert H. Lurie Children's Hospital of Chicago, Chicago, Illinois, USA

CANDACE MANNARINO, MD
Assistant Professor, Department of Pediatrics, Divisions of Cardiology and Critical Care Medicine, Ann & Robert H Lurie Children's Hospital of Chicago, Chicago, Illinois, USA

JOSEPH C. MANNING, PhD, RN
Clinical Associate Professor/Charge Nurse, Paediatric Critical Care Outreach, Nottingham Children's Hospital, Nottingham University Hospitals NHS Trust, Queens Medical Centre Campus, Associate Professor/Deputy Director, Centre for Children and Young People Health Research, School of Health Sciences, University of Nottingham, Nottingham, United Kingdom

MJAYE L. MAZWI, MBCHB
Department of Critical Care Medicine, Division of Cardiology, The Hospital for Sick Children, Toronto, Ontario, Canada

MARY E. McBRIDE, MD, MEd
Associate Professor of Pediatrics and Medical Education, Department of Pediatrics, Divisions of Cardiology and Critical Care Medicine, Ann & Robert H Lurie Children's Hospital of Chicago, Chicago, Illinois, USA

NDIDIAMAKA MUSA, MD
Professor, Division of Pediatric Critical Care, Seattle Children's Hospital, University of Washington School of Medicine, Seattle, Washington, USA

CARLIE MYERS, MD, MS
Instructor, Division of Critical Care Medicine, Cincinnati Children's Hospital Medical Center, University of Cincinnati, Cincinnati, Ohio, USA

MARIANNE NELLIS, MD, MS
Associate Professor, Department of Pediatrics, Division of Pediatric Critical Care Medicine, Weill Cornell Medicine, New York, New York, USA

AKIRA NISHISAKI, MD, MSCE
Division of Critical Care Medicine, Department of Anesthesiology and Critical Care Medicine, Children's Hospital of Philadelphia, University of Pennsylvania, Philadelphia, Pennsylvania, USA

JACQUELINE S.M. ONG, MB BChir (Cantab)
Division of Paediatric Critical Care, Khoo Teck Puat–University Children's Medical Institute, National University Hospital, Department of Paediatrics, Yong Loo Lin School of Medicine, National University of Singapore, Singapore

JENNA PACHECO, PharmD, BCPPS
Division of Palliative Care, Tufts Children's Hospital, Tufts Medical Center, Boston, Massachusetts, USA

ERIN T. PAQUETTE, MD
Division of Critical Care Medicine, Department of Pediatrics, Ann & Robert H. Lurie Children's Hospital of Chicago, Chicago, Illinois, USA

MARGARET PARKER, MD, MCCM
Department of Pediatrics, Stony Brook University, Easton, Maryland, USA

MALLORY A. PERRY-EADDY, PhD, RN, CCRN
Assistant Professor, Department of Pediatrics, University of Connecticut School of Nursing, Storrs, Connecticut, USA; Assistant Professor, Department of Pediatrics, University of Connecticut School of Medicine, Farmington, Connecticut, USA

BLYTHE E. POLLACK, MSN, CPNP-AC
Division of Pediatric Critical Care, University of Michigan Medical School, Ann Arbor, Michigan, USA

MICHELLE RAMIREZ, MD
Division of Pediatric Critical Care Medicine, Department of Pediatrics, NYU Langone Medical Center, Hassenfeld Children's Hospital, New York, New York, USA

THERESE S. RICHMOND, PhD, RN, FAAN
Andrea B. Laporte Professor of Nursing, Associate Dean for Research and Innovation, University of Pennsylvania School of Nursing, Philadelphia, Pennsylvania, USA

JULIANA ROMANO, MD
Department of Pediatrics, Division of Pediatric Critical Care Medicine, Weill Cornell Medicine, New York, New York, USA

SARA ROSS, MD
Associate Professor, Tufts University School of Medicine, Division of Pediatric Critical Care, Tufts Children's Hospital, Tufts Medical Center, Boston, Massachusetts, USA

LAZARO N. SANCHEZ-PINTO, MD, MBI, FAMIA
Department of Pediatrics, Ann and Robert H. Lurie Children's Hospital of Chicago,
Northwestern University Feinberg School of Medicine, Chicago, Illinois, USA

JENNIFER SHENKER, MD
Fellow in Pediatric Critical Care Medicine, Department of Pediatrics, NewYork
Presbyterian Hospital, Weill Cornell Medicine, New York, New York, USA

KATHERINE N. SLAIN, DO
Division of Pediatric Critical Care Medicine, University Hospitals Rainbow Babies &
Children's Hospital, Department of Pediatrics, Case Western Reserve University School
of Medicine, Cleveland, Ohio, USA

ANN THOMPSON, MD, MCCM
Department of Critical Care Medicine, Vice Dean, University of Pittsburgh, Pittsburgh,
Pennsylvania, USA

YUEN LIE TJOENG, MD, MS
Assistant Professor, Division of Pediatric Critical Care, Seattle Children's Hospital,
University of Washington School of Medicine, Seattle, Washington, USA

MEGAN TOAL, MD
Department of Pediatrics, Division of Pediatric Critical Care Medicine, Weill Cornell
Medicine, New York, New York, USA

CHANI TRAUBE, MD
Department of Pediatrics, Weill Cornell Medicine, New York, New York, USA

TAMARA VESEL, MD
Clinical Associate Professor of Medicine and Pediatrics, Tufts University School of
Medicine, Division of Palliative Care, Tufts Medical Center, Boston, USA

R. SCOTT WATSON, MD, MPH
Associate Division Chief, Division of Pediatric Critical Care Medicine, Children's Hospital,
Professor, Division of Pediatric Critical Care Medicine, University of Washington, Seattle,
Washington, USA

MARK D. WEBER, RN, CPNP-AC, FCCM
Division of Critical Care Medicine, Department of Anesthesiology and Critical Care
Medicine, Children's Hospital of Philadelphia, University of Pennsylvania, Philadelphia,
Pennsylvania, USA

KIMBERLY WHALEN, RN, MS, CCRN
Pediatric Intensive Care Unit, Mass General for Children, Boston, Massachusetts, USA

DEREK WHEELER, MD, MMM, MBA
Professor, Division of Critical Care, Ann & Robert H. Lurie Children's Hospital of Chicago,
Northwestern University Feinberg School of Medicine, Chicago, Illinois, USA

ERIC WILSTERMAN, MD
Department of Pediatrics, Division of Pediatric Critical Care Medicine, Weill Cornell
Medicine, New York, New York, USA

PHOEBE YAGER, MD
Assistant Professor, Harvard Medical School, Pediatric Intensive Care Unit, Mass General
for Children, Boston, Massachusetts, USA

JERRY J. ZIMMERMAN, MD, PHD, FCCM
Department of Pediatrics, Faculty, Pediatric Critical Care Medicine, Seattle Children's Hospital, Harborview Medical Center, University of Washington, School of Medicine, Seattle Children's Hospital, Seattle, Washington, USA

Contents

The transfusion of all blood components (red blood cells, plasma, and platelets) has been associated with increased morbidity and mortality in children. It is essential that pediatric providers weigh the risks and benefits before transfusing a critically ill child. A growing body of evidence has demonstrated the safety of restrictive transfusion practices in critically ill children.

Pediatric providers were called on to care for adult patients well beyond their typical scope of practice during the first surge of the SARS-CoV-2 pandemic. Here, the authors share novel viewpoints and innovations from the perspective of providers, consultants, and families. The authors enumerate several of the challenges encountered, including those faced by leadership in supporting teams, balancing competing responsibilities to children while caring for critically ill adult patients, preserving the model of interdisciplinary care, maintaining communication with families, and finding meaning in work during this unprecedented crisis.

Children who survive the pediatric intensive care unit (PICU) are at risk of developing post-intensive care syndrome in pediatrics (PICS-p). PICS-p, defined as new physical, cognitive, emotional, and/or social health dysfunction following critical illness, can affect the child and family. Historically, synthesizing PICU outcomes research has been challenging due to inconsistency in study design and in outcomes measurement. PICS-p risk may be mitigated by implementing intensive care unit best practices that limit iatrogenic injury and by supporting the resiliency of critically ill children and their families.

Literature suggests the pediatric critical care (PCC) workforce includes limited providers from groups underrepresented in medicine (URiM; African American/Black, Hispanic/Latinx, American Indian/Alaska Native, Native Hawaiian/Pacific Islander). Additionally, women and providers URiM hold fewer leadership positions regardless of health-care discipline or specialty. Data on sexual and gender minority representation and persons with different physical abilities within the PCC workforce are incomplete or unknown. More data are needed to understand the true landscape of the PCC workforce across disciplines. Efforts to increase representation, promote mentorship/sponsorship, and cultivate inclusivity must be prioritized to foster diversity and inclusion in PCC.

Social determinants of health (SDoH) play a significant role in the health and well-being of children in the United States. Disparities in the risk and outcomes of critical illness have been extensively documented but are yet to be fully explored through the lens of SDoH. In this review, we provide justification for routine SDoH screening as a critical first step toward understanding the causes of, and effectively addressing health disparities affecting critically ill children. Second, we summarize important aspects of SDoH screening that need to be considered before implementing this practice in the pediatric critical care setting.

Firearms are now the leading cause of death among youth in the United States, with rates of homicide and suicide rising even more steeply during the SARS-CoV-2 pandemic. These injuries and deaths have wide-ranging consequences for the physical and emotional health of youth and families. While pediatric critical care clinicians must treat the injured survivors, they can also play a role in prevention by understanding the risks and consequences of firearm injuries; taking a trauma-informed approach to the care of injured youth; counseling patients and families on firearm access; and advocating for youth safety policy and programming.

Simulation in health-care professions has grown in the last few decades. We provide an overview of the history of simulation in other fields, the trajectory of simulation in health professions education, and research in medical education, including the learning theories and tools to assess and evaluate simulation programs. We also propose future directions for simulation and research in health professions education.

Point-of-care ultrasound (POCUS) is now transitioning from an emerging technology to a standard of care for critically ill children. POCUS can provide immediate answers to clinical questions impacting management and outcomes within this fragile population. Recently published international guidelines specific to POCUS use in neonatal and pediatric critical care populations now complement previous Society of Critical Care Medicine guidelines. The authors review consensus statements within guidelines, identify important limitations to statements, and provide considerations for the successful implementation of POCUS in the pediatric critical care setting.

Mary Dahmer, Aimee Jennings, Margaret Parker, Lazaro N. Sanchez-Pinto, Ann Thompson, Chani Traube, and Jerry J. Zimmerman

Pediatric critical care addresses prevention, diagnosis, and treatment of organ dysfunction in the setting of increasingly complex patients, therapies, and environments. Soon burgeoning data science will enable all aspects of intensive care: driving facilitated diagnostics, empowering a learning health-care environment, promoting continuous advancement of care, and informing the continuum of critical care outside the intensive care unit preceding and following critical illness/injury. Although novel technology will progressively objectify personalized critical care, humanism, practiced at the bedside, defines the essence of pediatric critical care now and in the future.

CRITICAL CARE CLINICS

Preface

Looking Forward: Contemporary and Emerging Issues in Pediatric Critical Care Medicine

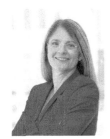   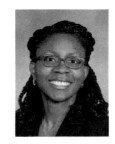

Lauren R. Sorce, PhD, RN, CPNP-AC/PC,   Joy D. Howell, MD, FAAP, FCCM
FCCM, FAAN

Editors

We are delighted to present this Pediatric issue of *Critical Care Clinics*. In this issue, you will find a variety of topics that address current and evolving issues relevant to the pediatric critical care team. This issue contains a few landscape reviews of old and new therapies, including a review of cardiovascular monitoring, advances in extracorporeal membrane oxygenation, and the application of CAR-T cell therapy for pediatric malignancies. To provide new perspectives on existing issues, we include content focused on transfusion medicine, experiences delivering critical care to adults during early waves of the pandemic, and pediatric critical care outcomes (beyond the traditional morbidity and mortality). There is content focused on social and societal issues that impact the health care and well-being of children, including discussions of workforce diversity, the benefits of social determinants of health screening in the PICU, and the impacts of gun violence. Last, as we look forward, we include discussions of simulation education, point-of-care ultrasound, and the future of Pediatric Critical Care Medicine.

To generate the highest-quality articles for this issue of *Critical Care Clinics*, we identified and invited a diverse group of authors with content expertise relative to the topics above. To demonstrate inclusive excellence, we fashioned writing teams that included authors from the different professions, at different stages of their careers, as well as reflecting the various nationalities and backgrounds presently represented within the pediatric critical care team.

During these tumultuous times and the changing landscape of health care around the world, we envision the opportunity to ground ourselves in our collective purpose of guiding children and their families through critical illness. As our specialty evolves,

Crit Care Clin 39 (2023) xv–xvi
https://doi.org/10.1016/j.ccc.2022.09.001
0749-0704/23/© 2022 Published by Elsevier Inc.

criticalcare.theclinics.com

we hope this issue provides readers with a broad overview of important topics that stimulate discussion, highlight areas ripe for further investigation, and inspire advocacy as we look forward to the future of pediatric critical care.

Lauren R. Sorce, PhD, RN, CPNP-AC/PC, FCCM, FAAN
Ann & Robert H. Lurie Children's Hospital of Chicago
Division of Pediatric Critical Care Medicine
Northwestern University, Feinberg School of Medicine
Pediatric Critical Care Nurse Practitioner
225 East Chicago Avenue
Chicago, IL 60611, USA

Joy D. Howell, MD, FAAP, FCCM
Weill Cornell Medicine
Department of Pediatrics
Division of Pediatric Critical Care Medicine
525 East 68th Street, M-508
New York, NY 10065, USA

E-mail addresses:
LSorce@luriechildrens.org (L.R. Sorce)
jdh2002@med.cornell.edu (J.D. Howell)

Beyond Conventional Hemodynamic Monitoring— Monitoring to Improve Our Understanding of Disease Process and Interventions

Michelle Ramírez, MD[a], Mjaye L. Mazwi, MBChB[b],
Ronald A. Bronicki, MD, FCCM[c], Paul A. Checchia, MD, FCCM[c],
Jacqueline S.M. Ong, MB BChir (Cantab)[d,e,*]

KEYWORDS

- Hemodynamic monitoring • Cardiac output • Data integration

KEY POINTS

- Hemodynamic monitoring is a fundamental component of intensive care and provides a vast amount of data from which clinicians can build an assessment of adequacy of cardiac output in patients.
- Hemodynamic monitoring ranges from basic techniques such as physical examination to advanced modalities requiring specific skills and technologies. Each modality has strengths and weaknesses.
- Each modality also provides a data stream over time, allowing the clinician to also evaluate change over a period of assessment.
- Integration of data is necessary to act in an anticipatory rather than reactionary manner— an ideal to which we aim in intensive care.

[a] Division of Pediatric Critical Care Medicine, Department of Pediatrics, New York University Langone Medical Center, Hassenfeld Children's Hospital, New York, NY 10016, USA; [b] Department of Critical Care Medicine, Division of Cardiology, The Hospital for Sick Children, 555 University Avenue, Toronto, Ontario M5G 1X8, Canada; [c] Division of Critical Care Medicine, Department of Pediatrics, Baylor College of Medicine, Texas Children's Hospital, 6621 Fannin, WT6-006, Houston, TX 77030, USA; [d] Division of Paediatric Critical Care, Khoo Teck Puat - University Children's Medical Institute, NUHS Tower Block Level 12, 1E Kent Ridge Road, Singapore 119228; [e] Department of Paediatrics, Yong Loo Lin School of Medicine, National University of Singapore, 21 Lower Kent Ridge Road, Singapore 119077
* Corresponding author. Division of Paediatric Critical Care, Khoo Teck Puat - University Children's Medical Institute, NUHS Tower Block Level 12, 1E Kent Ridge Road, Singapore 119228.
E-mail address: jacqueline_ong@nuhs.edu.sg

Crit Care Clin 39 (2023) 243–254
https://doi.org/10.1016/j.ccc.2022.09.002
0749-0704/23/© 2022 Elsevier Inc. All rights reserved.

INTRODUCTION

Critical care practitioners are compelled to monitor their patients. It is in our nature—the more parameters we see and measure, the better we feel about managing and supporting our patients. By definition, the intensive care unit (ICU) was established in order to monitor patients more closely and more specifically than other locations in the hospital.[1]

While the history of formal hemodynamic monitoring is relatively brief, an appreciation for the qualitative aspects of monitoring dates to ancient times. Hemodynamic monitoring is a natural extension of the physical examination, refuting or corroborating the findings, establishing a physiologic phenotype, and enabling the clinician to tailor therapy accordingly.

Nonetheless, all of this monitoring comes with a price: it provides an enormous quantity of data; some valuable, some artifact, and some noise. This data, coupled with the inherent limitations of our human cognitive abilities, leaves the critical care practitioner with the difficult task of prioritizing which monitors and information to observe, interpret, and act on while caring for each patient. We are left with the questions: What matters? Which monitor takes precedence? What story does the monitoring data tell us about the state of the patients in our care? Additionally, no single monitoring strategy can provide all of the information that is necessary to paint the entire picture of the state of the patient. Every bedside practitioner is forced to "fill in the gaps" of information through physical examination findings, individual experience and knowledge, thus producing their own understanding of the patient that may or may not be accurate or congruent with the assessment of other members of the team.

Furthermore, the data and information provided by various types of hemodynamic monitoring must be accurately interpreted by the bedside clinician. Studies have however repeatedly demonstrated that estimations of hemodynamic status based on the physical examination and interpretation of standard hemodynamic data is often discordant from objectively measured readings.[2,3] Although it would be easy to assume that experience can aid in the accuracy of data interpretation, several studies highlight that these discrepancies occur irrespective of experience and training.[4] Further, studies have shown that there are deficiencies in the knowledge necessary to accurately interpret hemodynamic data.[5-7]

Given such variability in data quality, quantity, and interpretation, we must remember that the goal of monitoring is not only to establish an accurate understanding of the hemodynamic state but also to guide action in an anticipatory rather than a reactionary manner. As the hemodynamic phenotype may vary considerably among patients, and within patients over time, a one-size-fits-all strategy in critical care has inherent shortcomings. Thus, the care of patients should be tailored appropriately as the patient's condition remains dynamic in the ICU. In order to examine the role of monitoring in the integration of data, we must first understand the current state of available monitoring approaches. This evolution of monitoring may be best demonstrated via the use of a clinical vignette.

CLINICAL VIGNETTE

A previously healthy adolescent male is assessed in the emergency room with fever, hypotension, and somnolence. Initial vital signs are a blood pressure (BP) 71/22 mm Hg (mean of 49 mm Hg), heart rate 140 beats per minute (bpm), pulse oximetry saturation (SpO$_2$) 100% on room air and temperature 102.5°F (39.2°C). Examination is remarkable for a flushed appearance, bounding pulses, and mild confusion. Sepsis is suspected and vascular access is established. He receives 40 mL/kg of fluid and broad-spectrum antibiotics and is transferred to the pediatric ICU (PICU).

BEDSIDE ASSESSMENT OF CARDIAC OUTPUT

As seen in the vignette, clinical parameters such as HR, BP, pulse oximetry, and this vignette demonstrates how HR, BP, pulse oximetry can provide data that, when combined with physical examination, inform the initial assessment of the patient's hemodynamic status. monitoring provide data that, when combined with the physical examination, provides an initial assessment of the patient's hemodynamic status. Other assessments such as the mental status of the child, urine output, and their trends over time contribute to establishing a patient's clinical trajectory. This first step in assessment is universal and remains an important aspect of evaluation. However, as discussed above, there is often a lack of correlation between estimations of hemodynamic parameters based on the physical examination and measured values (eg, cardiac output [CO] and systemic vascular resistance [SVR]). As with all parameters, the examination is one data point that should be incorporated into the whole and does not supersede the rest. Moreover, a "normal" finding in the bedside parameters or clinical examination equates neither to adequate CO nor to adequate tissue oxygenation.

CLINICAL VIGNETTE CONTINUED

In the PICU, an arterial line and central venous access are established. The initial central venous pressure (CVP) is 2 mm Hg with superior vena cava saturation 87% and a serum lactate 6 mmol/L. Cardiac ultrasonography during initial resuscitation shows hyperdynamic left ventricular (LV) systolic function (ejection fraction [EF] 70%) and a collapsed inferior vena cava. The CVP increases with the administration of 80 mL/kg of fluid but arterial pressure remains marginal. A vasopressor infusion is initiated, resulting in improved BP, mental status, and narrowing of the pulse pressure.

BASIC NONINVASIVE MEASURES OF CARDIAC OUTPUT
Venous Pressures and Oximetry

The presence of a central venous line (CVL) is not absolute in every critically ill child but is certainly a common practice.[8] Once the central line is transduced, it can provide continuous pressure readings. Commonly, CVP (or right atrial pressure—equivalent if there is a continuous column of fluid between measuring sites) is used to make inferences about the adequacy of VR to the heart. The CVP is the most commonly used variable to guide fluid resuscitation[9] because it is often used as a surrogate of intravascular volume and as such, an indicator of right ventricular end diastolic volume (RVEDV). Fluid administration can be titrated to CVP, to identify the optimal CO and "best" loading conditions for an individual patient.

There are, however, limitations to the use of the CVP. The relationship between the CVP and RVEDV compliance is complex, changes with other interventions (eg, ventilation mode) and is variable from patient to patient. The CVP also does not provide an accurate indication of LV filling pressure, and compliance of the LV is also unknown. This is likely the reason why the overall predictive value of the CVP as a measure of fluid responsiveness has been found to be poor.[10] Nevertheless, the CVP can provide meaningful data despite these challenges.

The CVL may also enable the clinician to assess the global oxygen supply/demand relationship if properly positioned. As shown in the clinical vignette, performing venous oximetry (from a CVL positioned in preferably in the right internal jugular vein, superior vena cava, or right atrium in the absence of an atrial level shunt) allows measurement of the (OER = SaO2-ScvO2/ SaO2), so as to provide an indication of the adequacy of systemic oxygen delivery (DO$_2$).[11] In this instance, the venous saturation of the sample is high (87%), reflective of a high CO and DO_2, depressed metabolic demand, and/or impaired oxygen extraction due to mitochondrial dysfunction or a disturbance of the microcirculation or a combination of both.

Oxygen extraction ratio versus lactate

Another advantage of monitoring the OER is that it increases well before lactate production. Lactate begins to accumulate when production exceeds its clearance, and thus this biomarker proves a relatively late indication of tissue hypoxia compared with venous oximetry. Further, lactate elevation may occur despite normal or elevated DO_2 in which case, increased tissue oxygen utilization is the issue.[12,13]

Near Infrared Spectroscopy

The technique of near infrared spectroscopy (NIRS) is worth mentioning because it is noninvasive and related to venous oximetry. NIRS uses different wavelengths of infrared light absorbed by oxygenated and deoxygenated hemoglobin in the microvasculature to assess regional tissue oxygenation. NIRS oximetry provides similar data points to those obtained from venous oximetry. Sensors are placed over the forehead to monitor cerebral regional oxygen saturation (rSO_2) and over the flank to monitor renal tissue oxygenation. The proprietary algorithms of NIRS oximetry assess the absorption of light by hemoglobin moieties in the nonpulsatile blood in contrast to pulse oximetry. Because the majority of blood in the nonpulsatile microcirculation is venous (some 70%–80%), the oxygen saturation is used as a surrogate for venous oxygen saturation of the interrogated tissue and may be used as an indicator of the adequacy global DO_2 (eg, cerebral oximetry).[14] Although this technology provides a continuous, noninvasive assessment of tissue oxygenation, it has limitations as well. Most notably, the values are calculated from an algorithm and not measured (a limitation shared with pulse oximetry) and the signal is mixed (venous and arterial) as opposed to pulse oximetry. Thus there may be, at times, considerable variation in the reading.

Echocardiography

The assessment of heart function is an essential component of the management of fragile hemodynamic states. Routine monitoring and biochemical parameters lack sensitivity and specificity to assess cardiac function.[15] When used as an adjunct to clinical examination and other cardiovascular monitoring modalities, bedside echocardiography provides real-time diagnostic information necessary for the management of unfavorable hemodynamic states.[16] It is important to understand that echocardiography assesses cardiac performance (elastance) of the heart under the conditions of preload and afterload that exist when the study is being performed.[17] Therefore, in patients with rapidly changing hemodynamic states, it may be useful to reassess cardiac performance when new loading conditions exist because cardiac performance may be substantially different. Understanding cardiac performance helps to guide choice of therapeutic agents to support fragile hemodynamic states, for example, the selection of an inotrope as well as a vasopressor if fluid refractory hypotension is associated with depressed myocardial function. Other useful information provided by echocardiography includes an assessment of volume status and loading conditions as well as excluding cardiac pathologic condition such as pericardial effusions that may contribute to fragile hemodynamic states.[18]

CLINICAL VIGNETTE CONTINUED

During the next 12 hours, our patient develops tachypnea and a new complaint of abdominal pain. Vital signs associated with these new symptoms include BP 88/64 mm Hg (mean 73 mm Hg), sinus tachycardia 125 bpm, SpO_2 94% on face-mask fractional inspired oxygen (F_iO_2) of 0.4, and temperature of 99°F (37.2°C). The physical examination 14 hours after admission is remarkable for a gallop rhythm, perfusion described as fair to poor, and tachypnea. A chest radiograph demonstrates cardiomegaly and diffuse interstitial pulmonary edema. A repeat echocardiogram now demonstrates severely depressed LV systolic function with an EF of 24% and minimally elevated LV end diastolic volume. The CVP is 12 mm Hg. The serum lactate level is normal with markedly elevated serum troponin level. The differential diagnosis is broadened to include myocarditis and sepsis-related myocardial dysfunction. Given the patient's rapidly changing clinical state, a discussion is held to determine if he might benefit from more advanced monitoring.

ADVANCED CARDIAC OUTPUT MONITORING
Invasive Assessment of Cardiac Output

Pulmonary artery catheter
There are several invasive technologies available for the measurement of CO. The thermodilution technique for determining CO uses the pulmonary artery (PA) catheter (the Swan-Ganz catheter). This technique uses cold water injection into the central circulation and venous return (CO) is estimated by examining the dilution of cold water to warm blood. The performance of such a measurement represents how the PA catheter can become a true CO monitor. Furthermore, it provides information on systemic and pulmonary vascular resistance, as well as PA occlusion pressure. Although controversies exist around the specific patient population benefitting most from the placement of the PA catheter and measurement of CO, it remains the gold standard by which other CO monitors are compared. Studies by Perkin and Anas[19] and Bronicki[11] included excellent reviews of the PA catheter technology and the thermodilution technique.

Transpulmonary thermodilution
Similarly, but less invasive in nature, transpulmonary thermodilution (TPTD) relies on the injection of ice-cold saline. This does not require insertion of a PA catheter because it can be performed through any CVL. An arterial line with a thermistor is required to measure temperature changes as the cold injectate flows from the venous to the arterial circulation. This technique allows for the continuous measurement of CO, but it has a higher propensity than PA catheter measurements to be affected by baseline drift and recirculation given that the time-temperature curves obtained are broader and lower in magnitude. Furthermore, similar to PA catheters, it can be affected by valvular insufficiency and intracardiac shunts. There are, however, multiple studies in both adult and pediatric populations, comparing TPTD and PA catheter CO measurements reporting a high degree of correlation between the two techniques across a variety of disease states.[19–22] Its biggest shortcoming is the need for frequent recalibration, particularly in shock states in children where pulmonary thermodilution may overestimate CO.[21,22] Probably the most commonly used device in the pediatric population using TPTD is the Pulse index Continuous Cardiac Output ([PiCCO] Monitor; Pulsion Medical Systems, Germany), further discussed below.

Pulse contour analysis
The invasive nature of PA catheters and the potential for serious complications has led to the development of several minimally/less invasive methods to determine CO. One such method is pulse contour analysis (PCA), which uses the area under the curve (AUC) of the systolic BP (**Fig. 1**), obtained from an arterial catheter, to determine the stroke volume (SV). The AUC is used to calculate CO (CO = HR × SV) through an algorithm providing continuous CO reading, as well as cardiac index (CI) and heart rate values. Devices using this technology can be either calibrated or uncalibrated. It is important to remember that

this technique converts a pressure reading (systolic BP) into a volume reading (SV); it is not a direct measurement of CO but rather a calculated value.

PCA has several limitations, including the need for frequent recalibration in certain devices, with accuracy decreasing if uncalibrated devices are used. Accuracy will be dependent on the quality of arterial line waveform, so over dampening or under dampening of arterial line systems will affect results. In addition, changes in SVR, particularly low SVR states, will affect accuracy of readings,[22] as will the presence of intra-aortic balloon pumps, aortic insufficiency, and arrhythmias.

If we focus on the relationship and accuracy between PCA and PA catheters, the gold standard for measuring CO, several studies offer conflicting evidence of accuracy with PCA. For example, a recent study looking at liver transplant recipients comparing PCA versus PA catheters found poor agreement between the CO measured by both techniques, with a high percentage error of 44% to 72%.[23]

Currently, there are several devices available using PCA technology, two such devices are the PiCCO (Pulsion Medical Systems, Munich, Germany) and the FloTrac (Edwards Lifesciences, Irvine, CA, USA) systems.

The PiCCO monitor requires placement of an arterial line with a thermistor on the tip and a standard CVL. To measure CO continuously via PCA, device calibration is required using TPTD with injection of a cold fluid through a CVL. Calibration is recommended once every 8 hours or with significant hemodynamic changes. As with any device using thermodilution, the presence of intracardiac shunts can affect accuracy.[24] Correlation studies of PiCCO monitor CO with standard PA catheters have shown good correlation, specifically in adults undergoing coronary bypass surgery,[25] single lung transplant,[26] and other cardiothoracic surgeries.[27] Other studies looking at patients undergoing off-pump coronary artery bypass surgery[28] have shown good correlation during periods of hemodynamic stability but large discrepancies at other points. Overall, this device seems to be a reasonable choice for measuring and trending CO in specific patient populations under certain physiologic states.

The FloTrac system uses a specialized sensor attached to a previously inserted arterial line catheter and connected to a monitor (Vigileo monitor). It does not require placement of a CVL, and it does not require external calibration. It provides values for CO, CI, SV, SVR, and stroke volume variation every 20 seconds via pulse contour analysis. Currently, in children undergoing cardiac surgery, the most recent generation of the FloTrac system lacked accuracy and trending ability when compared with PA catheters.[20,29] Similarly, in patients undergoing liver transplantation, there is large percentage error with the FloTrac system when compared with PA catheter-derived CI.[30] Although promising, current data indicates this device remains inferior to PA catheters for monitoring CO.

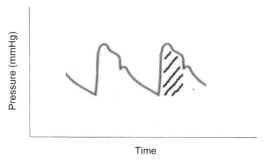

Fig. 1. AUC in blue, arterial waveform from invasive arterial line.

Noninvasive assessment of cardiac output

Naturally, noninvasive devices should provide values that are reliable, reproducible, and accurate (compared with the gold standard), continuously, across a variety of pathologic states. Unfortunately, many of these noninvasive options have conflicting evidence, may not be accurate across different pathophysiological states and may not provide interchangeable measurements when compared with standard methods. Studies evaluating percentage error have found some devices to have percentage errors greater than 30%, making many of these unreliable.

Electrical Bioreactance

Electrical bioreactance cardiometry consists of 4 dual electrodes placed on the upper and lower chest wall or neck and lower chest. An alternating current is released by each of the electrodes and the other electrode detects and interprets the return signal, which is created by opening of the aortic valve and resulting changes in erythrocyte orientation. Currently, the NICOM (Cheetah Medical, Newton Center, MA) and the Aesculon Electrical Cardiometry (Osypka Medical Gmbh, Berlin, Germany) devices are available for clinical use.

Several adult studies have shown promise of this noninvasive technology in post-cardiac surgical adults in the ICU, with acceptable accuracy in a range of circulatory states.[31,32] However, a small study[33] looking at 50 adult patients in cardiogenic shock and comparing NICOM values with those obtained via indirect Fick and thermodilution, showed NICOM was not a reliable measure of CO in patients presenting with decompensated heart failure and cardiogenic shock. In pediatrics, several studies have also shown conflicting results.[34–37] Overall, bioreactance may be valid for use in adults and older pediatric populations, but results are inconclusive for neonates, those with congenital heart disease and hemodynamically unstable patients.

PUTTING IT ALL TOGETHER: DATA INTEGRATION

As we return to the clinical vignette, we are left with the continued problem of integration of data at the bedside of a critically ill patient. The range of data that could be generated while monitoring patients represent observed variables assessing specific factors affecting cardiopulmonary function. Although we have described a variety of approaches for the measurement of CO, in everyday clinical practice, CO is often inferred at the bedside by the clinician rather than being directly measured or calculated by a monitoring device. Measured clinical variables provide data that aid this inference for a given patient (eg, a clinician may infer that CO is marginal because of a wide arteriovenous oxygen saturation [AVO_2] difference, narrow pulse pressure, poor urine output, and cool extremities). As a result of being inferred rather than directly measured, CO may be described as "latent" clinical variable.

As is true of CO when not directly measured, hemodynamic state must be inferred from the observed monitoring data.[38] The ability to accurately infer patient state from observed clinical monitoring data is the integrative cognitive exercise that is the hallmark of the expert critical care clinician. Typically, this exercise involves inferring variables, such as CO or SVR, from directly observed data and then integrating this information to determine whether the resultant hemodynamic state is favorable or unfavorable. The expert clinician may determine that a state of "cold shock" — measured by a wide AVO_2 difference, narrow pulse pressure, poor urine output, and elevated serum lactate — is the product of marginal CO and elevated SVR.[39] Identifying variables contributing to this unfavorable hemodynamic state allows targeted interventions to improve patient condition, for example, initiation of an inodilator to augment CO and decrease SVR. Conversely, early sepsis causing "warm shock" may be identified by a narrow AVO_2 difference, wide pulse pressure, and elevated serum lactate.[40] Recognizing that the main contributor to this unfavorable hemodynamic state is a pathologic decrease in SVR should prompt targeted vasoconstrictor therapy while increasing mean systemic venous pressure with volume to offset the effect of venodilation. In the case vignette above, the patient dynamically transitions between these states illustrating the importance of not only accurate inference at initial presentation but also longitudinal reassessment of monitoring parameters as the patient state changes. Ancillary testing modalities, including point of care ultrasonography and echocardiography, described in the vignette, support this exercise rather than fundamentally changing it.[41,42] The ability to recognize favorable and unfavorable hemodynamic states and identify contributing variables is required of critical care clinicians regardless of where they practice in the world or the complexity of monitoring modalities available.

Much of the data generated in the process of patient monitoring has the property of "time" series, or repeated measurement of the same variable over time.[43] This essential property of the data allows clinicians to gain an understanding of the direction, magnitude, and rate of change in both the specific measured variable and the underlying latent hemodynamic state. It also allows the critical care clinician to ascertain the trajectory of the patient through illness and assess the effect of therapeutic interventions.[44] This is essential in dynamic environments such as critical care, where patients experience significant changes in underlying state and risk frequently.

Part of the importance of understanding the cognitive exercise required of clinicians is that it helps identify the role and potential promise of novel approaches to patient monitoring. Some of these approaches aim to directly measure and represent latent patient state using analytical techniques such as machine learning.[45] Others leverage data visualization to more effectively present currently available clinical information in a manner that facilitates more accurate and reproducible identification of hemodynamic states[46,47] (**Fig. 2**). These approaches are not mutually exclusive, and it is likely

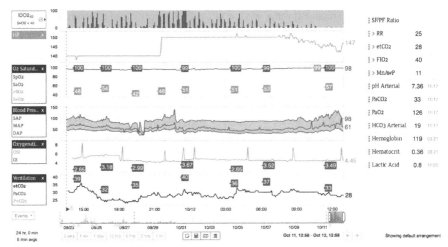

Fig. 2. The "Hemodynamic view" of the tracking, trajectory, and triggering (T3) application. This example of using data visualization represents the time series of monitoring data for a single patient in a customizable visual format that is intended to facilitate an appreciation of relevant relationships between monitored variables. The goal of representing the data in this manner is to facilitate correct clinician inference of hidden variables and hemodynamic state. (*Courtesy of* Etiometry Inc, Boston, MA; with permission.)

that a combination of analytical insights and data visualization will augment clinicians performing this fundamental critical care task in the future.

SUMMARY

Appropriate monitoring permits comprehension of etiologic and compensatory factors responsible for the patient's hemodynamic state. This allows clinicians to calculate secondary parameters as well as identify modifiable variables that can be targeted with therapeutic strategies. However, the primacy of monitoring lies in documentation of improved outcomes based on hemodynamic monitoring-driven treatments in controlled clinical studies. The clinician's focus should be on proper integration and interpretation of all of the available data to accurately identify hemodynamic states rather than chasing the perfect monitor.

Looking to the future, currently available wearable technology can already measure heart rate, detect some arrhythmias, and perform pulse oximetry. It is only a matter of time until advancements in biomedical engineering evolve to create wearable patches to directly measure complex hemodynamics.

CLINICS CARE POINTS

- Current hemodynamic monitoring modalities can provide important, yet at times, overwhelming amounts of information that make it hard to discern the important from the superfluous.

- Vital signs, central venous pressure, venous oximetry, near infra-red spectroscopy and echocardiography can provide preliminary information about cardiac output, but none of these are direct measurements.

- The pulmonary artery catheter remains the gold standard measurement for cardiac output, but due to its invasive nature can lead to complications.

- Current literature supports transpulmonary thermodilution and calibrated pulse contour analysis devices as the best less-invasive measures of cardiac ouput when compared to pulmonary artery catheters.

- Current non-invasive devices do not provide reliable cardiac output measurements at this time.

REFERENCES

1. Nightingale F. Notes on hospitals. 3rd edition. London, UK: Longman, Green, Longman, Roberts, and Green; 1863. p. 89.
2. Stevenson LW, Perloff JK. The limited reliability of physical signs for estimating hemodynamics in chronic heart failure. JAMA 1989;261(6):884–8.
3. Narang N, Chung B, Nguyen A, et al. Discordance between clinical assessment and invasive hemodynamics in patients with advanced heart failure. J Card Fail 2020;26(2):128–35.
4. Bronicki RA. Hemodynamic monitoring. Pediatr Crit care med 2016;17(8 Suppl 1):S207–14.
5. Gnaegi A, Feihl F, Perret C. Intensive care physicians' insufficient knowledge of right-heart catheterization at the bedside: time to act? Crit Care Med 1997; 25(2):213–20.
6. Iberti TJ, Fischer EP, Leibowitz AB, et al. A multicenter study of physicians' knowledge of the pulmonary artery catheter. JAMA 1990;264(22):2928–32.

7. Squara P, Bennett D, Perret C. Pulmonary artery catheter: does the problem lie in the users? Chest 2002;121(6):2009–15.
8. Derderian SC, Good R, Vuille-Ditbille RN, et al. Central venous lines in critically ill children: Thrombosis but not infection is site dependent. J Pediatr Surg 2019; 54(9):1740–3.
9. De Backer D, Vincent JL. Should we measure the central venous pressure to guide fluid management? Ten answers to 10 questions. Crit Care 2018;22(1):43.
10. Eskesen TG, Wetterslev M, Perner A. Systematic review including re-analyses of 1148 individual data sets of central venous pressure as a predictor of fluid responsiveness. Intensive Care Med 2016;42(3):324–32.
11. Bronicki RA. Venous oximetry and the assessment of oxygen transport balance. Pediatr Crit Care Med 2011;12(4 Suppl):S21–6.
12. Domico M, Checchia PA. Biomonitors of cardiac injury and performance: B-type natriuretic peptide and troponin as monitors of hemodynamics and oxygen transport balance. Pediatr Crit Care Med 2011;12(4 Suppl):S33–42.
13. Allen M. Lactate and acid base as a hemodynamic monitor and markers of cellular perfusion. Pediatr Crit Care Med 2011;12(4 Suppl):S43–9.
14. Ghanayem N, Hoffman G. Near infrared spectroscopy as a hemodynamic monitor in critical illness. Pediatr Crit Care Med 2016;17(8 Suppl):S201–6.
15. Noori S, Seri I. Evidence-based versus pathophysiology-based approach to diagnosis and treatment of neonatal cardiovascular compromise. Semin Fetal Neonatal Med 2015;20(4):238–45.
16. Tissot C, Singh Y, Sekarski N. Echocardiographic evaluation of ventricular function-for the neonatologist and pediatric intensivist. Front Pediatr 2018;6. https://doi.org/10.3389/fped.2018.00079.
17. Weber KT, Janicki JS, Hunter WC, et al. The contractile behavior of the heart and its functional coupling to the circulation. Prog Cardiovasc Dis 1982;24(5): 375–400.
18. Levitov A, Frankel HL, Blaivas M, et al. Guidelines for the appropriate use of bedside general and cardiac ultrasonography in the evaluation of critically ill patients—part II: cardiac ultrasonography. Crit Care Med 2016;44(6):1206–27.
19. Perkin RM, Anas N. Pulmonary artery catheters. Pediatr Crit Care Med 2011;12(4 Suppl):S12–20.
20. Mukkamala R, Kohl BA, Mahajan A. Comparison of accuracy of two uncalibrated pulse contour cardiac output monitors in off-pump coronary artery bypass surgery patients using pulmonary artery catheter-thermodilution as a reference. BMC Anesthesiol 2021;21(1):189.
21. Funk DJ, Moretti EW, Gan TJ. Minimally invasive cardiac output. Anesth Analg 2009;108(887–97). https://doi.org/10.1213/ane.0b013e31818ffd99.
22. Biais M, Mazocky E, Stecken L, et al. Impact of systemic vascular resistance on the accuracy of the pulsioflex device. Anesth Analg 2017;5(10):487–93.
23. Halemani K, Kumar L, Narayanan B, et al. Correlation of cardiac output by arterial contour-derived cardiac output monitor versus pulmonary artery catheter in liver transplant: experience at an Indian center. Turk J Anaesthesiol Reanim 2022; 50(2):135–41.
24. Genahr A, McLuckie A. Transpulmonary thermodilution in the critically ill. Br J Intensive Care 2004;14(1):6–10.
25. Buhre W, Weyland A, Kazmaier S, et al. Comparison of cardiac output assessed by pulse-contour analysis and thermodilution in patients undergoing minimally invasive direct coronary artery bypass grafting. J Cardiothorac Vasc Anesth 1999;13(4):437–40.

26. Della Rocca G, Costa MG, Coccia C, et al. Cardiac output monitoring: aortic transpulmonary thermodilution and pulse contour analysis agree with standard thermodilution methods in patients undergoing lung transplantation. Can J Anaesth 2003;50(7):707–11.
27. Goedje O, Hoeke K, Lichtwarck-Aschoff M, et al. Continuous cardiac output by femoral arterial thermodilution calibrated pulse contour analysis: comparison with pulmonary arterial thermodilution. Crit Care Med 1999;27(11):2407–12.
28. Halvorsen PS, Sokolov A, Cvancarova M, et al. Continuous cardiac output during off-pump coronary artery bypass surgery: pulse-contour analyses vs pulmonary artery thermodilution. Br J Anaesth 2007;99(4):484–92.
29. Kusaka Y, Ohchi F, Minami T. Evaluation of the fourth-generation FloTrac/Vigileo system in comparison with the intermittent bolus thermodilution method in patients undergoing cardiac surgery. J Cardiothorac Vasc Anesth 2019;33(4): 953–60.
30. Lee M, Weinberg L, Pearce B, et al. Agreement in hemodynamic monitoring during orthotopic liver transplantation: a comparison of FloTrac/Vigileo at two monitoring sites with pulmonary artery catheter thermodilution. J Clin Monit Comput 2017;31(2):343–51.
31. Squara P, Denjean D, Estagnasie P, et al. Noninvasive cardiac output monitoring (NICOM): a clinical validation. Intensive Care Med 2007;33(7):1191–4.
32. Raval NY, Squara P, Cleman M, et al. Multicenter evaluation of noninvasive cardiac output measurement by bioreactance technique. J Clin Monit Comput 2008;22(2):113–9.
33. Rali AS, Buechler T, Van Gotten B, et al. Non-invasive cardiac output monitoring in cardiogenic shock: the NICOM study. J Card Fail 2020;26(2):160–5.
34. Xu SH, Zhang J, Zhang Y, et al. Non-invasive cardiac output measurement by electrical cardiometry and M-mode echocardiography in the neonate: a prospective observational study of 136 neonatal infants. Transl Pediatr 2021;10(7): 1757–64.
35. Van Wyk L, Smith J, Lawrenson J, et al. Agreement of cardiac output measurements between bioreactance and transthoracic echocardiography in preterm infants during the transitional phase: a single-centre, prospective study. Neonatology 2020;117:271–8.
36. Weisz DE, Jain A, Ting J, et al. Non-invasive cardiac output monitoring in preterm infants undergoing patent ductus arteriosus ligation: a comparison with echocardiography. Neonatology 2014;106(4):330–6.
37. Mansfield RC, Kaza N, Charalambous A, et al. Cardiac output measurement in neonates and children using noninvasive electrical bioimpedance compared with standard methods: a systematic review and meta-analysis. Crit Care Med 2022;50(1):126–37.
38. Salkind N. Encyclopedia of Research Design. SAGE Publications Inc 2010. https://doi.org/10.4135/9781412961288.
39. Kissoon N, Orr RA, Carcillo JA. Updated American college of critical care medicine–pediatric advanced life support guidelines for management of pediatric and neonatal septic shock: relevance to the emergency care clinician. Pediatr Emerg Care 2010;26(11):867–9.
40. Brierley J, Peters MJ. Distinct hemodynamic patterns of septic shock at presentation to pediatric intensive care. Pediatrics 2008;122(4):752–9.
41. Bortcosh W, Shaahinfar A, Sojar S, et al. New directions in point-of-care ultrasound at the crossroads of paediatric emergency and critical care. Curr Opin Pediatr 2018;30(3):350–8.

42. Blanco P, Volpicelli G. Common pitfalls in point-of-care ultrasound: a practical guide for emergency and critical care physicians. Crit Ultrasound J 2016;8(1):15.
43. Cryer JD, Kung-Sik C. Time series analysis with applications in R. Available at: https://mybiostats.files.wordpress.com/2015/03/time-series-analysis-with-applications-in-r-cryer-and-chan.pdf. Accessed June 5, 2022.
44. Eytan D, Goodwin AJ, Greer R, et al. Distributions and behavior of vital signs in critically ill children by admission diagnosis. Pediatr Crit Care Med 2018;19(2):115–24.
45. Johnson AEW, Ghassemi MM, Nemati S, et al. Machine learning and decision support in critical care. Proc IEEE Inst Electr Electron Eng 2016;104(2):444–66.
46. Lowry AW, Futterman CA, Gazit AZ. Acute vital signs changes are underrepresented by a conventional electronic health record when compared with automatically acquired data in a single-center tertiary pediatric cardiac intensive care unit. J Am Med Inform Assoc 2022;29(7):1183–90.
47. Gaies M, Olive MK, Owens G, et al. Pediatric cardiac critical care outcomes improve following implementation of a commercial data aggregation and visualization software platform. J Am Coll Cardiol 2019;73(9):562.

Extracorporeal Membrane Oxygenation Then and Now; Broadening Indications and Availability

Blythe E. Pollack, MSN, CPNP-AC[a],*, Roxanne Kirsch, MD, MBE[b,c],
Rachel Chapman, MD[d,e], Robert Hyslop, RN[f],
Graeme MacLaren, MBBS, MSc[g], Ryan P. Barbaro, MD, MSc[a,h]

KEYWORDS

- Extracorporeal membrane oxygenation (ECMO) • Extracorporeal membrane oxygenation to support cardiopulmonary resuscitation (ECPR)
- Extracorporeal life support (ECLS) • Neonatal
- Pediatric acute respiratory distress syndrome (PARDS) • Cardiac failure

KEY POINTS

- Extracorporeal membrane oxygenation (ECMO) use is well established in congenital diaphragmatic hernia, meconium aspiration, pediatric acute respiratory distress syndrome (PARDS), postcardiac surgery, myocarditis, cardiomyopathy, and to support cardiopulmonary resuscitation. ECMO use is also increasingly reported in rare diseases, genetic syndromes, cancer, and hematopoietic stem cell transplant, traumatic or thermal injuries, and coronavirus disease 2019.
- Over time the mortality rate of children supported with ECMO has remained relatively stable but the pre-ECMO severity of illness and comorbidities have increased.
- The complexity around ECMO utilization increasingly demands high-quality research into ethical delivery of ECMO care.

Fig. 1 was produced for this article by Holly R Fischer at the direction of the coauthors and paid for using funds from the Elliott Deedler ECMO Scholar Fund.
[a] Division of Pediatric Critical Care, University of Michigan Medical School, 1500 E. Medical Center Drive, Ann Arbor, MI 48109, USA; [b] Division Cardiac Critical Care, Department Critical Care Medicine, 555 Univeristy Avenue, Toronto, ON, Canada M5G 1X8; [c] Department of Bioethics, The Hospital for Sick Children, 555 University Avenue, Toronto, ON, Canada M5G 1XB; [d] Department of Pediatrics, Division of Neonatology and the Fetal and Neonatal Institute, Children's Hospital, 4650 Sunset Blvd., Los Angeles, CA 90027, USA; [e] Department of Pediatrics, Keck School of Medicine of University of Southern California, 1975 Zonal Ave, Los Angeles, CA 90033, USA; [f] Heart Institute, Children's Hospital Colorado, 13123 E. 16th Ave, Aurora, CO 80045, USA; [g] Cardiothoracic Intensive Care Unit, National University Health System, 5 Lower Kent Ridge Rd, Singapore 119074, Singapore; [h] Susan B. Miester Child Health Evaluation and Research Center, Univeristy of Michigan, NCRC Building 16, 2800 Plymouth Road, Ann Arbor, MI 48109, USA
* Corresponding author.
E-mail address: bpollack@med.umich.edu

INTRODUCTION

Extracorporeal membrane oxygenation (ECMO) has now been successfully delivered to children[1] and young adults[2] for more than 50 years. ECMO is an invasive life support technology that requires a blood pump, membrane lung, and vascular cannula(s) to withdraw venous blood from the patient, add oxygen, remove carbon dioxide, and return the blood.[3,4] Since its initial applications, ECMO has been used to support respiratory failure (respiratory ECMO), cardiac failure (cardiac ECMO), and cardiac pulmonary resuscitation (extracorporeal cardiopulmonary resuscitation [ECPR]).[1,3]

The first decades of ECMO support were dominated by neonatal respiratory failure and limited to a few centers across the world.[5,6] In the 1990s, evidence for neonatal respiratory ECMO support increased[7,8] but the number of cases began to decline[9,10] as inhaled nitric oxide[11,12] and high-frequency oscillatory ventilation were applied for severe respiratory failure.[13] Meanwhile, pediatric cardiac ECMO[14] and ECPR[15,16] sustained steady growth[10,17] because congenital heart surgery programs grew.[18,19] In the years surrounding the 2009 influenza A (H1N1) pandemic, there were advances in ECMO technology (blood pumps, artificial lungs, and cannula),[17,20,21] evidence supporting ECMO use,[22–26] and a subsequent surge in adult ECMO use.[27] This adult-predominant growth in technology,[28] evidence,[29] centers,[30] and patients repeated itself in the years surrounding the coronavirus disease 2019 (COVID-19) pandemic caused by severe acute respiratory syndrome coronavirus 2 (SARS-CoV-2).[31,32]

This report aims to describe the diversity of ECMO support, underlying evidence, technologic advancement, broadening center distribution, expanding indications, and emerging controversies that have evolved during 5 decades of pediatric ECMO support.

DIVERSITY OF EXTRACORPOREAL MEMBRANE OXYGENATION SUPPORT
Respiratory Extracorporeal Membrane Oxygenation Support

Respiratory ECMO is initiated to support oxygenation and carbon dioxide removal in the setting of respiratory failure.[3] In children, respiratory ECMO support has been delivered via venoarterial (VA), venovenous (VV), or venopulmonary (VP) cannulation (**Fig. 1**).[3,4] In VA, VV, and VP ECMO blood is drained from a systemic vein or the right atrium. After gas exchange, the blood is then returned but the location differs by mode: a systemic artery in VA, a systemic vein or right atrium in VV, or the main pulmonary artery in VP.[3,4] In children outside of the neonatal period, three-fourths receive VV cannulation for respiratory support but in neonates, three-fourths receive VA cannulation for respiratory support.[33] VP ECMO for respiratory support is predominantly delivered to adolescents and largely emerged during the COVID-19 pandemic.[34] VP ECMO for respiratory support emerged because it was considered to reduce recirculation and thus improve the feasibility of patient mobility; it also provided right ventricular support in long ECMO runs where prolonged increase in pulmonary arterial pressures may strain the right heart over time.[28,34] In the neonatal period, respiratory ECMO support is deployed to support perinatal conditions such as congenital diaphragmatic hernia, meconium aspiration, and persistent pulmonary hypertension. In older children, the conditions leading to respiratory ECMO are heterogenous but approximately half are infectious causes that lead to severe hypoxemic respiratory failure, such as pneumonia.[17,35]

Cardiac Extracorporeal Membrane Oxygenation Support

Cardiac ECMO has always been closely tied to the development of cardiopulmonary bypass itself.[36] It is initiated for right, left, or biventricular failure or gas exchange in the

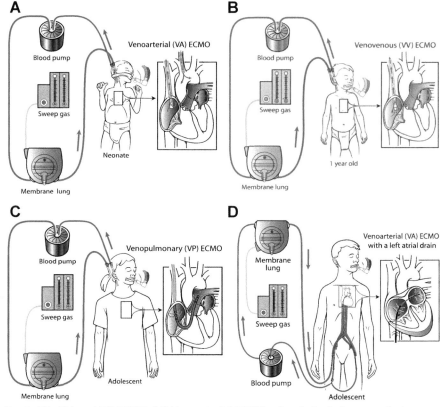

Fig. 1. VA, VV, and VP ECMO. (*A*) Venoarterial ECMO using 2 single lumen catheters, one placed in the RIJV draining form the right atrium and one placed in the right carotid artery, reinfusing just above the aortic arch. (*B*) VV ECMO using dual lumen catheter placed in the RIJV, draining from the superior vena cava and right atrium, reinfusing into the right atrium. (*C*) VP ECMO using a dual lumen catheter placed in the RIJV, draining from the right atrium and reinfusing into the main pulmonary artery. (*D*) VA ECMO using 2 single lumen catheters one placed in the right femoral vein, draining form the inferior vena cava and one placed in the right femoral artery, reinfusing into the aorta. In this picture also, a left atrial drain placed in the left formal vein and traversing the right atrium into the left atrium across a septostomy.

setting of cardiac failure. It is frequently used after cardiac surgery for congenital heart disease. Postcardiotomy support often uses a central VA cannulation strategy,[3,4] draining venous blood from the right atrium and returning it after gas exchange to the ascending aorta. Cardiac ECMO for medical diseases, such as those associated with arrhythmias, myocarditis, or cardiomyopathy,[17] is more likely to be delivered by peripheral cannulation. Common peripheral cannulation strategies[3,4] include using either the right internal jugular vein (RIJV) and carotid artery, or femoral vein and artery (see **Fig. 1**).

Extracorporeal Cardiopulmonary Resuscitation

ECPR is initiated during cardiopulmonary resuscitation that does not achieve sustained (≥20 minutes) return of spontaneous circulation.[3] In children, ECPR overwhelmingly follows in-hospital cardiac arrest and most frequently after cardiac surgery via central VA cannulation but it can also occur in association with arrhythmias, myocarditis, or cardiomyopathy, generally via peripheral VA cannulation.[17,37–41] Pediatric out of hospital cardiac arrest is often secondary respiratory failure, drowning or an acute life-threatening event.[42] Children with these conditions presenting in cardiac arrest with ongoing cardiopulmonary resuscitation are often considered poor candidates for ECPR[39–41,43] because the associated survival and neurologic outcomes are poor.[42] As a result, ECPR following out of hospital cardiac arrest occurs rarely in children but it is an area of growth and research in adult ECMO.[16,44] There is not consensus on when conventional cardiopulmonary resuscitation should transition to ECPR but a retrospective review identified refractory cardiopulmonary resuscitation to be 15 minutes.[45]

EVIDENCE, TECHNOLOGY, CARE

The first randomized clinical trial of ECMO versus conventional mechanical ventilation for adults with severe acute respiratory failure was published in 1979, and it reported more than 90% mortality in both groups.[46] During the next several decades, growth in ECMO support was dominated by the pediatric experience[47] and neonatal evidence in perinatal lung disease.[7,8] However, in the most recent 15 years, growth in ECMO use (**Fig. 2**) and evidence has been dominated by the adult experience.[9,16,22–25,29,48–50]

Initially, blood pumps were roller pumps, membrane lungs were made of silicone, limited cannula options for ECMO existed, and almost all ECMO systems relied on institutionally assembled pieces.[20] In 2011, the US Food and Drug Administration (FDA) classified the Cardiohelp system (Maquet Cardiopulmonary) as substantially equivalent to cardiopulmonary bypass devices (6 hours or less of use), catalyzing substantial expansion of the use of centrifugal pumps and polymethylpentene membrane lungs.[51] Coincident with growth in adult ECMO, there has been growth in centrifugal

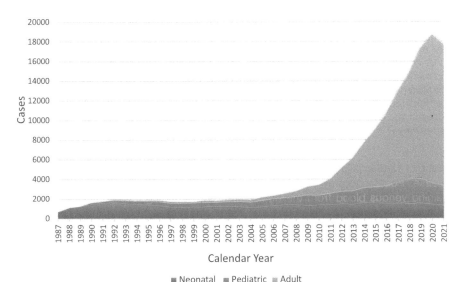

Fig. 2. Total ECMO runs from 1987 to 2021, including the adult, pediatric, and neonatal population. ECMO: neonatal = 0 to 28 days; pediatric = 29 days to 17 years old; adult aged 18 years or older. (*Data from* Extracorporeal Life Support Organizaiton (ELSO) Registry.[30])

blood pumps used for ECMO and ventricular assist devices (VADs),[26,52] membrane lungs,[20] ECMO cannulas,[21,53] and the development of integrated ECMO systems have further simplified the delivery of ECMO.

ECMO anticoagulation is an important facet of care, and it has seen the development of reduced anticoagulation monitoring protocols with preservation of outcomes.[54,55] There have also been increasing efforts to support early mobilization on ECMO, or awake ECMO. This is well reported in bridge-to-transplant populations[56–59] but it is also becoming increasingly reported as an aspect of ECMO care, including ECMO supported patients with COVID-19.[60–62] The process of mobilizing a patient with ECMO support is labor intensive and requires team-based care.[59] Multidisciplinary teams increasingly also participate broadly in patient selection and day-to-day management,[63] and centers are encouraged to benchmark outcomes and care practice against peer institutions.[64] Centers increasingly also recognize the importance of providing screening and potential follow-up for neurodevelopmental and rehabilitation for patients after ECMO support.[33,65] However, despite progress, complications remain common during pediatric ECMO support (Supplemental Table 1).

SHIFTING CARE, EXPANDING INDICATIONS, AND BROADENING CENTERS
Neonatal Respiratory Extracorporeal Membrane Oxygenation

In response to the negative 1979 adult clinical trial studying acute respiratory distress syndrome,[46] many ECMO leaders explicitly focused on ECMO in perinatal lung disease, such as meconium aspiration syndrome and persistent pulmonary hypertension of the newborn, where the natural history of the disease is rapid recovery (<5 days).[66] In 1985, Bartlett and colleagues described their threshold for transitioning from mechanical ventilation to ECMO support based on an oxygenation index (OI) as low as 25 or as high 40. In 1996, the UK Neonatal ECMO Clinical Trial was published, and solidified an OI of 40 as a common transition point to ECMO support for perinatal lung disease.[7]

Advancements in neonatal care have led to use of ECMO in neonates who failed multiple support strategies or therapies and thus are at greater risk for morbidity and mortality (**Fig. 3**). In the 1980s, the average duration of ECMO was 5 days and 81% survived; meconium aspiration comprising 43% of cases, congenital diaphragmatic hernia 17%, and persistent pulmonary hypertension of the newborn 14%.[5] More recently, the average ECMO run time was 9.2 days and 71% survived; congenital diaphragmatic hernia was the most common indication for neonatal ECMO support (31%), meconium aspiration the second most common indication (15%) and persistent pulmonary hypertension of the newborn (6%). Survival for meconium aspiration syndrome remains more than 90%.[30] Survival of congenital diaphragmatic hernia has remained relatively unchanged, hovering between 50% and 60% but with reports of higher survival rates at select centers.[67,68] Efforts to improve care have attempted to standardized pre-ECMO care such as permissive hypercapnia, and targeted management of pulmonary hypertension (**Table 1**).[69]

Clinical experience and focused retrospective reviews suggest ECMO support in neonates is expanding into increasingly complex conditions. For example, ECMO support for hypoxic ischemic encephalopathy-associated pulmonary hypertension,[70,71] airway anomalies or fetal thoracic masses threatening the airway,[72,73] and neonates with pulmonary hypoplasia and pulmonary hypertension in the setting of oligohydramnios related to renal and urologic anomalies.[74] ECMO use is also expanding into conditions some practitioners historically considered contraindications, such as smaller (down to 2 kg with consideration to 1.5 kg) and less mature (down to 34 weeks

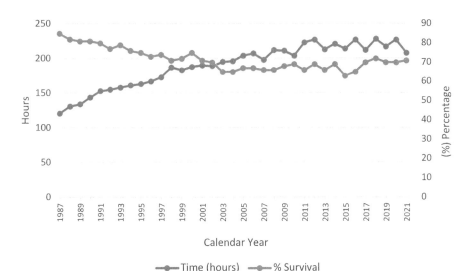

Fig. 3. Neonatal respiratory ECMO survival from 1987 through 2021. ECMO, neonatal = 0 to 28 days. (*Data from* Extracorporeal Life Support Organizaiton (ELSO) Registry. Available at https://www.elso.org/Registry/InternationalSummaryandReports/InternationalSummary. aspx.)

with consideration to 32 weeks gestational age) neonates as well as genetic syndromes (**Table 2**).[66,75–77]

Pediatric Respiratory Failure

There have been no clinical trials performed in pediatric ECMO for respiratory support[78] nor consensus statements established on when to initiate ECMO support.[79] Correspondingly, there are neither clear inclusion nor exclusion criteria for ECMO support in children outside of the neonatal period.[79] However, an examination of published literature demonstrates there has been a shift in pre-ECMO ventilator

Table 1
Guidelines for initiation of extracorporeal membrane oxygenation in neonates with congenital diaphragmatic hernia

Mechanical Support	OR Clinical Findings	OR Acute Deterioration
• CMV settings: PIP >26–28 cm H_2O, PEEP >6 cm H_2O, respiratory rate >50 bpm • HFOV settings: MAP >14 cm H_2O, Frequency <7 Hz, amplitude >40 cm H_2O	• pH < 7.2 with Pco_2 >70 mm Hg • SpO_2 <85% • Lactate >3 mmol/L • Fluid and vasoactive resistant hypotension • Pulmonary hypertension • Left ventricular failure	• SpO_2 <70%, unable to recover • Unstable hemodynamics

Abbreviations: CMV, conventional mechanical ventilation; HFOV, high-frequency oscillatory ventilation; MAP, mean airway pressure; Pco_2, arterial partial pressure of carbon dioxide; PEEP, positive end expiratory pressure; PIP, peak inspiratory pressure; SpO_2, peripherally measured percentage of oxygen-saturated hemoglobin.

From Guner Y, Jancelewicz T, Di Nardo M, et al. Management of Congenital Diaphragmatic Hernia Treated With Extracorporeal Life Support: Interim Guidelines Consensus Statement From the Extracorporeal Life Support Organization. ASAIO J. 2021;67(2); with permission.

Table 2
Neonatal complex conditions, survival outcomes following the use of extracorporeal membrane oxygenation support

Condition	Survival = %, Reported Cases = N	Reference
Meconium aspiration syndrome	91% (535/586)	ELSO Registry,[30] 2021
Persistent pulmonary hypertension of the newborn	73% (199/272)	ELSO Registry,[30] 2021
Congenital diaphragmatic hernia	58% (715/1222)	ELSO Registry,[30] 2021
Hypoxic ischemic encephalopathy-associated pulmonary hypertension	80% (16/20)	Agarwal [71] 2019
Airway anomalies and fetal thoracic masses threatening the airway	100% (3/3)	Krunisaki,[72] 2006 Straughan,[73] 2021
Neonates with pulmonary hypoplasia and pulmonary hypertension in the setting of oligohydramnios related to renal and urologic anomalies	42% (19/45)	Bagdure,[74] 2017
Trisomy 13	53% (8/15)[a]	Alore,[76] 2021
Trisomy 18	38% (5/13)[b]	Alore,[76] 2021

[a] 1 d to 6.8 y of life included in this study.
[b] 0 d to 2.2 y of life included in this study.

settings, greater tolerance of respiratory acidosis before transition to ECMO support (**Table 3**)[35,80] and an increase in the proportion of children with comorbidities (from 19% in 1993 to 47% in 2007).[35,81] Nonetheless, mortality was relatively stable.[81]

Although it remains an uncommon indication, 2022 consensus statements provide guidance for the consideration of pediatric respiratory ECMO support after hematopoietic cell transplantation and immune effector cell therapy (**Table 4**).[82] Specific recommendations were provided regarding neutrophil count, engraftment, graft function, complications, and overall goals of care. Moreover, the use of ECMO support in children with neoplasms has increased 3-fold in the ELSO Registry when comparing 2000 to 2009 with 2010 to 2019, whereas survival has remained relatively static at approximately 40%.[83] Additionally, ECMO support has increased in other immune-mediated diseases,[84] burn and inhalational injury,[85] trauma,[86] acute poisonings,[87] and as a bridge to lung transplant (**Table 5**).[88]

In 2020, the SARS-CoV-2 pandemic challenged health-care systems globally.[89] The potential effectiveness of ECMO during a viral pandemic was demonstrated with the 2009 influenza pandemic.[23,24] The contagious spread, heavy resource consumption, and long hospitalizations associated with COVID-19 challenged the role of ECMO but observational studies demonstrated its feasibility[90,91] and potential benefit.[48,49] Unlike the adult population, the pediatric population was not as heavily affected, allowing for the adult experience to inform pediatric care.[92] VP ECMO for respiratory support largely emerged during the SARS-CoV-2 pandemic but it is limited to near adult-sized children due to the size of currently available cannulas.[34,61] Additionally, some children who had COVID-19 later developed myocardial failure related to multisystem inflammatory syndrome in children[93] and required cardiac ECMO.[94]

Cardiac Extracorporeal Membrane Oxygenation

Survival after cardiac ECMO support has improved slightly in the most recent era (**Fig. 4**).[30] Since 1989, ELSO reports the average survival after cardiac ECMO to be

Table 3
Precannulation trends early extracorporeal membrane oxygenation data versus recent extracorporeal membrane oxygenation data

	Survivors	Nonsurvivors
pH		
1993–1995	7.36 (7.27–7.45)	7.33 (7.22–7.41)
1999–2001	7.32 (7.20–7.43)	7.26 (7.18–7.36)
2005–2007	7.26 (7.14–7.37)	7.23 (7.10–7.33)
2009–2012	7.23 (7.11–7.34)	7.19 (7.07–7.30)
PaCO$_2$		
1993–1995	48 (37–62)	50 (40–63)
1999–2001	51 (40–72)	57 (44–76)
2005–2007	60 (45–82)	60 (46–81)
2009–2012	64 (48–87)	65 (51–86)
HCO$_3$		
1993–1995	26 (21–32)	24 (20–30)
1999–2001	26 (22–32)	25 (20–33)
2005–2007	26 (21–32)	25 (20–31)
2009–2012	26 (21–32)	25 (20–31)

Abbreviations: HCO$_3$, bicarbonate; Paco$_2$, Partial pressure of carbon dioxide. Comorbidity including 1 or more of the 11 diagnoses: Renal failure, chronic lung disease, congenital heart disease (2 ventricles), congenital heart disease (1 ventricle), cardiac arrest, cancer, solid organ transplant, cardiomyopathy/myocarditis, primary immunodeficiency, liver failure, hematopoietic stem cell transplantation.
Data from Zabrocki LA, Brogan TV, Statler KD, Poss WB, Rollins MD, Bratton SL. Extracorporeal membrane oxygenation for pediatric respiratory failure: Survival and predictors of mortality. Crit Care Med. Feb 2011;39(2):364-70.

44% and 54% for children 0 to 28 days and those 29 days to 17 years, respectively. More recently, between 2017 and 2021, ELSO reports the average survival to be 52% and 60% for children 0 to 28 days and those 29 days to 17 years, respectively.[30] The utilization of cardiac ECMO has become a postoperative standard of care, and it is used as a bridge to recovery after cardiopulmonary bypass, for unremitting low cardiac output state. A relatively short duration of ECMO is usually required, focused on maximizing myocardial perfusion, addressing residual lesions, treating arrhythmias, and improving end organ function.[95,96] Some case series have demonstrated the role in ECMO in children with refractory cardiogenic shock[97] or acute fulminant myocarditis.[98]

Improved mortality outcomes with cardiac ECMO are associated with weight greater than 3.3 kg, biventricular anatomy, low vasoactive inotrope score,[99] lactate clearance less than 24 hours after initiation, absent renal failure, good hemostasis, lack of chromosomal anomalies, elective ECMO initiation rather than ECPR, and ability to separate in less than 5 days.[100,101] Nonetheless, cardiac programs are more likely to consider 2 to 3 kg neonates for cardiac ECMO than in past eras.[102] Although single ventricle circulations were historically regarded as a contraindication to ECMO support, there has been growing use of ECMO in this population.[103,104] ECMO use for children with cavopulmonary connections[105,106] has included VV-ECMO support to improve oxygenation in the setting of lung disease or elevated pulmonary vascular resistance, or VA-ECMO support to stabilize before surgical revision.

Clinicians have found an association between early ventricular decompression and improved outcome.[107,108] It is thought the already inadequately ejecting systemic ventricle is exposed to increased afterload because of VA ECMO. The afterload

Table 4
Extracorporeal membrane oxygenation candidacy and management in patients receiving hematopoietic cell transplantation

Candidacy	• ECMO candidacy should be determined by a multidisciplinary team • Consider prognosis of the primary disease • Consideration should evaluate if the child is likely to recover (generally in 2–3 wk) • ECMO should be considered in survivors more than 2 y post-HCT who remain in remission of their primary disease and without secondary cancers or chronic graft vs host failure • Consider with caution if the prognosis of the primary disease is poor • Consider with caution if there are associated comorbidities or HCT-specific complications • Consider the number of injured organs with more organ injuries increasing caution regarding recovery • Extreme caution if neutrophils have not recovered and engraftment has not occurred, primary graft failure or rejection
ECMO management	• Initiate early if a patient is determined to be a candidate • High flow rates in order to reduce anticoagulation need • Target platelets count at least >40,000μL • Fibrinogen >200 mg/dL • Normal ATIII 80%–100% • Use of coated circuits and oxygenators with a limited number of connectors • High vigilance for infection • Lung rest ventilator settings • Initiate RRT when (a) acute kidney injury reaches Kidney Disease Improving Global Outcomes > stage 2; (b) fluid overload more than 10% and refractory to diuretics; (c) refractory electrolyte abnormalities; and (d) hyperammonemia (serum ammonia >250 mmol/L) • ECMO management should be by a multidisciplinary team

Abbreviations: ATIII, antithrombin III; ECMO, extracorporeal membrane oxygenation; HCT, hematopoietic cell transplantation; RRT; renal replacement therapy.

Recommendations adapted from Di Nardo M, Ahmad AH, Merli P, et al. Extracorporeal membrane oxygenation in children receiving haematopoietic cell transplantation and immune effector cell therapy: an international and multidisciplinary consensus statement. Lancet Child Adolesc Health. Feb 2022;6(2):116-128; with permission.

increases systemic ventricle congestion, which in turn negatively affect subendocardial perfusion, function, and recovery of the myocardium, and can additionally lead to pulmonary edema or hemorrhage.[107,108] As a result, experts have advocated for early left atrial decompression.[109] Left atrial decompression is most commonly a catheter-based approach such as balloon septoplasty or a left atrial drain placement (see **Fig. 1**). More recently,[107] the use of a percutaneous microaxial VAD has emerged as alternative route for decompression among older children.[110,111] Increasingly, ECMO is used as a bridge to alternate durable mechanical circulatory support or transplant if there is a lack of recovery.[112]

Extracorporeal Cardiopulmonary Resuscitation

In the earliest reports of ECMO in children, ECMO was reported as being deployed to patients receiving cardiopulmonary resuscitation.[1] The ELSO registry reports survival to discharge following ECPR as approximately 40% in children, with minimal variation

Table 5
Pediatric complex conditions, survival outcomes following the use of extracorporeal membrane oxygenation support

Condition	Survival = %, Reported cases = N	Reference
Bronchiolitis	78% (256/329)	Barbaro,[35] 2016
Viral or bacterial pneumonia	65% (385/595)	Barbaro,[35] 2016
Nonpulmonary infections	52% (146/281)	Barbaro,[35] 2016
Neoplasms	42% (376/902)	Suzuki,[83] 2022
Hematopoietic cell transplant	25% (4/16)	Bridges,[135] 2021, Maue,[136] 2019
Immune-mediated diseases	50% (104/207)[a]	Barreto,[84] 2022
Burn and inhalational injury	46% (43/93)[b]	Suzuki,[85] 2022
Trauma	63% (362/573)[c]	Behr,[86] 2020
Acute poisonings	86% (12/14)[d]	De Lange,[87] 2013
Bridge to lung transplant	84% (57/68)[e]	Thompson,[88] 2022

[a] As young as 2 mo included in this study.
[b] As young as 0 d included in this study, median age 2 years old.
[c] Data reported in discontinued reason, 63% being expected recovery, 34% with death or poor.
[d] Age not defined.
[e] 19 y of age included in this study.

over time (**Table 6**).[17,30] The American Heart Association and International Consensus on Cardiopulmonary Resuscitation guidelines recommended ECPR be considered for children with known cardiac diagnoses and in-hospital cardiac arrest.[38,40,41] Coinciding with increasing research in ECPR, there has been increasing use of ECPR

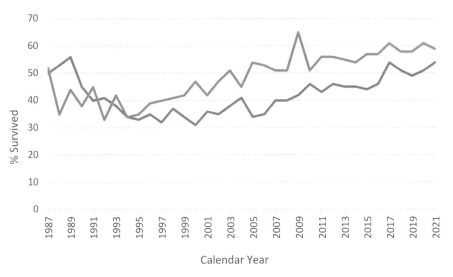

Fig. 4. Pediatric cardiac ECMO survival 1987 through 2021. ECMO: neonatal = 0 to 28 days; pediatric = 29 days to 17 years old. (*Data from* Extracorporeal Life Support Organizaiton (ELSO) Registry. Available at https://www.elso.org/Registry/InternationalSummaryand Reports/InternationalSummary.aspx.)

Table 6
Extracorporeal cardiopulmonary resuscitation cases and survival children

	Total Runs	Survived (#:%)
Neonatal		
1994–2003	158	63 (40%)
2004–2013	964	397 (39%)
2014–2021	1298	571 (44%)
Pediatric		
1992–2001	162	56 (35%)
2002–2011	1512	629 (42%)
2012–2021	4457	1911 (43%)

ECMO to support cardiopulmonary resuscitation (ECPR); neonatal = 0 to 28 days old; pediatric = 29 d to 17 years old.
Data from Extracorporeal Life Support Organizaiton (ELSO) Registry. Available at https://www.elso.org/Registry/InternationalSummaryandReports/InternationalSummary.aspx.

reported to the ELSO Registry (**Fig. 5**).[30] Additionally, ECMO can be considered to support the postcardiac arrest patient in the setting of persistent cardiorespiratory instability despite escalation of usual intensive care medical supports.[38]

ETHICAL DILEMMAS

The expanded indications for ECMO have prompted focused studies in the ethical domain.[52,113,114] The ethical dilemmas faced in ECMO are shared with other technologic supports such as dialysis and ventilators including: end-of-life considerations,

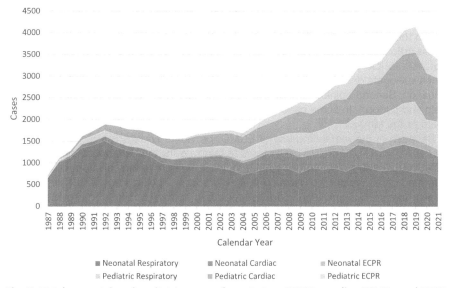

Fig. 5. Total neonatal and pediatric cases of respiratory ECMO, cardiac ECMO, and ECPR from 1987 to 2021. ECMO, ECMO to support cardiopulmonary resuscitation (ECPR): neonatal = 0 to 28 days; pediatric = 29 days to 17 years old. (*Data from* Extracorporeal Life Support Organizaiton (ELSO) Registry. Available at https://www.elso.org/Registry/InternationalSummaryandReports/InternationalSummary.aspx.)

initiation of new technology, treatment decisions, cessation of support, organ dona-tion considerations, moral distress of intensive care staff, and palliative care proced-ures.[115–117] Similarly, recent reviews on ethics in ECMO reveal issues to those of other life-sustaining therapies including consent, decisional authority, resource allocation, equitable access, and research ethics.[114,118–120] Consequently, many of the estab-lished clinically applied ethics frameworks and tools can be adapted to ECMO.

A recent narrative review of pediatric ECMO demonstrates 3 key domains requiring further guidance and support: communication/decision-making, ethics, and end-of-life care provision.[114] Current recommendations suggest iterative discussions with a surrogate decision-maker.[121–123] Tailoring communication for longer courses of ECMO (months) requires similar attention to transparency, clear communication, and attendance to team dynamics,[124] as well as burdens and benefits of the therapy.

Equitable offering and delivery of ECMO support is both imperative and difficult due to few absolute contraindications in the current era. Unconscious biases have been demonstrated in disparate utilization and outcomes of ECMO in racial and ethnic groups of all ages.[125–127] A robust decision-making process is necessary to ensure all children have equal opportunity to receive potentially beneficial ECMO support and avoid exposure when it is not beneficial.[126] ECMO requires resources that during high demand can be scarce: intensive human and material resources. The SARS-CoV-2 pandemic forced reconsideration of restricted utilization of ECMO even in resource replete countries.[128,129] Historically, rationing of medical care and devices has been avoided in the United States; this avoidance impedes engagement in discourse around systemic accountability for use. Appropriate resource consideration would include therapies across the spectrum of health-care delivery for a region to fairly allo-cate ECMO.[130]

Recently published guidance on the practicalities of compassionate decannulation from ECMO can aid teams in the required steps accompanying these difficult deci-sions.[131] The ethical underpinnings for ECMO remain the same as withdrawal of other life-sustaining therapies and are legally supported in many countries across Europe, and in the United States, Canada, and elsewhere.[132–134] Although outside the scope of this article, expanding use in countries where withdrawal of life-sustaining therapy is not permissible presents additional ethical challenges. Often teams are burdened when surrogate decision-makers do not accept a recommendation for ECMO discon-tinuation. Second opinions, mediated solutions, and bioethics consultation can be of help and support. In some cases, legal recourse is required by either the health-care team or the family.[122,133]

Because of the expanding use of ECMO, providers and institutions encounter an increasing demand to build procedures to facilitate the ethical application of this life support technology. Communication strategies, inherent to ethical informed consent, informed care, and shared decision-making warrant ongoing study. The interface be-tween human lives and technologic support has and will continue to provide ethical dilemmas demanding attention, study, and application of ethical justification among current norms and contexts.

SUMMARY

For the last 50 years, ECMO has been a life support technology provided to children when health-care providers find conventional management to be insufficient and thought a patient is at risk of death. Over time, ECMO has shifted from an experi-mental therapy to a standard of care in certain conditions. Nonetheless, ECMO ev-idence and consensus guidance in children is relatively limited. During the next decades, continued advancement of ECMO will hopefully result in evidence refining care delivery, limiting complications, improving both survival and the quality of life for survivors.

CLINICS CARE POINTS

- When neonates reach an oxygenation index of 40 or higher there is evidence that instituting ECMO support can reduce mortality, and survivors have at least equivalent neurodevelopment outcomes and respiratory morbidity compared to conventional management without ECMO support.
- Patient and mechanical complications are relatively common among ECMO supported patients, and survivors of critical illness severe enough to require ECMO will commonly experience deficits in neuromotor ability, reading comprehension, communication, and visual-spatial ability. Health care teams should have strategies to attempt to minimize, detect and manage of complications as well as follow-up care plans to identify and support disabilities.

DISCLOSURE

G. MacLaren is a member of the board of directors of the Extracorporeal Life Support Organization (ELSO). R.P. Barbaro is the ELSO Registry Chair and receives support unrelated to this study from the National Institutes of Health, United States, R01 HL153519; K12 HL138039.

SUPPLEMENTARY DATA

Supplementary data related to this article can be found online at https://doi.org/10.1016/j.pmr.2016.04.003.

REFERENCES

1. Bartlett RH, Gazzaniga AB, Jefferies MR, et al. Extracorporeal membrane oxygenation (ECMO) cardiopulmonary support in infancy. Trans Am Soc Artif Intern Organs 1976;22:80–93.
2. Hill JD, O'Brien TG, Murray JJ, et al. Prolonged extracorporeal oxygenation for acute post-traumatic respiratory failure (shock-lung syndrome). Use of the Bramson membrane lung. N Engl J Med 1972;286(12):629–34.
3. Conrad SA, Broman LM, Taccone FS, et al. The extracorporeal life support organization maastricht treaty for nomenclature in extracorporeal life support. A position paper of the extracorporeal life support organization. Am J Respir Crit Care Med 2018;198(4):447–51.
4. Broman LM, Taccone FS, Lorusso R, et al. The ELSO Maastricht Treaty for ECLS Nomenclature: abbreviations for cannulation configuration in extracorporeal life support - a position paper of the Extracorporeal Life Support Organization. Crit Care 2019;23(1):36.
5. Toomasian JM, Snedecor SM, Cornell RG, et al. National experience with extracorporeal membrane oxygenation for newborn respiratory failure. Data from 715 cases. ASAIO J 1988;34(2):140–7.
6. Stolar CJ, Delosh T, Bartlett RH. Extracorporeal life support organization 1993. ASAIO J 1993;39(4):976–9.

7. UK collaborative randomised trial of neonatal extracorporeal membrane oxygenation. UK Collaborative ECMO Trail Group. Lancet 1996;348(9020): 75–82.

8. Mugford M, Elbourne D, Field D. Extracorporeal membrane oxygenation for severe respiratory failure in newborn infants. Cochrane Database Syst Rev 2008; 16(3):CD001340.

9. Barbaro RP, Odetola FO, Kidwell KM, et al. Association of hospital-level volume of extracorporeal membrane oxygenation cases and mortality. Analysis of the extracorporeal life support organization registry. Am J Respir Crit Care Med 2015;191(8):894–901.

10. Conrad SA, Rycus PT, Dalton H. Extracorporeal life support registry report 2004. ASAIO J 2005;51(1):4–10.

11. Inhaled nitric oxide in full-term and nearly full-term infants with hypoxic respiratory failure. N Engl J Med 1997;336(9):597–604.

12. Roberts JD Jr, Fineman JR, Morin FC 3rd, et al. Inhaled nitric oxide and persistent pulmonary hypertension of the newborn. The Inhaled Nitric Oxide Study Group. N Engl J Med 1997;336(9):605–10.

13. Hintz SR, Suttner DM, Sheehan AM, et al. Decreased use of neonatal extracorporeal membrane oxygenation (ECMO): how new treatment modalities have affected ECMO utilization. Pediatrics 2000;106(6):1339–43.

14. Booth KL, Roth SJ, Thiagarajan RR, et al. Extracorporeal membrane oxygenation support of the Fontan and bidirectional Glenn circulations. Ann Thorac Surg 2004;77(4):1341–8.

15. Thiagarajan RR, Laussen PC, Rycus PT, et al. Extracorporeal membrane oxygenation to aid cardiopulmonary resuscitation in infants and children. Circulation 2007;116(15):1693–700.

16. Belohlavek J, Smalcova J, Rob D, et al. Effect of intra-arrest transport, extracorporeal cardiopulmonary resuscitation, and immediate invasive assessment and treatment on functional neurologic outcome in refractory out-of-hospital cardiac arrest: a randomized clinical trial. JAMA 2022;327(8):737–47.

17. Barbaro RP, Paden ML, Guner YS, et al. Pediatric extracorporeal life support organization registry international report 2016. ASAIO J 2017;63(4):456–63.

18. van der Linde D, Konings EE, Slager MA, et al. Birth prevalence of congenital heart disease worldwide: a systematic review and meta-analysis. J Am Coll Cardiol 2011;58(21):2241–7.

19. Global, regional. And national burden of congenital heart disease, 1990-2017: a systematic analysis for the Global Burden of Disease Study 2017. Lancet Child Adolesc Health 2020;4(3):185–200.

20. Hayes MM, Fallon BP, Barbaro RP, et al. Membrane lung and blood pump use during prolonged extracorporeal membrane oxygenation: trends from 2002 to 2017. ASAIO J 2021;67(9):1062–70.

21. Wang D, Zhou X, Liu X, et al. Wang-Zwische double lumen cannula-toward a percutaneous and ambulatory paracorporeal artificial lung. ASAIO J 2008; 54(6):606–11.

22. Peek GJ, Mugford M, Tiruvoipati R, et al. Efficacy and economic assessment of conventional ventilatory support versus extracorporeal membrane oxygenation for severe adult respiratory failure (CESAR): a multicentre randomised controlled trial. Lancet 2009;374(9698):1351–63.

23. Noah MA, Peek GJ, Finney SJ, et al. Referral to an extracorporeal membrane oxygenation center and mortality among patients with severe 2009 influenza A(H1N1). JAMA 2011;306(15):1659–68.

24. Davies A, Jones D, Bailey M, et al. Extracorporeal membrane oxygenation for 2009 influenza A(H1N1) acute respiratory distress syndrome. JAMA 2009; 302(17):1888–95.

25. Chen YS, Lin JW, Yu HY, et al. Cardiopulmonary resuscitation with assisted extracorporeal life-support versus conventional cardiopulmonary resuscitation in adults with in-hospital cardiac arrest: an observational study and propensity analysis. Lancet 2008;372(9638):554–61.

26. Fraser CD Jr, Jaquiss RD, Rosenthal DN, et al. Prospective trial of a pediatric ventricular assist device. N Engl J Med 2012;367(6):532–41.

27. Thiagarajan RR, Barbaro RP, Rycus PT, et al. Extracorporeal life support organization registry international report 2016. ASAIO J 2017;63(1):60–7.

28. Mustafa AK, Alexander PJ, Joshi DJ, et al. Extracorporeal membrane oxygenation for patients with COVID-19 in severe respiratory failure. JAMA Surg 2020; 155(10):990–2.

29. Combes A, Hajage D, Capellier G, et al. Extracorporeal membrane oxygenation for severe acute respiratory distress syndrome. N Engl J Med 2018;378(21): 1965–75.

30. Extracorporeal life support Organizaiton (ELSO) registry. 2022. Available at: https://www.elso.org/Registry/InternationalSummaryandReports/International Summary.aspx. Accessed July 29, 2022.

31. Barbaro RP, MacLaren G, Boonstra PS, et al. Extracorporeal membrane oxygenation for COVID-19: evolving outcomes from the international extracorporeal life support organization registry. Lancet 2021;398(10307):1230–8.

32. Barbaro RP, MacLaren G, Boonstra PS, et al. Extracorporeal membrane oxygenation support in COVID-19: an international cohort study of the Extracorporeal Life Support Organization registry. Lancet 2020;396(10257):1071–8.

33. Barbaro RP, Brodie D, MacLaren G. Bridging the gap between intensivists and primary care clinicians in extracorporeal membrane oxygenation for respiratory failure in children: a review. JAMA Pediatr 2021;175(5):510–7.

34. Saeed O, Stein LH, Cavarocchi N, et al. Outcomes by cannulation methods for venovenous extracorporeal membrane oxygenation during COVID-19: a multicenter retrospective study. Artif Organs 2022;46(8):1659–68.

35. Barbaro RP, Boonstra PS, Paden ML, et al. Development and validation of the pediatric risk estimate score for children using extracorporeal respiratory support (Ped-RESCUERS). Intensive Care Med 2016;42(5):879–88.

36. Stoney WS. Evolution of cardiopulmonary bypass. Circulation 2009;119(21): 2844–53.

37. Kane DA, Thiagarajan RR, Wypij D, et al. Rapid-response extracorporeal membrane oxygenation to support cardiopulmonary resuscitation in children with cardiac disease. Circulation 2010;122(11 Suppl):S241–8.

38. Topjian AA, de Caen A, Wainwright MS, et al. Pediatric post-cardiac arrest care: a scientific statement from the American heart association. Circulation 2019; 140(6):e194–233.

39. Holmberg MJ, Geri G, Wiberg S, et al. Extracorporeal cardiopulmonary resuscitation for cardiac arrest: a systematic review. Resuscitation 2018;131:91–100.

40. Maconochie IK, Aickin R, Hazinski MF, et al. Pediatric life support: 2020 international consensus on cardiopulmonary resuscitation and emergency cardiovascular care science with treatment recommendations. Circulation 2020; 142(16_suppl_1):S140–84.

41. Marino BS, Tabbutt S, MacLaren G, et al. Cardiopulmonary resuscitation in infants and children with cardiac disease: a scientific statement from the American heart association. Circulation 2018;137(22):e691–782.

42. Meert KL, Telford R, Holubkov R, et al. Pediatric out-of-hospital cardiac arrest characteristics and their association with survival and neurobehavioral outcome. Pediatr Crit Care Med 2016;17(12):e543–50.

43. Nguyen DA, De Mul A, Hoskote AU, et al. Factors associated with initiation of extracorporeal cardiopulmonary resuscitation in the pediatric population: an international survey. ASAIO J 2022;68(3):413–8.

44. Meert KL, Guerguerian AM, Barbaro R, et al. Extracorporeal cardiopulmonary resuscitation: one-year survival and neurobehavioral outcome among infants and children with in-hospital cardiac arrest. Crit Care Med 2019;47(3):393–402.

45. Conrad SA, Rycus PT. Extracorporeal membrane oxygenation for refractory cardiac arrest. Ann Card Anaesth 2017;20(Supplement):S4–10.

46. Zapol WM, Snider MT, Hill JD, et al. Extracorporeal membrane oxygenation in severe acute respiratory failure. A randomized prospective study. JAMA 1979; 242(20):2193–6.

47. Paden ML, Conrad SA, Rycus PT, et al. Extracorporeal life support organization registry report 2012. ASAIO J 2013;59(3):202–10.

48. Shaefi S, Brenner SK, Gupta S, et al. Extracorporeal membrane oxygenation in patients with severe respiratory failure from COVID-19. Intensive Care Med 2021;47(2):208–21.

49. Urner M, Barnett AG, Bassi GL, et al. Venovenous extracorporeal membrane oxygenation in patients with acute covid-19 associated respiratory failure: comparative effectiveness study. BMJ 2022;377:e068723.

50. Bréchot N, Hajage D, Kimmoun A, et al. Venoarterial extracorporeal membrane oxygenation to rescue sepsis-induced cardiogenic shock: a retrospective, multicentre, international cohort study. Lancet 2020;396(10250):545–52.

51. (k) Premarket Notification. U.S. Food & Drug Administration. 2022. Available at: https://www.accessdata.fda.gov/scripts/cdrh/cfdocs/cfpmn/pmn.cfm?ID=K102 726. Accessed July 28, 2022.

52. Combes A, Price S, Slutsky AS, et al. Temporary circulatory support for cardiogenic shock. Lancet 2020;396(10245):199–212.

53. Ravichandran AK, Baran DA, Stelling K, et al. Outcomes with the tandem protek duo dual-lumen percutaneous right ventricular assist device. ASAIO J 2018; 64(4):570–2.

54. Yu JS, Barbaro RP, Granoski DA, et al. Prospective side by side comparison of outcomes and complications with a simple versus intensive anticoagulation monitoring strategy in pediatric extracorporeal life support patients. Pediatr Crit Care Med 2017;18(11):1055–62.

55. Ozment CP, Scott BL, Bembea MM, et al. Anticoagulation and transfusion management during neonatal and pediatric extracorporeal membrane oxygenation: a survey of medical directors in the United States. Pediatr Crit Care Med 2021; 22(6):530–41.

56. Schmidt F, Jack T, Sasse M, et al. Awake veno-arterial extracorporeal membrane oxygenation" in pediatric cardiogenic shock: a single-center experience. Pediatr Cardiol 2015;36(8):1647–56.

57. Turner DA, Rehder KJ, Bonadonna D, et al. Ambulatory ECMO as a bridge to lung transplant in a previously well pediatric patient with ARDS. Pediatrics 2014;134(2):e583–5.

58. Fuehner T, Kuehn C, Hadem J, et al. Extracorporeal membrane oxygenation in awake patients as bridge to lung transplantation. Am J Respir Crit Care Med 2012;185(7):763–8.

59. Abrams D, Garan AR, Brodie D. Awake and fully mobile patients on cardiac extracorporeal life support. Ann Cardiothorac Surg 2019;8(1):44–53.

60. Abrams D, Madahar P, Eckhardt CM, et al. Early mobilization during extracorporeal membrane oxygenation for cardiopulmonary failure in adults: factors associated with intensity of treatment. Ann Am Thorac Soc 2022;19(1):90–8.

61. Gurnani PK, Michalak LA, Tabachnick D, et al. Outcomes of extubated COVID and non-COVID patients receiving awake venovenous extracorporeal membrane oxygenation. ASAIO J 2022;68(4):478–85.

62. Nelson-McMillan K, Vricella LA, Stewart FD, et al. Recovery from total acute lung failure after 20 Months of extracorporeal life support. ASAIO J 2020;66(1):e11–4.

63. DellaVolpe J, Barbaro RP, Cannon JW, et al. Joint society of critical care medicine-extracorporeal life support organization task force position paper on the role of the intensivist in the initiation and management of extracorporeal membrane oxygenation. Crit Care Med 2020;48(6):838–46.

64. Dhar AV, Morrison T, Barbaro RP, et al. Starting and sustaining an extracorporeal membrane oxygenation program. ASAIO J 2022. https://doi.org/10.1097/MAT.0000000000001783.

65. Ijsselstijn H, Schiller RM, Holder C, et al. Extracorporeal life support organization (ELSO) guidelines for follow-up after neonatal and pediatric extracorporeal membrane oxygenation. ASAIO J 2021;67(9):955–63.

66. Bartlett RH, Gazzaniga AB, Toomasian J, et al. Extracorporeal membrane oxygenation (ECMO) in neonatal respiratory failure. 100 cases. Ann Surg 1986;204(3):236–45.

67. Kays DW. ECMO in CDH: is there a role? Semin Pediatr Surg 2017;26(3):166–70.

68. Kays DW, Talbert JL, Islam S, et al. Improved survival in left liver-up congenital diaphragmatic hernia by early repair before extracorporeal membrane oxygenation: optimization of patient selection by multivariate risk modeling. J Am Coll Surg 2016;222(4):459–70.

69. Guner Y, Jancelewicz T, Di Nardo M, et al. Management of congenital diaphragmatic hernia treated with extracorporeal life support: Interim guidelines consensus statement from the extracorporeal life support organization. ASAIO J 2021;67(2):113–20.

70. Weems MF, Upadhyay K, Sandhu HS. Survey of ECMO practices for infants with hypoxic ischemic encephalopathy. J Perinatol 2018;38(9):1197–204.

71. Agarwal P, Altinok D, Desai J, et al. In-hospital outcomes of neonates with hypoxic-ischemic encephalopathy receiving extracorporeal membrane oxygenation. J Perinatol 2019;39(5):661–5.

72. Kunisaki SM, Fauza DO, Barnewolt CE, et al. Ex utero intrapartum treatment with placement on extracorporeal membrane oxygenation for fetal thoracic masses. J Pediatr Surg 2007;42(2):420–5.

73. Straughan AJ, Mulcahy CF, Sandler AD, et al. Tracheal agenesis: vertical division of the native esophagus - a novel surgical approach and review of the literature. Ann Otol Rhinol Laryngol 2021;130(6):547–62.

74. Bagdure D, Torres N, Walker LK, et al. Extracorporeal membrane oxygenation for neonates with congenital renal and urological anomalies and pulmonary hypoplasia: a case report and review of the extracorporeal life support organization registry. J Pediatr Intensive Care 2017;6(3):188–93.

75. Kuo KW, Barbaro RP, Gadepalli SK, et al. Should extracorporeal membrane oxygenation Be offered? An Int Surv J Pediatr 2017;182:107–13.

76. Alore EA, Fallon SC, Thomas JA, et al. Outcomes after extracorporeal life support cannulation in pediatric patients with trisomy 13 and trisomy 18. J Surg Res 2021;257:260–6.

77. Morrison WE, Kirsch R. Pushing the ECMO envelope for children with genetic conditions. Pediatr Crit Care Med 2017;18(9):896–7.

78. Fackler JC, Bohn D, Green T, et al. Stopping a RCT. Abstr Am J Respir Crit Care Med 1997;155:A504.

79. Dalton HJ, Macrae DJ. Extracorporeal support in children with pediatric acute respiratory distress syndrome: proceedings from the Pediatric Acute Lung Injury Consensus Conference. Pediatr Crit Care Med 2015;16(5 Suppl 1): S111–7.

80. Moler FW, Palmisano J, Custer JR. Extracorporeal life support for pediatric respiratory failure: predictors of survival from 220 patients. Crit Care Med 1993; 21(10):1604–11.

81. Zabrocki LA, Brogan TV, Statler KD, et al. Extracorporeal membrane oxygenation for pediatric respiratory failure: survival and predictors of mortality. Crit Care Med 2011;39(2):364–70.

82. Di Nardo M, Ahmad AH, Merli P, et al. Extracorporeal membrane oxygenation in children receiving haematopoietic cell transplantation and immune effector cell therapy: an international and multidisciplinary consensus statement. Lancet Child Adolesc Health 2022;6(2):116–28.

83. Suzuki Y, Cass SH, Kugelmann A, et al. Outcome of extracorporeal membrane oxygenation for pediatric patients with neoplasm: an extracorporeal life support organization database study (2000-2019). Pediatr Crit Care Med 2022;23(5): e240–8.

84. Barreto JA, Mehta A, Thiagarajan RR, et al. The use of extracorporeal life support in children with immune-mediated diseases. Pediatr Crit Care Med 2022; 23(1):e60–5.

85. Suzuki Y, Williams TP, Patino J, et al. Extracorporeal membrane oxygenation for pediatric burn patients: is management improving over time? ASAIO J 2022; 68(3):426–31.

86. Behr CA, Strotmeyer SJ, Swol J, et al. Characteristics and outcomes of extracorporeal life support in pediatric trauma patients. J Trauma Acute Care Surg 2020; 89(4):631–5.

87. de Lange DW, Sikma MA, Meulenbelt J. Extracorporeal membrane oxygenation in the treatment of poisoned patients. Clin Toxicol (Phila) 2013;51(5):385–93.

88. Thompson K, Staffa SJ, Nasr VG, et al. Mortality after lung transplantation for children bridged with extracorporeal membrane oxygenation. Ann Am Thorac Soc 2022;19(3):415–23.

89. Supady A, Combes A, Barbaro RP, et al. Respiratory indications for ECMO: focus on COVID-19. Intensive Care Med 2022;48(10):1326–37.

90. Ramanathan K, Antognini D, Combes A, et al. Planning and provision of ECMO services for severe ARDS during the COVID-19 pandemic and other outbreaks of emerging infectious diseases. Lancet Respir Med 2020;8(5):518–26.

91. MacLaren G, Fisher D, Brodie D. Treating the most critically ill patients with COVID-19: the evolving role of extracorporeal membrane oxygenation. JAMA 2022;327(1):31–2.

92. Brodie D, Abrams D, MacLaren G, et al. Extracorporeal membrane oxygenation during respiratory pandemics: past, present, and future. Am J Respir Crit Care Med 2022;205(12):1382–90.

93. Son MBF, Murray N, Friedman K, et al. Multisystem inflammatory syndrome in children - initial therapy and outcomes. N Engl J Med 2021;385(1):23–34.

94. Miller AD, Zambrano LD, Yousaf AR, et al. Multisystem inflammatory syndrome in children-United States, february 2020-July 2021. Clin Infect Dis 2022; 75(1):186.

95. Lorusso R, Raffa GM, Kowalewski M, et al. Structured review of post-cardiotomy extracorporeal membrane oxygenation: Part 2-pediatric patients. J Heart Lung Transpl 2019;38(11):1144–61.

96. Salvin JW, Laussen PC, Thiagarajan RR. Extracorporeal membrane oxygenation for postcardiotomy mechanical cardiovascular support in children with congenital heart disease. Paediatr Anaesth 2008;18(12):1157–62.

97. Brown KL, Ichord R, Marino BS, et al. Outcomes following extracorporeal membrane oxygenation in children with cardiac disease. Pediatr Crit Care Med 2013; 14(5 Suppl 1):S73–83.

98. Rajagopal SK, Almond CS, Laussen PC, et al. Extracorporeal membrane oxygenation for the support of infants, children, and young adults with acute myocarditis: a review of the Extracorporeal Life Support Organization registry. Crit Care Med 2010;38(2):382–7.

99. Gaies MG, Gurney JG, Yen AH, et al. Vasoactive-inotropic score as a predictor of morbidity and mortality in infants after cardiopulmonary bypass. Pediatr Crit Care Med 2010;11(2):234–8.

100. Merrill ED, Schoeneberg L, Sandesara P, et al. Outcomes after prolonged extracorporeal membrane oxygenation support in children with cardiac disease–Extracorporeal Life Support Organization registry study. J Thorac Cardiovasc Surg 2014;148(2):582–8.

101. Roeleveld PP, Mendonca M. Neonatal cardiac ECMO in 2019 and beyond. Front Pediatr 2019;7:327.

102. Bhat P, Hirsch JC, Gelehrter S, et al. Outcomes of infants weighing three kilograms or less requiring extracorporeal membrane oxygenation after cardiac surgery. Ann Thorac Surg 2013;95(2):656–61.

103. Sherwin ED, Gauvreau K, Scheurer MA, et al. Extracorporeal membrane oxygenation after stage 1 palliation for hypoplastic left heart syndrome. J Thorac Cardiovasc Surg 2012;144(6):1337–43.

104. Misfeldt AM, Kirsch RE, Goldberg DJ, et al. Outcomes of single-ventricle patients supported with extracorporeal membrane oxygenation. Pediatr Crit Care Med 2016;17(3):194–202.

105. Allan CK, Thiagarajan RR, del Nido PJ, et al. Indication for initiation of mechanical circulatory support impacts survival of infants with shunted single-ventricle circulation supported with extracorporeal membrane oxygenation. J Thorac Cardiovasc Surg 2007;133(3):660–7.

106. Hoskote A, Bohn D, Gruenwald C, et al. Extracorporeal life support after staged palliation of a functional single ventricle: subsequent morbidity and survival. J Thorac Cardiovasc Surg 2006;131(5):1114–21.

107. Zampi JD, Alghanem F, Yu S, et al. Relationship between time to left atrial decompression and outcomes in patients receiving venoarterial extracorporeal membrane oxygenation support: a multicenter pediatric interventional cardiology early-career society study. Pediatr Crit Care Med 2019;20(8):728–36.

108. Sperotto F, Polito A, Amigoni A, et al. Left atrial decompression in pediatric patients supported with extracorporeal membrane oxygenation for failure to wean from cardiopulmonary bypass: a propensity-weighted analysis. J Am Heart Assoc 2022;e023963. https://doi.org/10.1161/JAHA.121.023963.

109. Brown G, Moynihan KM, Deatrick KB, et al. Extracorporeal life support organization (ELSO): guidelines for pediatric cardiac failure. ASAIO J 2021;67(5): 463–75.

110. Parekh D, Jeewa A, Tume SC, et al. Percutaneous mechanical circulatory support using impella devices for decompensated cardiogenic shock: a pediatric heart center experience. ASAIO J 2018;64(1):98–104.

111. Meuwese CL, de Haan M, Zwetsloot PP, et al. The hemodynamic effect of different left ventricular unloading techniques during veno-arterial extracorporeal life support: a systematic review and meta-analysis. Perfusion 2020;35(7): 664–71.

112. Dipchand AI, Kirk R, Naftel DC, et al. Ventricular assist device support as a bridge to transplantation in pediatric patients. J Am Coll Cardiol 2018;72(4): 402–15.

113. Bein T, Brodie D. Understanding ethical decisions for patients on extracorporeal life support. Intensive Care Med 2017;43(10):1510–1.

114. Moynihan KM, Dorste A, Siegel BD, et al. Decision-making, ethics, and end-of-life care in pediatric extracorporeal membrane oxygenation: a comprehensive narrative review. Pediatr Crit Care Med 2021;22(9):806–12.

115. Skillman JJ. Ethical dilemmas in the care of the critically ill. Lancet 1974;2(7881): 634–7.

116. Searle JF. Ethical problems in intensive care. Br J Anaesth 1978;50(12):1265–6.

117. Schneiderman LJ, Spragg RG. Ethical decisions in discontinuing mechanical ventilation. N Engl J Med 1988;318(15):984–8.

118. Courtwright AM, Robinson EM, Feins K, et al. Ethics committee consultation and extracorporeal membrane oxygenation. Ann Am Thorac Soc 2016;13(9): 1553–8.

119. Wirpsa MJ, Carabini LM, Neely KJ, et al. Mitigating ethical conflict and moral distress in the care of patients on ECMO: impact of an automatic ethics consultation protocol. J Med Ethics 2021;2020:106881.

120. Schou A, Mølgaard J, Andersen LW, et al. Ethics in extracorporeal life support: a narrative review. Crit Care 2021;25(1):256.

121. Moynihan KM, Purol N, Alexander PMA, et al. A communication guide for pediatric extracorporeal membrane oxygenation. Pediatr Crit Care Med 2021;22(9): 832–41.

122. Kirsch R, Munson D. Ethical and end of life considerations for neonates requiring ECMO support. Semin Perinatol 2018;42(2):129–37.

123. Stephens AL, Bruce CR. Setting expectations for ECMO: improving communication between clinical teams and decision makers. Methodist Debakey Cardiovasc J 2018;14(2):120–5.

124. Barbaro RP, Annich G, Kirsch R. Extracorporeal life support. In: Krishnan H, Fine-Goulden MR, Raman S, et al, editors. Challenging concepts in paediatric critical care: cases with expert commentary. United Kingdom: Oxford University Press; 2020.

125. Chan T, Barrett CS, Tjoeng YL, et al. Racial variations in extracorporeal membrane oxygenation use following congenital heart surgery. J Thorac Cardiovasc Surg 2018;156(1):306–15.

126. Moynihan KM, Jansen M, Siegel BD, et al. Extracorporeal membrane oxygenation candidacy decisions: an argument for a process-based longitudinal approach. Pediatr Crit Care Med 2022;23(9):e434–9.
127. Cleveland Manchanda EC, Sanky C, Appel JM. Crisis standards of care in the USA: a systematic review and implications for equity amidst COVID-19. J Racial Ethn Health Disparities 2021;8(4):824–36.
128. Ehmann MR, Zink EK, Levin AB, et al. Operational recommendations for scarce resource allocation in a public health crisis. Chest 2021;159(3):1076–83.
129. MacLaren G, Fisher D, Brodie D. Preparing for the most critically ill patients with COVID-19: the potential role of extracorporeal membrane oxygenation. JAMA 2020;323(13):1245–6.
130. White DB, Lo B. A framework for rationing ventilators and critical care beds during the COVID-19 pandemic. JAMA 2020;323(18):1773–4.
131. Machado DS, Garros D, Montuno L, et al. Finishing well: compassionate extracorporeal membrane oxygenation discontinuation. J Pain Symptom Manage 2022;63(5):e553–62.
132. Cantor NL. Twenty-five years after Quinlan: a review of the jurisprudence of death and dying. J L Med Ethics Summer 2001;29(2):182–96.
133. Kirsch RE, Balit CR, Carnevale FA, et al. Ethical, cultural, social, and individual considerations prior to transition to limitation or withdrawal of life-sustaining therapies. Pediatr Crit Care Med 2018;19(8S Suppl 2):S10–8.
134. Brodie D, Curtis JR, Vincent JL, et al. Treatment limitations in the era of ECMO. Lancet Respir Med 2017;5(10):769–70.
135. Bridges BC, Kilbaugh TJ, Barbaro RP, et al. Veno-venous extracorporeal membrane oxygenation for children with cancer or hematopoietic cell transplant: a ten center cohort. ASAIO J 2021;67(8):923–9.
136. Maue DK, Hobson MJ, Friedman ML, et al. Outcomes of pediatric oncology and hematopoietic cell transplant patients receiving extracorporeal membrane oxygenation. Perfusion 2019;34(7):598–604.

Cytokine Release Syndrome in the Pediatric Population and Implications for Intensive Care Management

Juliana Romano, MD*, Eric Wilsterman, MD, Megan Toal, MD, Christine Joyce, MD

KEYWORDS

- CAR-T • Cytokine release syndrome (CRS) • Pediatric intensive care

KEY POINTS

- Immune effector cell therapies have led to significantly improved survival in relapsed, refractory leukemias and lymphomas and have increased cancer survival rates in pediatric patients.
- Cytokine release syndrome (CRS) represents an immune hypersensitivity syndrome that can lead to profound multiorgan system failure and death.
- A universal grading system for CRS allows clinicians to accurately diagnose and initiate treatment regimens.

INTRODUCTION

Although leukemia remains the most common pediatric cancer, improvements in treatment have led to improved survival. For pediatric patients with acute lymphoblastic leukemia (ALL), survival rates approach 90%. However, survival rates for patients who have a relapse are significantly lower, with 5-year overall survival rates ranging from 19% to 52%, depending on ALL type.[1,2] A variety of new treatment modalities are available, among them new treatments in immunotherapy, using the body's own immune system to target malignant cells.[3,4] Tisagenlecleucel, the first chimeric antigen receptor (CAR) T cell to be approved by the Food and Drug Administration (FDA), demonstrated 90% remission in relapsed and refractory ALL. Recent studies show long-term disease-free survival in pediatric patients treated with CAR T cells as high as 60% at a median of 4.8 years out.[3,5] Although CAR T cell therapy has yet to be FDA approved in other pediatric cancers, treatment of B-cell non-

Department of Pediatrics, Division of Pediatric Critical Care Medicine, Weill Cornell Medicine, 525 East 68th Street, M508, New York, NY 10065, USA
* Corresponding author.
E-mail address: jur9084@nyp.org

Crit Care Clin 39 (2023) 277–285
https://doi.org/10.1016/j.ccc.2022.09.004
0749-0704/23/© 2022 Elsevier Inc. All rights reserved.

criticalcare.theclinics.com

Hodgkin lymphoma, mantle cell lymphoma, follicular lymphoma, and multiple myeloma are approved in ages 18 years and older and clinical trials are ongoing for other pediatric cancers.[6,7] Although these agents have the potential to revolutionize therapeutic options, they also come with their own set of toxicities, which in the most extreme form can lead to life threatening multiorgan system failure.[3,4,8] In this review article, we focus on the diagnosis and management of cytokine release syndrome (CRS).

Chimeric Antigen Receptor T-cells and Development of Cytokine Release Syndrome

Before understanding the pathophysiology behind CRS, an understanding of the therapy inciting it is necessary. CAR T cells represent one of several types of adoptive cell transfer, an immunotherapeutic approach whereby a patient's own cells are collected and used to target cancer cells. Following a blood draw, T cells are separated out and genetically engineered to produce receptors on their surface called CARs. This allows the T cells to recognize and attach to antigens on cancer cells. Once engineered to express the antigen-specific CAR, the T cells are expanded into the hundreds of millions. Patients undergo lymphodepletion and are then infused with the engineered CAR T cells.[9] There are currently 6 FDA-approved CAR T cells, all of which target either CD-19 or B-cell maturation antigen. Of these, only tisagenlecleucel, which targets CD-19, is FDA-approved in children.[9,10]

Once infused, CAR T cells recognize the antigen, resulting in CAR T proliferation, cytokine release, and immune cell activation.[11,12] Following activation, the CAR T cells produce interferon (IFN)-γ, tumor necrosis factor (TNF)-α, and granulocyte-macrophage colony-stimulating factor, which further activate monocyte and macrophages to secrete interleukin (IL)-1, IL-6, and inducible nitric oxide synthase.[12–14] It is this immune response that enables the patient's own immune system to fight against their cancer. However, when the above response is exaggerated, these immune effector cells are hyperactivated by excessive release of inflammatory mediators. This overactivation of this immune response leads to CRS.

Although recognized early as a side effect of CAR T therapy, it was not until 2018 when the American Society for Transplantation and Cell Therapy (ASTCT) convened an expert panel, that a uniform definition and grading system was created for CRS. Widely accepted, the ASTCT criteria define CRS as a "supraphysiologic response following any immune therapy that results in the activation or engagement of endogenous or infused T cells and/or other immune effector cells. Symptoms can be progressive, must include fever at the onset, and may include hypotension, capillary leak (hypoxia) and end organ dysfunction."[15]

Although most well recognized in CAR T therapy, it is important to note that CRS has also been described in the treatment with blinatumomab, a bispecific T cell engaging antibody, and following haploidentical hematopoietic stem cell transplant.[16,17]

Epidemiology and Predictors of Disease Severity

CRS exists along a spectrum of diseases with similar symptomology to macrophage activation syndrome and hemophagocytic lymphohistiocytosis (HLH).[18] The clinical syndrome of CRS can range from mild flulike symptoms to multisystem organ failure and death, and awareness and early recognition are key to management.[14,19] The incidence of CRS following CAR T cell therapy for relapsed/refractory ALL has been reported as high as 100% for all grades of CRS but falls slightly less than 70% for grades 3 or 4 CRS.[20] In children and young adults, CRS symptoms usually occur between 0 and 10 days after CAR T cell infusion, with a mean onset of 4 days for mild/moderate and 1 day for severe CRS.[20]

As previously mentioned, patients with CRS have elevated plasma level IFN-γ, IL-6, IL-10, IL-2, and TNF-α as well as C-reactive protein (CRP) and ferritin.[12] Elevated CRP levels have been shown to correlate with disease severity, although no specific thresholds for prediction of disease severity have been reproducibly established.[16,19] Similarly, no other biomarker or combination of biomarkers has been found to predict disease severity because most peak after patients become acutely ill.[18,21] The timing and magnitude of immune cell activation seems to coincide with maximal in vivo T cell expansion and correlate with disease burden and therefore likely high levels of T cell activation.[15] Higher dose level of CAR T cells also correlates with risk of developing CRS.[22]

Diagnosis

Presenting symptoms of CRS are relatively nonspecific and may impact every organ system (**Table 1**). Fever greater than 38°C is a requirement for diagnosis.[15] Patients may present with rigors, malaise, fatigue, myalgias, nausea vomiting, and headache. Respiratory involvement may present as tachypnea and hypoxemia progressing to acute hypoxemic respiratory failure. Patients may have cardiac insufficiency with tachycardia, arrhythmia, or progression to shock. Other signs of end-organ dysfunction may include renal dysfunction and azotemia, hepatic dysfunction with transaminitis and hyperbilirubinemia, and frank disseminated intravascular coagulation (DIC).

Grading is broken into 4 categories based on the ASTCT criteria and are outlined in **Table 2**. For these symptoms to be included in the grading scheme, they cannot be attributed to other causes. All grades involve fever greater than 38°C (unless patients have received antipyretic or anticytokine therapy, in which case fever is not required for diagnosis). From there, grading severity increases based on severity of respiratory and cardiovascular dysfunction.[15] Notably, there are no laboratory criteria for the diagnosis of CRS.

As symptoms of CRS are relatively nonspecific to CRS, caution should be taken to exclude other causes, particularly sepsis. Sepsis may occur concurrently with CRS or even be mistaken for CRS.

Clinical Management

Critical to proper management of CRS is awareness of its prevalence, high degree of clinical suspicion, and cardiopulmonary monitoring. The expert consensus document

Table 1	
Signs and symptoms of CRS	
Organ System	**Symptoms**
Constitutional	Fever, rigors, malaise, fatigue, anorexia, myalgias
Neurologic	Headache, mental status changes, confusion, delirium, hallucinations, tremor, altered gait, seizures
Cardiovascular	Tachycardia, widened pulse pressure, hypotension, cardiomyopathy
Respiratory	Tachypnea, hypoxemia, pulmonary edema, pneumonitis, ARDS*
Gastrointestinal	Nausea, vomiting, diarrhea, ascites
Renal	Acute kidney injury, renal failure
Hepatic	Hepatomegaly, transaminitis, hyperbilirubinemia, cholestasis, liver failure
Skin	Rash, edema
Coagulation	Elevated D-dimer, hypofibrinogenemia, bleeding
Rheumatologic	Vasculitis, arthralgias

* Acute Respiratory Distress Syndrome

Table 2
Grading and management of CRS

	Grade 1 CRS	Grade 2 CRS	Grade 3 CRS	Grade 4 CRS
Signs and symptoms	• Temperature ≥38°C[a] • No hypotension • No hypoxia	• Temperature ≥38°C[a] with • Not requiring vasopressors and/or[b] • Requiring low-flow nasal cannula[c] or blow by	• Temperature ≥38°C[a] with • Requiring a vasopressor with or without vasopressin and/or[b] • Requiring high-flow nasal casual[c], facemask, nonrebreather mask or Venturi mask	• Temperature ≥38°C[a] with • Requiring multiple vasopressors (excluding vasopressin) and/or[b] • Requiring positive pressure (eg, CPAP, BiPAP, intubation, and mechanical ventilation)
Management	• Acetaminophen, as needed, for fever • Evaluate for infectious causes • Consider broad-spectrum antibiotics and filgrastim (if patient is neutropenic) • Assess for adequate hydration • Consider anti-IL-6 therapy for persistent or refractory fever[d] • Supportive care	• Manage according to recommendations for grade 1 CRS (if applicable) • IV fluid bolus as needed to maintain normotension for age • For hypotension refractory to fluid boluses or hypoxia, consider anti-IL-6 therapy with i.v. tocilizumab (12 mg/kg for patients weighing <30 kg or 8 mg/kg for those weighing ≥30 kg, to a maximum of 800 mg per dose) repeat dose every 8 h for up to 3 doses within 24 h (but titrate frequency according to response) • If hypotension persists after 2 fluid boluses and anti-IL-6 therapy, start vasopressors,	• Manage according to recommendations for grades 1 and 2 CRS • Transfer patient to PICU and obtain echocardiogram, if not performed already • Administer i.v.dexamethasone 0.5 mg/kg (maximum 10 mg per dose) every 6 h; can increase dose to maximum of 20 mg every 6 h if patient is refractory to lower dose (alternatively methylprednisolone 1–2 mg/kg/ d divided every 6–12 h can be used)[f]	• Administer i.v. fluids, anti-IL-6 therapy, corticosteroids, and vasopressors and perform hemodynamic monitoring as described for grades 1, 2, or 3 CRS • If low doses of corticosteroids do not lead to clinical improvement, consider high-dose methylprednisolone (1g daily for 3 d followed by rapid taper on the basis of clinical response)

transfer patient to PICU, and obtain echocardiogram

• For patients at high risk or severe CRS[e], if hypotension persists after anti-IL-6 therapy, or there are signs of hypoperfusion or rapid deterioration, use stress-dose hydrocortisone (12.5–25 mg/m²/d divided every 6 h; i.v. dexamethasone 0.5 mg/kg(maximum 10 mg per dose) every 6 h; or methylprednisolone 1–2 mg/kg/d divided every 6–12 h)

Early recognition of CRS and appropriate intervention are essential to avoid life-threatening complications of this toxicity. CRS should be suspected if any of the above listed signs and symptoms are present within the first 3 wk after CAR T cell therapy. CRS grading should be performed at least twice a day and when a change in the patient's clinical status occurs.

[a] Fever is defined as temperature 38°C or greater not attributable to any other cause. In patients who have CRS then receive antipyretic or anticytokine therapy such as tocilizumab or steroids, fever is no longer required to grade subsequent CRS severity. In this case, CRS grading is driven by hypotension and/or hypoxia.

[b] CRS grade is determined by the more severe event: hypotension or hypoxia not attributable to any other cause. For example, a patient with temperature of 39.5°C, hypotension requiring 1 vasopressor, and hypoxia requiring low-flow nasal cannula is classified as grade 3 CRS.

[c] Low-flow nasal cannula is defined as oxygen delivered at 6 L/min or greater. Low flow also includes blow-by oxygen delivery, sometimes used in pediatrics. High-flow nasal cannula is defined as oxygen delivered at greater than 6 L/min.

[d] For example, persistent fever lasting more than 3 d or fever with a temperature of 39°C or greater for 10 h that is unresponsive to acetaminophen.

[e] Patients with early onset of CRS signs and symptoms (within 3 d of cell infusion), bulky disease, and comorbidities are at high risk of developing severe CRS.

[f] Simultaneous administration of corticosteroids and anti-IL-6 therapy or waiting to see if the patient responds to anti-IL-6 monotherapy before administering corticosteroids are both reasonable approaches (strategy used might vary depending on the CAR T cell products and/or risk factors).

Adapted from Mahadeo KM, Khazal SJ, Abdel-Azim H, et al. Management guidelines for paediatric patients receiving chimeric antigen receptor T cell therapy. Nat Rev Clin Oncol. 2019;16(1):45-63. https://doi.org/10.1038/s41571-018-0075-2.

for management of pediatric patients receiving CAR T therapy recommends strong consideration of inpatient monitoring for a minimum of 3 to 7 days, as well as reassessment of CRS grading at a minimum of every 12 hour and more frequently with any change. Postinfusion, the guidelines recommend a minimum of daily monitoring of CBC, hepatic function, CRP, ferritin, and evaluation for both DIC and tumor-lysis syndrome as CRS can result in both of these conditions.[23] Low threshold for admission to the pediatric intensive care unit (PICU) is reasonable, given up to 50% of CRS patients require critical care services. The most common indications for admission to the PICU are hemodynamic instability, respiratory insufficiency, and neurologic deterioration.[12,24]

Once the diagnosis of CRS is made, treatment focuses on mitigating the exaggerated immune response, both through broad strategies of immunosuppression, as well as focused therapies targeting specific cytokines.[19] This immunosuppression, however, may also negatively affect the efficacy of the originally intended treatment. The goal, therefore, is to balance administration of immunosuppressive therapy to adequately control the CRS but not completely extinguish the intended therapeutic effect of the immunotherapy.[18] The development of the CRS severity stratification system has helped to optimize this balance.

Initial evaluation of a patient with suspected CRS must include consideration of other diagnoses, followed by appropriate evaluation and diagnosis. Most notably, given that fever is a hallmark CRS symptom, infectious causes must be especially considered in this vulnerable population. It is recommended that blood cultures be drawn in all patients and empiric antibiotics initiated. This is particularly important in neutropenic patients.[12,23]

Once a diagnosis of CRS is established, the mainstays of management include supportive care with goal of symptom relief, as well as immune suppression.

In general, fever and malaise associated with CRS should be managed with standard antipyretic therapies. As previously mentioned, all patients should undergo a thorough infectious evaluation and receive broad spectrum antibiotics. Close attention should be given to hydration status, avoiding fluid overload. Cardiovascular involvement may manifest as tachycardia, arrhythmias, or shock, which may be vasodilatory, cardiogenic, or mixed vasodilatory and cardiogenic shock. As such, frequent hemodynamic assessments, including serial blood pressure measurements, facilitate early recognition of cardiovascular involvement. Predictors of development of hypotension requiring vasopressor support include those with leukemic blast count greater than 25% pretreatment, or preexisting cardiac dysfunction.[24] This is especially important to note given a significant percentage of the patients receiving these therapies are already at increased risk for cardiac dysfunction due to exposure to cardiotoxic medications such as anthracyclines, and/or radiation exposure as part of their prior treatment regimen.[24] For patients with suspected adrenal insufficiency, stress dose hydrocortisone should be administered.

Involvement of the respiratory system may lead to respiratory insufficiency, ranging from mild hypoxia to severe pediatric acute respiratory distress syndrome (PARDS).[25] The cause of respiratory failure in CRS is largely believed to be a result of pulmonary edema from capillary leak.[26] Respiratory support should be escalated as needed, and managed according to PARDS guidelines.[12,27]

Providers should also be aware of potential involvement of gastrointestinal and renal systems, and liver and renal function should be monitored. Fluid overload and/or renal insufficiency may require dialysis.

In addition to supportive care, specific treatment of CRS involves the use of anti-IL6 therapies and corticosteroids. Tocilizumab, a monoclonal antibody that works by blocking the IL-6 receptor, was approved by the FDA for treatment of CRS in 2018.[27] Timing of use depends largely on the severity of CRS as discussed below. Fortunately, although remarkably effective at treating CRS, tocilizumab has not been shown to have an impact on long-term efficacy of CAR T cells.[16]

For most cases of Grade 1 and 2 CRS, the use of anti-IL-6 therapy and/or corticosteroids are not usually recommended, unless other comorbidities are present, or symptoms persist for 3 or more days (see **Table 2**). For grade 3 or 4 CRS, treatment generally begins with tocilizumab at a dose of 8 mg/kg, up to 3 doses. If CRS persists, corticosteroids may be added, typically as dexamethasone 0.5 mg/kg (up to 10 mg) every 6 hours or methylprednisolone 1 to 2 mg/kg/d divided every 6 hours for continued symptoms. In patients with grade 4 CRS who are unresponsive to prescribed therapies, consideration may be given to high dose methylprednisolone followed by a rapid taper once clinical improvement is achieved.[23] For patients unresponsive to management with tocilizumab and corticosteroids, the addition of other anticytokine agents may be considered, such as siltuximab, anakinra, ruxolitinib, or cyclophosphamide. For patients refractory to all of the above therapies, an alternate diagnosis, such as HLH, should be reconsidered.[23]

Complications and Immune Effector Cell-Associated Neurotoxicity Syndrome

Immune effector cell-associated neurotoxicity syndrome (ICANS) refers to a neurotoxicity syndrome that develops following the administration of CAR T cell therapy. Although it is related to CRS, the term ICANS refers to a separate, independent disease process. It is fairly common and can be seen in 25% to 44% of treated patients.[2] ICANS typically presents in patients who have had precedent CRS, usually within the first 7 to 10 days following administration of CAR T cell therapy. Common symptoms include confusion, language disturbance, and altered mental status. More severe presentations may include the development of seizures or coma and have been described in 10% to 20% of patients with ICANS. On the most severe end of the spectrum, patients can develop rapidly progressive cerebral edema, which may result in death. Associated risk factors for the development of severe ICANS include high tumor burden, severe CRS, neurologic comorbidities, high CAR T cell doses, and high peak levels of CAR T cell expansion. The presence of active or previously treated CNS disease has not been shown to be associated with the development of severe ICANS.[2]

All patients who received CAR T cell therapies should be monitored closely for the development of neurologic symptoms with validated screening tools.[24] The ASTCT guidelines recommend using the Immune Effector-Cell Encephalopathy score for children aged greater than 12 years, and the Cornell Assessment of Pediatric Delirium for those aged less than 12 years.[11,25] Patients with a positive screen should be considered for the diagnosis of ICANS.

There are no consensus guidelines on the treatment of ICANS. There have been descriptions of grading systems similar to that used with CRS, where ICANS severity is graded on a scale from 1 to 4. First-line therapy for all patients includes supportive care. The need for CNS imaging with CT scan or MRI should be considered, as well as EEG monitoring for seizure development and consideration of the use of prophylactic antiepileptic therapies. Tocilizumab does not cross the blood–brain barrier and is therefore not a therapeutic option in the treatment of ICANS. Patients may be treated with corticosteroids such as dexamethasone. The use of the IL-1 receptor antagonist anakinra is an active area of research at this time.

Typically, patients will have resolution of ICANS symptoms within 28 days of CAR T cell therapy. Long-term neurocognitive outcomes in patients who have received CAR T cell therapy remains an active area of study.

SUMMARY

The development of immune effector cell therapies has led to tremendous strides in the treatment of refractory pediatric ALL. CAR T cells have helped turn relapsed, refractory ALL from an entity with high mortality to one where many patients go on to long-term survival. CRS represents a potentially life-threatening complication of CAR T therapy. Providers caring for patients receiving CAR T cells should maintain a high index of suspicion as prompt recognition and intervention is critical to reduce morbidity and mortality.

CLINICS CARE POINTS

- Our understanding of cytokine release syndrome and its management continue to evolve as this remains an active area of research.
- A diagnosis of cytokine release syndrome should be strongly considered in any patient who develops a fever following treatment with CAR T cells.
- Management of cytokine release syndrome depends on disease severity, and ranges from supportive care to use of corticosteroids and anti-IL6 therapies.

CONFLICTS OF INTEREST

None.

REFERENCES

1. Rheingold SR, Ji L, Xu X, et al. Prognostic factors for survival after relapsed acute lymphoblastic leukemia (ALL): a Children's Oncology Group (COG) study. Am Soc Clin Oncol 2019;37(15_suppl):10008–10008.
2. Shalabi H, Gust J, Taraseviciute A, et al. Beyond the storm - subacute toxicities and late effects in children receiving CAR T cells. Nat Rev Clin Oncol 2021; 18(6):363–78.
3. Grupp SA, Kalos M, Barrett D, et al. Chimeric antigen receptor-modified T cells for acute lymphoid leukemia. N Engl J Med 2013;368(16):1509–18.
4. Mackall CL, Merchant MS, Fry TJ. Immune-based therapies for childhood cancer. Nat Rev Clin Oncol 2014;11(12):693–703.
5. Shah NN, Lee DW, Yates B, et al. Long-term follow-up of CD19-CAR T-cell therapy in children and young adults with B-all. J Clin Oncol 2021;39(15):1650–9.
6. Ramos CA, Heslop HE, Brenner MK. CAR-T cell therapy for lymphoma. Annu Rev Med 2016;67:165–83.
7. Marofi F, Rahman HS, Achmad MH, et al. A deep insight into CAR-T cell therapy in non-hodgkin lymphoma: application, opportunities, and future directions. Front Immunol 2021;12:681984.
8. Davila ML, Riviere I, Wang X, et al. Efficacy and toxicity management of 19-28z CAR T cell therapy in B cell acute lymphoblastic leukemia. Sci Transl Med 2014;6(224):224ra25.
9. National Cancer Institute, CAR T. Cells: engineering patients' immune cells to treat their cancers. Available at: https://www.cancer.gov/about-cancer/treatment/research/car-t-cells. Accessed June 18th, 2022.
10. June CH, Sadelain M. Chimeric antigen receptor therapy. N Engl J Med 2018; 379(1):64–73.

11. Fajgenbaum DC, June CH. Cytokine storm. N Engl J Med 2020;383(23):2255–73.
12. Baumeister SHC, Mohan GS, Elhaddad A, et al. Cytokine release syndrome and associated acute toxicities in pediatric patients undergoing immune effector cell therapy or hematopoietic cell transplantation. Front Oncol 2022;12:841117.
13. DeAngelo D.J., Ghobadi A., Park J.H., et al. Clinical outcomes for the phase 2, single-arm, multicenter trial of JCAR015 in adult B-ALL (ROCKET Study). Presented at: 32nd Annual SITC Meeting, National Harbor, MD, November 8-12. Poster P217.
14. Maude SL, Laetsch TW, Buechner J, et al. Tisagenlecleucel in children and young adults with B-cell lymphoblastic leukemia. N Engl J Med 2018;378(5):439–48.
15. Lee DW, Santomasso BD, Locke FL, et al. ASTCT consensus grading for cytokine release syndrome and neurologic toxicity associated with immune effector cells. Biol Blood Marrow Transpl 2019;25(4):625–38.
16. Klinger M, Brandl C, Zugmaier G, et al. Immunopharmacologic response of patients with B-lineage acute lymphoblastic leukemia to continuous infusion of T cell-engaging CD19/CD3-bispecific BiTE antibody blinatumomab. Blood 2012;119(26):6226–33.
17. Imus PH, Blackford AL, Bettinotti M, et al. Severe cytokine release syndrome after haploidentical peripheral blood stem cell transplantation. Biol Blood Marrow Transpl 2019;25(12):2431–7.
18. Lee DW, Gardner R, Porter DL, et al. Current concepts in the diagnosis and management of cytokine release syndrome. Blood 2014;124(2):188–95.
19. Maude SL, Barrett D, Teachey DT, et al. Managing cytokine release syndrome associated with novel T cell-engaging therapies. Cancer J 2014;20(2):119–22.
20. Teachey DT, Lacey SF, Shaw PA, et al. Identification of predictive biomarkers for cytokine release syndrome after chimeric antigen receptor T-cell therapy for acute lymphoblastic leukemia. Cancer Discov 2016;6(6):664–79.
21. Sheth VS, Gauthier J. Taming the beast: CRS and ICANS after CAR T-cell therapy for ALL. Bone Marrow Transpl 2021;56(3):552–66.
22. Kadauke S, Myers RM, Li Y, et al. Risk-adapted preemptive tocilizumab to prevent severe cytokine release syndrome after CTL019 for pediatric B-cell acute lymphoblastic leukemia: a prospective clinical trial. J Clin Oncol 2021;39(8):920–30.
23. Mahadeo KM, Khazal SJ, Abdel-Azim H, et al. Management guidelines for paediatric patients receiving chimeric antigen receptor T cell therapy. Nat Rev Clin Oncol 2019;16(1):45–63.
24. Shalabi H, Sachdev V, Kulshreshtha A, et al. Impact of cytokine release syndrome on cardiac function following CD19 CAR-T cell therapy in children and young adults with hematological malignancies. J Immunother Cancer 2020;8(2).
25. Fitzgerald JC, Weiss SL, Maude SL, et al. Cytokine release syndrome after chimeric antigen receptor T cell therapy for acute lymphoblastic leukemia. Crit Care Med 2017;45(2):e124–31.
26. Gutierrez C, McEvoy C, Munshi L, et al. Critical care management of toxicities associated with targeted agents and immunotherapies for cancer. Crit Care Med 2020;48(1):10–21.
27. Pediatric acute lung injury consensus conference G. Pediatric acute respiratory distress syndrome: consensus recommendations from the pediatric acute lung injury consensus conference. Pediatr Crit Care Med 2015;16(5):428–39.

Transfusion Strategies in the 21st Century

A Case-Based Narrative Report

Jennifer Shenker, MD[a], Hiba Abuelhija, MD[b],
Oliver Karam, MD, PhD[c], Marianne Nellis, MD, MS[d],*

KEYWORDS

- Transfusion • Critical illness • Children

KEY POINTS

- In addition to the risk of transfusion-transmitted infection, the transfusion of blood components is associated with lung injury, circulatory overload, and immunomodulation.
- The TAXI and TAXI-CAB recommendations provide guidance to clinicians on the appropriate thresholds for the transfusion of RBCs, plasma, and platelets. Restrictive transfusion practices may be considered.
- Viscoelastic testing should be considered to evaluate the hemostatic balance in critically ill children and alternative therapies to transfusion, such as antifibrinolytic therapy, may be considered in certain subgroups of critically ill children.

INTRODUCTION

Though the transfusion of blood has been documented in Western medicine as early as the 17th century, the practice of transfusing blood components, most commonly red blood cells (RBCs), plasma, and/or platelets, is comparatively new, beginning in the 1940s. Each component has unique features and indications.

RBC transfusions are typically prescribed to increase hemoglobin and improve oxygen delivery. Despite their intended benefit, studies have not been able to confirm increased oxygen consumption following RBC transfusion.[1] This finding may be related to the changes that occur in stored red cells which decreases their microcirculatory flow.[2,3]

[a] Department of Pediatrics, New York Presbyterian Hospital – Weill Cornell Medicine, 525 East 68th Street, M508, New York, NY 10065, USA; [b] Pediatric Critical Care, Hadassah University Medical Center, Hadassah Ein Kerem, POB 12000, Jerusalem 911200, Israel; [c] Department of Pediatrics, Yale School of Medicine, 333 Cedar Street, New Haven, CT 06520, USA; [d] Department of Pediatrics, Division of Pediatric Critical Care Medicine, Weill Cornell Medicine, 525 East 68th Street, M512, New York, NY 10065, USA
* Corresponding author.
E-mail address: man9026@med.cornell.edu

https://doi.org/10.1016/j.ccc.2022.09.005
0749-0704/23/© 2022 Elsevier Inc. All rights reserved.
criticalcare.theclinics.com

Plasma transfusions contain coagulation factors, fibrin, immunoglobulins, anti-thrombin, protein C, and protein S and are most commonly prescribed to either prevent or treat bleeding.[4] However, studies in both adults and children have shown that plasma rarely corrects the international normalized ratio (INR), the test which most clinicians use to guide plasma transfusions.[4–6] Plasma transfusions given in models of endothelial dysfunction have been shown to support the glycocalyx and possibly restore endothelial integrity.[7,8]

Platelets are an essential component of primary hemostasis and therefore platelet transfusions, like plasma, are prescribed to either prevent or treat bleeding. A recent randomized controlled trial of platelet transfusion thresholds in neonates showed that babies transfused to maintain higher platelet counts actually had more bleeding and/or mortality.[9] In addition, observational studies of children supported by extracorporeal membrane oxygenation have reported an association with increased bleeding on the day following a platelet transfusion.[10] While the exact mechanism is unclear, the inflammatory cytokines in stored platelets may play a role.[11,12]

In addition to the possible unintended consequences described above, the transfusion of all blood components has been associated with acute lung injury, acute circulatory overload, and immunomodulation.[13–17] With these risks in mind, it is essential that the pediatric provider weigh the risks and benefits before transfusing a critically ill child. In this review, we provide a series of common case scenarios encountered in the pediatric intensive care unit (PICU) and discuss the current evidence for and against the transfusion of blood components.

CASE 1: NEW ONCOLOGIC DIAGNOSIS
Case Scenario

A 5-year-old female with newly diagnosed acute lymphocytic leukemia is admitted to the PICU because of the risk of tumor lysis syndrome. On day 2, her hemoglobin (Hb) is 5.7 g/dL, platelet count is 17×10^9/L and INR is 1.6. She is not bleeding and is hemodynamically stable. A lumber puncture is scheduled for that afternoon. Are blood products indicated and if so, why?

Red Blood Cell Transfusion Strategy

RBCs are frequently transfused to oncology patients. Data from 4766 children with oncology and hematopoietic stem cell transplant (HSCT) diagnoses, recently published by Goel and colleagues, showed that RBCs were transfused in 32% of the patients.[18] Children between 1 and 6 years of age were the most frequently transfused. When looking at the pretransfusion Hb level, Goel showed the median (IQR) pretransfusion Hb was 7.5 (6.9–8) g/dL.[18] However, the current evidence suggests that even in critically ill children, a transfusion threshold below 7 g/dL is safe.[19] It is also known that RBC transfusions are associated with worse outcomes in critically ill children, including oncology patients.[20]

In 2018, the Transfusion and Anemia Expertise Initiative (TAXI) published recommendations on RBC transfusions specific to pediatric oncology patients.[21] They made a weak recommendation that in children with oncologic diagnoses who are critically ill or at risk for critical illness and are hemodynamically stable, a Hb concentration of 7 to 8 g/dL could be considered a threshold for RBC transfusion. The rationale for the strength of the recommendation was based on strong evidence that a threshold of 7 g/dL is safe for the general population of critically ill children[19] without an abundance of specific studies in the oncology population. Therefore, most clinicians will aim for an

Hb level above 7 g/dL in oncology patients, although there is no evidence to suggest that a slightly lower threshold is harmful.

Platelet Transfusion Strategy

Platelets are also frequently transfused to oncology patients. In a single-center study, 39% of all pediatric oncology patients will receive at least one platelet transfusion.[22] In the Goel study referenced above, platelets were transfused in 23% of patients.[18] Several studies have reported pretransfusion platelet counts. In a single-center study of 144 children who received platelets, approximately one-fifth of the time the pre-transfusion platelet count was $\leq 10 \times 10^9$/L.[22] Goel and colleagues showed the median pretransfusion platelet count was $\leq 10 \times 10^9$/L in 18% of the cases and between 10 and 20 $\times 10^9$/L in 34% of the cases.[18]

Randomized controlled trials performed in older children and adults demonstrated a prophylactic platelet transfusion threshold of 10 $\times 10^9$/L did not lead to worse outcomes as compared with a threshold of 20 $\times 10^9$/L.[23–25] Similar to the TAXI RBC guidelines, the Transfusion and Anemia Expertise Initiative-Control/Avoidance of Bleeding (TAXI-CAB) guidelines provide some clarity, although the level of evidence is overall lower.[26] In critically ill pediatric oncology patients, the experts suggest that prophylactic (ie, to prevent bleeding) platelet transfusions might be considered for a platelet count less than 10 $\times 10^9$/L.

Regarding the platelet transfusion strategy before lumbar punctures (LP), a single-center study evaluated transfusions before LPs in adults and children with cancer.[27] The authors described 354 LPs whereby the preprocedure platelet count was less than 50x10^9/L. Eighty-nine percent received at least one platelet transfusion to achieve a higher platelet count before the procedure. Of those who were transfused, one-third still had a platelet count less than 50x10^9/L after the transfusion and the LP. In the 11% that were not transfused, the median platelet count was 31x10^9/L (range 2–49). Notably in all patients, the proportion of traumatic taps was higher in the group with pre-LP platelet count was less than 50$\times$10^9/L (18% vs 4%, P <.001).

Therefore, it seems that in patients who are not experiencing significant bleeding, a platelet transfusion threshold of 10x10^9/L is sufficient to avoid spontaneous bleeding. The appropriate platelet transfusion threshold before procedures remains unclear, although there is no evidence it should be higher than 50x10^9/L.

Plasma Transfusion Strategy

Plasma transfusions are the least frequently transfused blood products in children with oncologic diagnoses. In the Goel study, plasma was transfused in 2% of the patients, with those less than 1 year being the most frequently transfused (6%).[18] Goel et al also described the pretransfusion coagulation tests, measured in 340 oncology children.[18] The median (IQR) INR was 1.7 (1.5–2.0). Whereas 25% of the plasma was given at an INR $\leq$ 1.5, only 15% was given at an INR $\geq$ 2.5. In a larger international study of 442 critically ill children (including oncology patients) receiving plasma transfusions, plasma transfusions were not able to correct an INR$\leq$ 2.5.[4] Similar to RBCs and platelets, plasma transfusions have also been independently associated with worse clinical outcomes in critically ill adults and children.[28]

Here too, the TAXI-CAB guidelines provide some clarity, although the level of evidence is overall lower.[26] In critically ill pediatric oncology patients with minor coagulopathy, defined as an INR$\leq$ 1.5 or an activated partial thromboplastin time (aPTT) $\leq$ 1.5 times the normal value, the experts state that prophylactic plasma transfusions may not be beneficial.

In summary, there is currently no evidence that plasma transfusions can correct moderately abnormal coagulation tests or that treating mildly abnormal coagulation tests improves outcomes. There is evidence, however, that plasma transfusions are associated with worse outcomes and as a result, oncology patients are seldomly transfused plasma.

CASE 2: FOLLOWING CARDIOPULMONARY BYPASS
Case Scenario

A 14-month-old female with a postnatal diagnosis of Tetralogy of Fallot, pulmonary atresia, and major aortopulmonary collateral arteries underwent multistage repair. She is admitted to the PICU after the unifocalization surgery. No major bleeding was reported during the operative course. She received 20 mL/kg of RBCs, 10 mL/kg platelets, and 10 mL/kg of plasma in the operating room. Heparin was reversed with protamine at the end of surgery. During the first 2 hours after admission, she developed excessive postoperative bleeding with chest tube drainage of 6 mL/kg/h for 2 consecutive hours without significant hemodynamic instability. Are blood products indicated and, if so, why?

This case scenario of bleeding following cardiopulmonary bypass (CPB) is common, though due to a variety of definitions of bleeding, has a wide range of incidence between 8% and 25%.[29] Bleeding following CPB is independently associated with increased mortality in infants.[30] Many factors contribute to the risk of bleeding and include low preoperative body weight, cyanotic heart disease, platelet dysfunction induced by the circuit, hemodilution, immaturity of the hemostatic system and hypofibrinogenemia.[31–34]

Platelet Transfusion Strategy

While there may be mild thrombocytopenia in some infants secondary to hemodilution, the issue following cardiopulmonary bypass is more of a qualitative problem with platelet dysfunction resulting from contact of the blood with an artificial circuit.[35] Platelet transfusion is common following CPB. In a recent database study of 882 children undergoing surgery with CPB and receiving at least one blood component, over three-quarters of children received a platelet transfusion following bypass.[36]

No recommendations exist to guide the prescription of platelet transfusions to children with bleeding following CPB. The TAXI-CAB group, after conducting a systematic review and screening nearly 3000 abstracts, concluded that there is insufficient evidence to support a platelet transfusion strategy or recommended a threshold.[37] While further research is clearly indicated in this area, given the risk of platelet dysfunction in the case described above and the significant bleeding, a platelet transfusion should be considered.

Plasma Transfusion Strategy

Though the level of coagulation factors decreases in children immediately following the initiation of CPB, the levels increase following the cessation of CPB and reversal of heparin with protamine.[38] Despite this, plasma is the most common blood component transfused in children following CPB.[36] Children with cyanotic disease, like the child in the case scenario, are two times more likely to receive plasma transfusions.[39] Similar to the oncologic population, epidemiologic studies have shown that children following CPB are transfused plasma at relatively low INR values (median 1.8).[36]

Similar to the guidance for platelet transfusions, TAXI-CAB reported that there is insufficient evidence to make recommendations for the transfusion of plasma to children with bleeding following CPB and clinical judgment must be used.[37] It is important to note, however, that the experts suggested that plasma should not be given for volume expansion.[40] Given the evidence for other hemostatic interventions mentioned below, plasma should not be considered a first-line treatment of bleeding in the patient presented.

Other Considerations

Though little evidence exists to establish transfusion thresholds for platelet and/or plasma in bleeding children following CPB, the TAXI-CAB group was able to make 2 clinical recommendations regarding the postoperative management of these children. First, given the complexity of the hemostatic system and its derangements following CPB, in addition to standard laboratory testing, viscoelastic testing, such as thromboelastography (TEG) or rotational thromboelastometry (ROTEM), may be considered to help guide transfusion decisions (Grade 2B).[37] Second, the use of postoperative transfusion algorithms may be considered to decrease overall exposure to blood products (Grade 2B).[37]

Other blood components may be considered to treat bleeding in this case scenario and early evidence suggests potential benefit. Cryoprecipitate transfusion should be considered in ongoing hemorrhage and hypofibrinogenemia and small observational studies suggest cryoprecipitate is more efficacious than plasma in this scenario.[41] Fibrinogen concentrate administered at the end of CPB may negate the need for cryoprecipitate and/or plasma.[42] Furthermore, prothrombin complex concentrates, in combination with fibrinogen concentrate, may be considered as a safe and more effective alternative than plasma.[43,44]

CASE 3: ACUTE LIVER FAILURE
Case Scenario

A 6-week-old female presents with jaundice, acholic stools, dark urine, and hepatomegaly and is found to have biliary atresia. On day 3 of hospitalization, laboratory assays are remarkable for a platelet count of 35x10^9/L and an INR of 1.7 without evidence of clinical bleeding. Are blood products indicated and, if so, why?

The coagulopathy seen in pediatric acute liver failure (PALF) is complex. Coagulation studies may not accurately assess the risk of bleeding in PALF due to a "rebalanced hemostasis."[45] Specifically with regard to primary hemostasis modulated by platelet adhesion and clot formation, there is compensation. Despite the thrombocytopenia and decreased platelet function seen in PALF, there are elevations in von Willebrand factor (vWF) that supports platelet adhesion and decreased ADAMTS-13.[46–48] In secondary hemostasis whereby coagulation factors are responsible for the creation of a stable clot, there is both a reduction in the procoagulant factors II, V, VII, IX, X, XI, and XIII and a reduction in anticoagulant proteins such as antithrombin, Protein C and Protein S.[49] Yet, children with acute liver failure are actually at higher risk of thrombosis as compared with bleeding.[45] The risk of any significant spontaneous bleeding is estimated to occur in less than 5% of PALF.[50]

Platelet Transfusion Strategy

Apart from those undergoing liver transplantation, very little epidemiologic information is known about the incidence of platelet transfusion in children with PALF. If needed, platelets must be transfused with extreme caution. Animal models have shown that platelet transfusions are involved in reperfusion injury of the liver[51] and observational data have demonstrated an independent association between platelet transfusion and decreased 1-year survival in children undergoing liver transplantation.[52] Therefore, the expert consensus from the TAXI-CAB group recommends against prophylactic platelet transfusions, restricting product administration to cases of clinically significant bleeding.[26]

Plasma Transfusion Strategy

Like platelets, the epidemiology of plasma transfusion, outside of therapeutic plasma exchange, is not well known. Although a defining feature of PALF, an INR greater than 1.5 should not be used to direct plasma transfusions in the absence of bleeding. Laboratory studies such as INR that measure the procoagulants, but not the anticoagulants, can be of limited use in cases of PALF and are not predictive of bleeding.[50] Similar to children following CPB, viscoelastic testing may be more helpful. Due to these limitations, and the known morbidities associated with plasma transfusion,[28] TAXI-CAB expert consensus was in favor of restricting the consideration of plasma transfusion only to children with PALF and active bleeding.[26] Therefore, in the case scenario described above, it is reasonable to hold on the transfusion of any blood products.

CASE 4: TRAUMA
Case Scenario

A 14-year-old male struck by a car as a pedestrian presents with a level one trauma activation is intubated in the field and has tachycardia and hypotension. Primary survey is notable for free fluid in the pelvis on FAST examination and a displaced femoral fracture. Hemoglobin on arterial blood gas is noted to be 7.5 g/dL. What is the best transfusion strategy?

The clinical scenario described above is concerning massive bleeding with hemorrhagic shock. Rather than resuscitation with crystalloid, patients with hemorrhagic shock should be resuscitated with blood products. Both the TAXI and TAXI-CAB programs support a balanced transfusion strategy using a 2:1:1 or 1:1:1 ratio of RBCs, plasma and platelets until the bleeding is no longer life threatening.[53,54] This recommendation is primarily based on data from adults,[55] as few prospective studies in children with massive bleeding have been performed. The balanced ratio recommended with component therapy is an attempt to recapitulate whole blood. Studies of resuscitation strategies in both adults and children have shown whole blood to be safe and associated with improved outcomes as compared with component therapy.[56-58]

A recent multicentered observational study in children began to explore the epidemiology and associated outcomes of massive bleeding in children.[59] Nearly half of massive bleeding events in children were secondary to trauma with a 28-day mortality rate of 36%. A secondary analysis of the database reported that children who received a high plasma: RBC ratio (>1:2) had higher survival at 6 hours postbleed.[60] In addition, there was increased early mortality in those with platelet or plasma deficit after initial resuscitation. Additionally, there is emerging evidence supporting the use of antifibrinolytic therapy in severely bleeding children. From the same dataset, the use of antifibrinolytic therapy was associated with decreased 6-h and 24-h mortality when given as part of the initial resuscitation.[61] Further interventional studies are needed before these observational findings can be recommended in all massively bleeding children.

In the case described above, the patient should be transfused with whole blood or component therapy in a balanced ratio until the bleeding is no longer life-threatening. If viscoelastic testing is available, it can be used to more directly guide the ratios of component therapy.

CASE 5: SEPSIS/DISSEMINATED INTRAVASCULAR COAGULOPATHY
Case Scenario

A 2-week-old male was admitted to the PICU due to suspected septic shock and uro-sepsis. He was sedated and mechanically ventilated, required inotropic support, and received broad spectrum antimicrobials. Shortly after admission, he develops thrombo-cytopenia and petechiae with guaiac-positive stools. Laboratory assays are significant for a platelet count of 68x10^9/L and an INR of 1.9. What is the best transfusion strategy?

Disseminated intravascular coagulopathy (DIC), most commonly associated with infection or trauma in children,[62] is the result of a procoagulant state that may para-doxically lead to bleeding. Excessive thrombin generation leads to microthrombi which can involve platelet consumption and subsequent thrombocytopenia. In adults, the incidence of DIC in patients with septic shock is as high as 73%.[63] Scoring sys-tems have been developed in adults[64,65] and trialed in children.[66]

Platelet and Plasma Transfusion Strategy

The most important aspect in the management of DIC is the treatment of the underly-ing cause. In addition to the general risks of plasma and platelet transfusions, one must be cautious in that both products are proinflammatory and prothrombotic and may continue to drive forward the pathophysiologic process of DIC described above. Therefore, both the Surviving Sepsis and TAXI-CAB recommendations encourage providers against both platelet and plasma transfusions in children with sepsis and/ or DIC unless the child has moderate to severe bleeding present.[26,67] Again in this pa-tient population, standard laboratory assays are not predictive of bleeding and visco-elastic testing may provide additional information.[68]

SUMMARY

While the transfusion of blood components may be life-saving in certain clinical cases, such as massive bleeding as described above, one must carefully weigh the risks and benefits of the blood product, specific to the clinical context and informed by current evidence. Standard laboratory testing alone should not be the impetus to transfuse. Viscoelastic testing should be considered in bleeding patients. A growing body of ev-idence has demonstrated the safety of restrictive transfusion practices.

CLINICS CARE POINTS

- When considering red blood cell transfusions, in the general critically ill child without cyanotic heart disease, typically transfusing when the hemoglobin is above 7 g/dL is not recommended.
- It is important to consider the clinical context of the child and other markers of tissue perfusion and not transfuse red blood cells based on hemoglobin alone.
- Though there is far less evidence for or against certain platelet transfusion thresholds in critically ill children, typically transfusing when the patient is not bleeding and the platelet count is above 100 x 10^9/L is not recommended.
- The international normlized ratio (INR) is a poor predictor of bleeding and minor abnormalities (INR < 2.0) are difficult to correct with plasma transfusion.

DISCLOSURE

The authors have nothing to disclose.

REFERENCES

1. Napolitano LM, Kurek S, Luchette FA, et al. Clinical practice guideline: red blood cell transfusion in adult trauma and critical care. Crit Care Med 2009;37(12): 3124–57.
2. van Bommel J, de Korte D, Lind A, et al. The effect of the transfusion of stored RBCs on intestinal microvascular oxygenation in the rat. Transfusion 2001; 41(12):1515–23.
3. Raat NJ, Verhoeven AJ, Mik EG, et al. The effect of storage time of human red cells on intestinal microcirculatory oxygenation in a rat isovolemic exchange model. Crit Care Med 2005;33(1):39–45 [discussion: 238-239].
4. Karam O, Demaret P, Shefler A, et al. Indications and Effects of plasma transfusions in critically ill children. Am J Respir Crit Care Med 2015;191(12):1395–402.
5. Abdel-Wahab OI, Healy B, Dzik WH. Effect of fresh-frozen plasma transfusion on prothrombin time and bleeding in patients with mild coagulation abnormalities. Transfusion 2006;46(8):1279–85.
6. Holland LL, Brooks JP. Toward rational fresh frozen plasma transfusion: the effect of plasma transfusion on coagulation test results. Am J Clin Pathol 2006;126(1): 133–9.
7. Haywood-Watson RJ, Holcomb JB, Gonzalez EA, et al. Modulation of syndecan-1 shedding after hemorrhagic shock and resuscitation. PLoS One 2011;6(8): e23530.
8. Kozar RA, Peng Z, Zhang R, et al. Plasma restoration of endothelial glycocalyx in a rodent model of hemorrhagic shock. Anesth Analg 2011;112(6):1289–95.
9. Curley A, Stanworth SJ, Willoughby K, et al. Randomized trial of platelet-transfusion thresholds in neonates. N Engl J Med 2019;380(3):242–51.
10. Cashen K, Dalton H, Reeder RW, et al. Platelet transfusion practice and related outcomes in pediatric extracorporeal membrane oxygenation. Pediatr Crit Care Med 2020;21(2):178–85.
11. Cognasse F, Garraud O. Cytokines and related molecules, and adverse reactions related to platelet concentrate transfusions. Transfus Clin Biol 2019;26(3):144–6.
12. Zhao J, Sun Z, You G, et al. Transfusion of cryopreserved platelets exacerbates inflammatory liver and lung injury in a mice model of hemorrhage. J Trauma Acute Care Surg 2018;85(2):327–33.
13. Politis C, Wiersum-Osselton J, Richardson C, et al. Adverse reactions following transfusion of blood components, with a focus on some rare reactions: reports to the International Haemovigilance Network Database (ISTARE) in 2012-2016. Transfus Clin Biol 2022;29(3):243–9.
14. Tung JP, Chiaretti S, Dean MM, et al. Transfusion-related acute lung injury (TRALI): potential pathways of development, strategies for prevention and treatment, and future research directions. Blood Rev 2022;53:100926.
15. Bulle EB, Klanderman RB, Pendergrast J, et al. The recipe for TACO: a narrative review on the pathophysiology and potential mitigation strategies of transfusion-associated circulatory overload. Blood Rev 2022;52:100891.
16. Muszynski JA, Spinella PC, Cholette JM, et al. Transfusion-related immunomodulation: review of the literature and implications for pediatric critical illness. Transfusion 2017;57(1):195–206.
17. Remy KE, Hall MW, Cholette J, et al. Mechanisms of red blood cell transfusion-related immunomodulation. Transfusion 2018;58(3):804–15.
18. Goel R, Nellis ME, Karam O, et al. Transfusion practices for pediatric oncology and hematopoietic stem cell transplantation patients: data from the National heart

lung and blood Institute Recipient epidemiology and Donor evaluation study-III (REDS-III). Transfusion 2021;61(9):2589–600.

19. Lacroix J, Hébert PC, Hutchison JS, et al. Transfusion strategies for patients in pediatric intensive care units. N Engl J Med 2007;356(16):1609–19.

20. Bateman ST, Lacroix J, Boven K, et al. Anemia, blood loss, and blood transfusions in North American children in the intensive care unit. Am J Respir Crit Care Med 2008;178(1):26–33.

21. Steiner ME, Zantek ND, Stanworth SJ, et al. Recommendations on RBC transfusion support in children with Hematologic and oncologic diagnoses from the pediatric critical care transfusion and anemia Expertise initiative. Pediatr Crit Care Med 2018;19(9S Suppl 1):S149–56.

22. Lieberman L, Liu Y, Barty R, et al. Platelet transfusion practice and platelet refractoriness for a cohort of pediatric oncology patients: a single-center study. Pediatr Blood Cancer 2020;67(12):e28734.

23. Rebulla P, Finazzi G, Marangoni F, et al. The threshold for prophylactic platelet transfusions in adults with acute myeloid leukemia. Gruppo Italiano Malattie Ematologiche Maligne dell'Adulto. N Engl J Med 1997;337(26):1870–5.

24. Heckman KD, Weiner GJ, Davis CS, et al. Randomized study of prophylactic platelet transfusion threshold during induction therapy for adult acute leukemia: 10,000/microL versus 20,000/microL. J Clin Oncol 1997;15(3):1143–9.

25. Zumberg MS, del Rosario ML, Nejame CF, et al. A prospective randomized trial of prophylactic platelet transfusion and bleeding incidence in hematopoietic stem cell transplant recipients: 10,000/L versus 20,000/microL trigger. Biol Blood Marrow Transpl 2002;8(10):569–76.

26. Lieberman L, Karam O, Stanworth SJ, et al. Plasma and platelet transfusion strategies in critically ill children with Malignancy, acute liver failure and/or liver transplantation, or sepsis: from the transfusion and anemia EXpertise Initiative-Control/Avoidance of bleeding. Pediatr Crit Care Med 2022;23(13 Suppl 1 1S):e37–49.

27. Chung HH, Morjaria S, Frame J, et al. Rethinking the need for a platelet transfusion threshold of 50 × 10(9)/L for lumbar puncture in cancer patients. Transfusion 2020;60(10):2243–9.

28. Karam O, Lacroix J, Robitaille N, et al. Association between plasma transfusions and clinical outcome in critically ill children: a prospective observational study. Vox Sang 2013;104(4):342–9.

29. Bercovitz RS, Shewmake AC, Newman DK, et al. Validation of a definition of excessive postoperative bleeding in infants undergoing cardiac surgery with cardiopulmonary bypass. J Thorac Cardiovasc Surg 2018;155(5):2112–24, e2112.

30. Wolf MJ, Maher KO, Kanter KR, et al. Early postoperative bleeding is independently associated with increased surgical mortality in infants after cardiopulmonary bypass. J Thorac Cardiovasc Surg 2014;148(2):631–6, e631.

31. Savan V, Willems A, Faraoni D, et al. Multivariate model for predicting postoperative blood loss in children undergoing cardiac surgery: a preliminary study. Br J Anaesth 2014;112(4):708–14.

32. Faraoni D, Willems A, Savan V, et al. Plasma fibrinogen concentration is correlated with postoperative blood loss in children undergoing cardiac surgery. A retrospective review. Eur J Anaesthesiol 2014;31(6):317–26.

33. Henriksson P, Värendh G, Lundström NR. Haemostatic defects in cyanotic congenital heart disease. Br Heart J 1979;41(1):23–7.

34. Bønding Andreasen J, Hvas AM, Ravn HB. Marked changes in platelet count and function following pediatric congenital heart surgery. Paediatr Anaesth 2014; 24(4):386–92.

35. Epstein D, Vishnepolsky A, Bolotin G, et al. Effect of Prolonged Hypothermic cardiopulmonary bypass, heparin, and protamine on platelet: a small-group study. Thorac Cardiovasc Surg 2021;69(8):719–22.
36. Hanson SJ, Karam O, Birch R, et al. Transfusion practices in pediatric cardiac surgery requiring cardiopulmonary bypass: a secondary analysis of a clinical database. Pediatr Crit Care Med 2021;22(11):978–87.
37. Cholette JM, Muszynski JA, Ibla JC, et al. Plasma and platelet transfusions strategies in neonates and children undergoing cardiac surgery with cardiopulmonary bypass or neonates and children supported by extracorporeal membrane oxygenation: from the transfusion and anemia EXpertise Initiative-Control/Avoidance of bleeding. Pediatr Crit Care Med 2022;23(13 Supple 1 1S):e25–36.
38. Chan AK, Leaker M, Burrows FA, et al. Coagulation and fibrinolytic profile of paediatric patients undergoing cardiopulmonary bypass. Thromb Haemost 1997;77(2):270–7.
39. Willems A, Patte P, De Groote F, et al. Cyanotic heart disease is an independent predicting factor for fresh frozen plasma and platelet transfusion after cardiac surgery. Transfus Apher Sci 2019;58(3):304–9.
40. Nellis ME, Karam O, Valentine SL, et al. Executive summary of recommendations and expert consensus for plasma and platelet transfusion practice in critically ill children: from the transfusion and anemia EXpertise Initiative-Control/Avoidance of bleeding (TAXI-CAB). Pediatr Crit Care Med 2022;23(1):34–51.
41. Miller BE, Mochizuki T, Levy JH, et al. Predicting and treating coagulopathies after cardiopulmonary bypass in children. Anesth Analg 1997;85(6):1196–202.
42. Tirotta CF, Lagueruela RG, Gupta A, et al. A randomized Pilot trial assessing the role of human fibrinogen concentrate in decreasing cryoprecipitate Use and blood loss in infants undergoing cardiopulmonary bypass. Pediatr Cardiol 2022;43(7):1444–54.
43. Velik-Salchner C, Tauber H, Rastner V, et al. Administration of fibrinogen concentrate combined with prothrombin complex maintains hemostasis in children undergoing congenital heart repair (a long-term propensity score-matched study). Acta Anaesthesiol Scand 2021;65(9):1178–86.
44. Harris AD, Hubbard RM, Sam RM, et al. A retrospective analysis of the Use of 3-factor prothrombin complex concentrates for Refractory bleeding after cardiopulmonary bypass in children undergoing heart surgery: a matched Case-Control study. Semin Cardiothorac Vasc Anesth 2020;24(3):227–31.
45. Bulut Y, Sapru A, Roach GD. Hemostatic balance in pediatric acute liver failure: epidemiology of bleeding and thrombosis, Physiology, and current strategies. Front Pediatr 2020;8:618119.
46. Lisman T, Stravitz RT. Rebalanced hemostasis in patients with acute liver failure. Semin Thromb Hemost 2015;41(5):468–73.
47. Lisman T, Porte RJ. Pathogenesis, prevention, and management of bleeding and thrombosis in patients with liver diseases. Res Pract Thromb Haemost 2017;1(2):150–61.
48. Hugenholtz GC, Adelmeijer J, Meijers JC, et al. An unbalance between von Willebrand factor and ADAMTS13 in acute liver failure: implications for hemostasis and clinical outcome. Hepatology 2013;58(2):752–61.
49. Agarwal B, Wright G, Gatt A, et al. Evaluation of coagulation abnormalities in acute liver failure. J Hepatol 2012;57(4):780–6.
50. Munoz SJ, Stravitz RT, Gabriel DA. Coagulopathy of acute liver failure. Clin Liver Dis 2009;13(1):95–107.

51. Sindram D, Porte RJ, Hoffman MR, et al. Platelets induce sinusoidal endothelial cell apoptosis upon reperfusion of the cold ischemic rat liver. Gastroenterology 2000;118(1):183–91.

52. de Boer MT, Christensen MC, Asmussen M, et al. The impact of intraoperative transfusion of platelets and red blood cells on survival after liver transplantation. Anesth Analg 2008;106(1):32–44, table of contents.

53. Karam O, Russell RT, Stricker P, et al. Recommendations on RBC transfusion in critically ill children with Nonlife-threatening bleeding or hemorrhagic shock from the pediatric critical care transfusion and anemia Expertise initiative. Pediatr Crit Care Med 2018;19(9S Suppl 1):S127–32.

54. Russell R, Bauer DF, Goobie SM, et al. Plasma and platelet transfusion strategies in critically ill children following severe trauma, traumatic Brain injury, and/or Intra-cranial hemorrhage: from the transfusion and anemia EXpertise Initiative-Control/Avoidance of bleeding. Pediatr Crit Care Med 2022;23(13 Suppl 1 1S):e14–24.

55. Holcomb JB, Tilley BC, Baraniuk S, et al. Transfusion of plasma, platelets, and red blood cells in a 1:1:1 vs a 1:1:2 ratio and mortality in patients with severe trauma: the PROPPR randomized clinical trial. Jama 2015;313(5):471–82.

56. Lee JS, Khan AD, Wright FL, et al. Whole blood versus Conventional blood component massive transfusion Protocol therapy in Civilian trauma patients. Am Surg 2022;88(5):880–6.

57. Leeper CM, Yazer MH, Morgan KM, et al. Adverse events after low titer group O whole blood versus component product transfusion in pediatric trauma patients: a propensity-matched cohort study. Transfusion 2021;61(9):2621–8.

58. Duchesne J, Smith A, Lawicki S, et al. Single Institution trial comparing whole blood vs balanced component therapy: 50 Years Later. J Am Coll Surg 2021; 232(4):433–42.

59. Leonard JC, Josephson CD, Luther JF, et al. Life-threatening bleeding in children: a prospective observational study. Crit Care Med 2021;49(11):1943–54.

60. Spinella PC, Leonard JC, Marshall C, et al. Transfusion ratios and deficits in injured children with life-threatening bleeding. Pediatr Crit Care Med 2022; 23(4):235–44.

61. Spinella PC, Leonard JC, Gaines BA, et al. Use of antifibrinolytics in pediatric life-threatening hemorrhage: a prospective observational multicenter study. Crit Care Med 2022;50(4):e382–92.

62. Oren H, Cingöz I, Duman M, et al. Disseminated intravascular coagulation in pe-diatric patients: clinical and laboratory features and prognostic factors influ-encing the survival. Pediatr Hematol Oncol 2005;22(8):679–88.

63. Fourrier F, Lestavel P, Chopin C, et al. Meningococcemia and purpura fulminans in adults: acute deficiencies of proteins C and S and early treatment with anti-thrombin III concentrates. Intensive Care Med 1990;16(2):121–4.

64. Toh CH, Hoots WK. The scoring system of the Scientific and Standardisation Committee on disseminated intravascular coagulation of the international Society on thrombosis and Haemostasis: a 5-year overview. J Thromb Haemost 2007; 5(3):604–6.

65. Gando S. The utility of a diagnostic scoring system for disseminated intravascular coagulation. Crit Care Clin 2012;28(3):373–88, vi.

66. Soundar EP, Jariwala P, Nguyen TC, et al. Evaluation of the International Society on Thrombosis and Haemostasis and institutional diagnostic criteria of dissemi-nated intravascular coagulation in pediatric patients. Am J Clin Pathol 2013; 139(6):812–6.

67. Weiss SL, Peters MJ, Alhazzani W, et al. Surviving sepsis Campaign international guidelines for the management of septic shock and sepsis-associated Organ dysfunction in children. Pediatr Crit Care Med 2020;21(2):e52–106.
68. Müller MCA, Meijers JC, van Meenen DM, et al. Thromboelastometry in critically ill patients with disseminated intravascular coagulation. Blood Coagul Fibrinolysis 2019;30(5):181–7.

Voices of Pandemic Care: Perspectives from Pediatric Providers During the First SARS-CoV-2 Surge

Lisa DelSignore, MD[a], Phoebe Yager, MD[b],
Kimberly Whalen, RN, MS, CCRN[b], Jenna Pacheco, PharmD, BCPPS[c],
Tamara Vesel, MD[d], Sara Ross, MD[a],*

KEYWORDS

- Pandemic • Perspectives • Critical care • Scope of practice • Palliative care
- Interdisciplinary care

KEY POINTS

- Strong physician and nursing leadership with focus on provider well-being was essential to providing care during the pandemic.
- With proper supervision and support, scope of practice can be expanded to deliver effective and safe care.
- The rapid onslaught of the first SARS-CoV-2 surge created opportunities for pediatric care innovation and exceptional interdisciplinary teamwork.
- Palliative care is well-positioned to bridge the gap between care teams and families while providing emotional support to providers and patients, alike.

INTRODUCTION

Pediatric providers were called on to care for patients outside their typical scope of practice during the first surge of the SARS-CoV-2 pandemic. Providers were forced to think creatively while working within established hospital systems and to use resources collaboratively across units and teams. Already published in the literature are examples of collaboration between pediatric and adult critical care groups,

---

None of the authors have commercial or financial conflicts of interest to disclose.
[a] Division of Pediatric Critical Care, Tufts Children's Hospital, Tufts Medical Center, 800 Washington Street, Box 93, Boston, MA 02111, USA; [b] Pediatric Intensive Care Unit, Mass General for Children, 55 Fruit Street, Boston, MA 02114, USA; [c] Tufts Children's Hospital, Tufts Medical Center, 800 Washington Street, #420, Boston, MA 02111, USA; [d] Division of Palliative Care, Tufts Medical Center, 800 Washington Street, South Building 7th Floor, Boston, MA 02111, USA
* Corresponding author.
E-mail address: sross3@tuftsmedicalcenter.org

Crit Care Clin 39 (2023) 299–308
https://doi.org/10.1016/j.ccc.2022.09.006
0749-0704/23/© 2022 Elsevier Inc. All rights reserved.

descriptions of how pediatric intensive care units (PICUs) were repurposed to safely care for adults including triage paradigms and care team structures, observations of staffing challenges and resource allocation, along with demographic and outcome data.[1-8] Our collective aim is not to duplicate what has been described elsewhere, but to supplement it by providing perspectives from interdisciplinary pediatric critical care team providers, consultants, and families impacted by the first SARS-CoV-2 surge.

The authorship team is composed of pediatric providers from two Boston hospital systems: Tufts Children's Hospital (TCH) and Mass General for Children (MGfC), both pediatric hospitals within larger academic medical centers providing care to patients of all ages. We share our perspectives bourn of our collective experiences during the first SARS-CoV-2 surge acknowledging that our PICUs approached care of critically ill adults similarly. Our perspectives are informed by challenges and imperatives faced, including the need to lead and support teams through change, balancing long-standing duty to children while contributing to the care of critically ill adults, preserving interdisciplinary care and connection to families while expanding scope of practice, and the need to find meaning in our work.

CARING FOR PATIENTS BY CARING FOR THE TEAMS

Shortly after New York, Massachusetts experienced its first wave of SARS-CoV-2 in March 2020, forcing hospitals to rapidly redeploy resources and alter organizational structure to accommodate the torrent of acutely ill patients, primarily adults. Overwhelmed by the volume of patients requiring intensive care unit (ICU)-level care, Mass General Hospital announced its decision to convert MGfCs 14-bed PICU to an adult ICU. This decision sparked a host of reactions for staff—anxiety, fear, pride, grief, and anger. Faced with the dual challenges of transitioning from treating children to treating adults *and* implementing dynamic COVID-19 care recommendations, PICU leadership strongly advocated to preserve the PICU nurse–physician team rather than to redeploy providers to other units. This allowed us to capitalize on years of established trust in a familiar environment facilitating rapid adjustment and preserving morale.

Despite recognized gaps in knowledge and experience specific to adult critical care, consensus yielded the decision to have the pediatric intensivist serve as a primary physician for adult patients. To address these gaps, we expanded our team to include internal medicine and combined internal medicine–pediatric residents and an adult intensivist consulted on every patient. The adult intensivist reviewed care plans with the team twice daily and was available to field questions at any time. Subspecialty consultation was delivered by adult providers. To extend the expertise of PICU nurses, nurse dyads composed of a PICU nurse and an adult medical/surgical nurse were created to jointly care for two patients. The PICU and adult nurses partnered, complementing one another's experience and skill set. Together they boosted one another's confidence in their ability to care for patients beyond the normal scope of practice. Delivering care in a familiar environment with trusted physicians and leadership promoted a sense of security for PICU nurses during this unfamiliar experience.

One of the core questions asked of PICU leadership was, "What does the team need to provide safe care?" It was recognized that unless providers believed they were safe themselves, it would be extremely difficult for them to provide safe care. Standard morning nurses' huddle (which predated the pandemic) organically morphed into a full team huddle, including physicians, respiratory therapists, nurses, and unit leadership. Time was dedicated to review, demonstrate, and practice donning and doffing procedures. Important updates were shared, and feedback was solicited from bedside providers to optimize workflows. The nurse–resident team caring for each patient was specified, and new members of the team were formally introduced including their home unit and typical scope of practice to accomplish an explicit welcome. In this way, the huddle prioritized team member safety, empowered team members to speak-up when concerns arose, defined limits of expertise, and ensured a shared mental model for the day ahead.

Knowledge is power, and thus there was ample attention paid to education. Much of the fear initially harbored by the team stemmed from uncertainty regarding how SARS-CoV-2 is spread and lack of experience donning and doffing personal protective equipment (PPE). The presence of nursing and physician leadership on the unit every day was important in addressing serious concerns of personal safety. This promoted bidirectional communication and solidarity and care for the team. Before receiving the first adult patient, PICU nurses floated to the adult ICUs to observe typical bedside care and familiarize themselves with other aspects of adult ICU nursing workflow. Dual-sided pocket guides with adult medication dosing on one side and local ICU COVID-19 management guidelines on the other were created and distributed. In response to the lack of advanced cardiovascular life support (ACLS) certification among some members of the team, an ACLS-certified provider reviewed the universally recognized algorithms with providers, and each provider was given an ACLS pocket guide.

With respect to patient selection, there were several considerations to be addressed, including whether to admit critically ill adult patients with COVID-19 versus without, to define age limits for patients cared for by pediatric providers, and whether to preferentially accept lateral transfers from legacy ICUs versus newly admitted patients directly from the emergency department who had not yet been stabilized. Ultimately, it was decided the best approach was to have the pediatric team focus on a single disease entity, that being COVID-19 acute respiratory distress syndrome, especially since that was the population with the greatest clinical need. Although the original plan was to limit care to younger adult patients, ultimately the age limit was abandoned as there was a team preference for caring older patients with fewer comorbidities by comparison to younger patients with significant comorbidities, including cardiac disease.

The long-standing role of the MGfCs PICU in the Northeast Regional Biothreats Team played a critical role in enabling a safe and rapid redirection to caring for adults with a high-consequence infectious disease like COVID-19. Many nurses and physicians on the team had already been trained to respond to such a threat. These individuals assumed leadership roles within the PICU and institution using expertise in infection control concepts while helping to oversee much of the institutional response to the pandemic. These relationships served as the basis for critical communication and promoted safe and efficient transition to adult care.

Family-centered care is the generally accepted standard in pediatric critical care. Although family members were not allowed at the bedside during the first SARS-CoV-2 wave, we applied our family-centered culture of care to our adult patients as best we could. We encouraged family members to help us complete "All About Me" posters to display at their loved one's bedside. This added a human element and helped our team know each patient behind the tubes and devices. It brought greater meaning to our work. This also conveyed our attempt to grasp and respect the personhood of each patient and our singular goal to return them to their families. When this was not possible, we ensured and communicated to families that their loved one did not die alone.

Of course, the physical and emotional stress placed on health care workers during this pandemic has been enormous. Stretching beyond the typical scope of practice is sufficiently difficult, but doing so while concerned for personal safety and the health of one's own family and loved ones compounds the challenge. This prompted deliberate attention to the well-being of the team and its individual members. In addition to the team huddle, pediatric psychiatrists and members of our palliative care team visited the unit daily to check-in and provide support. They held resiliency rounds on a regular basis. The institution established a peer-to-peer warm line to coach ICU and non-ICU providers preparing to have anticipated difficult conversations with families and to offer emotional support to any team member in need during these dark times. Celebrating the everyday successes, like extubation and discharges, also helped to lift the team's spirits.

Strong nurse and physician leadership played a significant role in the transition to caring for adult critically ill patients. Beyond ensuring that providers had the necessary supplies and medications needed to care for this new patient population, active presence on the unit and timely engagement, and responsiveness to articulated needs were crucial to team success. There was consistent adherence to the grounding principle that to provide safe and effective care, the team needed to feel safe and supported; we believe this principle was critical to sustaining the team and facilitating ongoing excellent care.

Although planning and preparation consumed the attention of numerous stakeholders, individual team members had their own personal concerns to reconcile with professional duties. Some had personal medical conditions that put them at risk of developing severe COVID illness. Others had difficulty managing the increased shift lengths required to staff additional teams. Importantly, we welcomed dialogue regarding individual limitations and found creative ways to mitigate risk and extend and sustain our human resources. For example, at TCH, one of our pregnant providers took the lead in our satellite PICU caring for pediatric non-COVID patients while liaising with our medical intensive care colleagues via phone to expedite transfer of adult patients to the repurposed PICU. Roles and responsibilities were creatively redesigned to reconcile personal safety while allowing individual team members to contribute meaningfully.

Maintaining Care of Pediatric Patients

In early March 2020, the TCH PICU wrestled with the duty to continue to provide care to critically ill children while preparing for the first wave of critically ill adults. Early data suggested that COVID-19 disease in children was less severe than in adults, and with the public health guidance intended to limit transition, we anticipated a low volume of critically ill pediatric COVID-related respiratory illness. That being said, we needed to maintain access to critical care resources for vulnerable populations of children (eg, those with chronic illnesses, technology dependence, immunosuppression). This was all the more imperative given that two of the four local tertiary and quaternary PICUs, including MGfC, had been fully transitioned to care for critically ill adults at the surge onset.

To maintain capacity to care for critically ill children, a satellite PICU space (five virtual beds with the ability to flex to eight beds) was created on an existing inpatient pediatric ward at TCH. We effectively began sharing this unit, which included not only bed spaces, but nursing staff and other resources. This required many hours of planning and preparation with key stakeholders from interdisciplinary groups (physicians, nursing, pharmacy, respiratory therapy, infection prevention, environmental services, and telecommunications) before admission of the first adult COVID-19 positive patient into this satellite PICU. Several adaptations to the environment were required to accommodate ICU level patients.

As an interdisciplinary team, the group obtained and reformatted portable patient monitors to approximate ICU monitoring capabilities, including the ability to display end-tidal CO_2, arterial line, and central venous pressure waveforms. We positioned these monitors strategically to be viewable from the central nursing station as these rooms did not have central monitoring. Emergency airway and other supplies were distributed to each room to mimic resources available in standard PICU rooms. Emergency responses were simulated, and the nomenclature of our units was adjusted to ensure responders arrived to the "new" space easily and in a timely fashion. Telecommunications created a new centralized phone number so that calls dispatched through the operator and paging systems were directed appropriately. Pharmacy updated the medication dispensing units to include medications readily available in our standard PICU in addition to those routinely available on the ward.

To staff the satellite PICU, the expertise of PICU nursing staff was used by integrating floor level nurses, supported by a PICU nurse, into the bedside staffing model. To balance the acuity and needs of all units, a flexible resident staffing model was adopted and the cadre of residents were shared by the pediatric floor, satellite PICU, and the newly repurposed adult COVID PICU. Both of these PICUs (adult COVID PICU and satellite PICU) remained staffed and supervised by pediatric ICU care providers. After admission of the first patient into the satellite PICU, feedback was collected daily during morning interdisciplinary bedside safety huddles to ensure that unanticipated needs were addressed and that a high degree of situational awareness was maintained while delivering safe and effective care for all of the patients.

By all measures, the satellite PICU was a success. At the height of the SARS-CoV-2 pandemic, there were 2 to 4 critically ill pediatric patients receiving care in the satellite space. This preserved access to critical care services for children within our referral network, provided ongoing exposure to pediatric patients for trainees, and taught team members how to work creatively and collaboratively to make the most of pooled resources.

INNOVATIONS IN INTERDISCIPLINARY CARE DELIVERY

Clinical pharmacists are among the numerous nonphysician providers who contribute to the work of an ICU on a daily basis. Over the last decade, the recognition of pediatric clinical pharmacists as essential members of the multidisciplinary care team in PICUs has expanded as the standardization of education and infrastructure for training pediatric clinical pharmacists has evolved.[9,10] At TCH, the pediatric clinical pharmacists round daily with the inpatient teams, gathering and analyzing the most up-to-date scientific and clinical information on how to deliver safe and effective pharmacotherapy.

When the TCH PICU transitioned to care for critically ill adults (both COVID-positive and non-COVID), pediatric clinical pharmacists remained the key members of the interdisciplinary care team. The pediatric clinical pharmacists continued to support care of pediatric patients in the satellite PICU while collaborating with adult clinical pharmacists to ensure appropriate management of adults beyond the typical scope of practice.

Before the first critically ill adult with COVID-19 was admitted to the PICU, the pediatric clinical pharmacists worked closely with pharmacy leadership and adult critical care clinical pharmacists to ensure continuity in the medication use process and standardization of educational content for clinicians. High-yield adult critical care pharmacy content, including common medications and dosing, was curated and made accessible to all house staff via physical binders housed in the PICU and electronically in a centralized repository that could be easily accessed while rounding. Frequent meetings with this group were held throughout the pandemic to advise physicians about anticipated drug shortages and the use of alternate medications as we continued to maintain supply.

To facilitate appropriate exchange of expertise inherent to the interdisciplinary team while acknowledging social distancing requirements and the need to conserve PPE, a hybrid rounding system was piloted using Health Insurance Portability and Accountability Act-compliant video conferencing alongside an in-person skeleton rounding team. Pediatric clinical pharmacists, palliative care physicians, adult physician consultants, and residents tending to order entry were some of the remote participants. A substantial amount of time was expended to operationalize hybrid rounding teams. Strategies contributing to the success of the model included the use of personal devices and headphones, limiting background noise by keeping everyone but the presenter muted, using the chat feature to minimize interruptions, and having a designated individual to display laboratories and other portions of the electronic health record to the entire group. With ongoing iterative feedback, we were able to effectively streamline hybrid rounds and expand to include other consulting providers from outside of the PICU who could weigh-in with recommendations when relevant.

Despite the success of the hybrid rounding format and the safety that provided team members during the uncertainty of the pandemic, the constraints of providing remote pharmacy support were significant. The successful practice of a critical care pharmacist relies on situational awareness gathered through the sight and sound of being present on the unit, whether that be visually assessing a patient, providing a timely response to a drug information question, or anticipating how a patient's therapeutic drug profile may need to change based on their clinical status. As such, there was a greater demand placed on bedside providers, who were also adapting to this new patient population, to be in more consistent communication throughout the day with remote consultative pharmacists.

Although pharmacy support was consistently remote and allowed for meaningful contribution to the team, the opportunity to experience the comradery typical of an inclusive multidisciplinary team was diminished. Nevertheless, invaluable lessons were learned including the importance of being part of a creative team and the experience of expanding expertise beyond the typical scope of practice.

PERSPECTIVES OF PEDIATRIC TRAINEES

The ways in which scope of practice were challenged in response to depleted resources during the pandemic are numerous, as providers in nearly all disciplines were expected to expand their competency and consider deployment to care for patients in ways they had not to date. In response, noninternal medicine trainees, attendings, and nurses were among the first to be considered for deployment to care for the overwhelming influx of adult patients at teaching hospitals. At both institutions, pediatric intensivists expressed concerns regarding potential exposure to medico-legal action from practicing outside one's scope. Fortunately, through meetings with hospital counsel, emergency privilege extensions and federal and state liability protections were provided to pediatric health care workers. Indemnifying pediatric providers, however, was only one hurdle to expanding scope of practice. Several models of redeployment of pediatric providers and resources have been described in the literature,[1–8] but only a few articles include the perspectives of pediatric trainees.[11–13] As published by

Kazmerski and colleagues, with 72% of pediatric faculty and trainees categorizing pediatric trainees as essential personnel during the pandemic, the perspectives of pediatric trainees are underreported, especially given the response of this group in the face of tremendous societal need.[12] The perspectives of two pediatric residents were captured for the purposes of this article.

Redeployed residents noted that although care for adults with multiple complex comorbidities was a departure from normal, the relative proximity to the broad and largely adult-based medical school curriculum was helpful. Furthermore, working in a familiar environment relying on established relationships, teams and processes allowed for the focus of the trainee to be merely on gaining comfort and competence with the expanding clinical medicine. Working with baseline interprofessional team members, such as pediatric nurses, palliative care, social workers, and pharmacists allowed for streamlined communication and care delivery. The addition of a weekly interdisciplinary debrief to discuss practices and processes that were working well and identify where care could improve may have further contributed to all providers feeling more aligned in our approach to caring for patients outside our typical scope of practice.

Naturally, fear of medical errors and harm to patients secondary to lack of established competence in caring for adult patients was pervasive among pediatric trainees. Although efforts were made to address knowledge gaps while the first surge was anticipated, uncertainty and anxiety persisted. Trainees derived a sense of security from shared decision-making between PICU and adult pulmonary critical care providers.

Finally, trainees with exposure to models of care in other countries recalled a generally larger scope of practice abroad with the expectation that physicians of all specialties maintain a broad understanding of medical modalities. Acceptance and routine exposure to a broad and varied patient population contributes to a less restrictive personal definition of scope of practice. There has been an increase in the number of trainees entering pediatric fellowship programs in addition to growth in the proportion of dual-trained providers working in niche subspecialty units, such as adult and pediatric cardiac and neuro ICUs.[14,15] Advantages to cohorted ICUs include improved interdisciplinary education/training, dedicated expertise, interservice communication, and streamlined development/implementation of guidelines and protocols.[16,17] These factors together, however, introduce the question of whether over time the US health care system will be disadvantaged relative to other countries in the ability of providers to be clinically nimble during a global pandemic, as we call on more specialized providers to harken back to their broad-based undergraduate training.

PALLIATIVE CARE: EASING THE BURDEN

The COVID-19 pandemic led to a surge in critically ill and end-of-life patients around the world. With specialization in communication, decision-making, and symptom management in critical illness, palliative care at TMC rapidly recognized the need to fill gaps that would inherently exist between the care teams and patients' families. Through in-person and remote consultation, members of the palliative care team were successfully embedded into all ICUs, including the repurposed PICU caring for critically ill adults. Given the nature of the hybrid-rounding model in the PICU, the pediatric palliative care physician would join rounds remotely each morning and liaise with families in the afternoons. Some of the functions of the palliative care team during this time were to:

- Obtain additional personal history of patients
- Provide frequent updates on patient condition and care plan to families given visitation limitations

- Provide guidance on anticipatory grief, hope, and realistic goals of care to families
- Provide a consistent point of contact for patients who moved between several units during extended hospitalizations
- Support complicated health care proxy (HCP) scenarios, including identifying the HCP and moderating difficult family decisions
- Provide grief and bereavement support to staff

After the first phase of the pandemic, the palliative care research team was interested in the research question, "How has the COVID-19 pandemic led to changes in the utilization, perceptions, and understanding of palliative care among critical care physicians, hospital leaders, and spiritual care providers?" Twenty-five in-depth interviews were conducted between August and October 2020. Qualitative findings indicated the pandemic reinforced positive perceptions of palliative care and palliative care connected providers, patients, and families, supported providers, and contributed to hospital efficiency.[18]

Providers identified collaboration with palliative care to have relieved some of the workload and reduced emotional burden by taking the lead in time-consuming, emotionally draining discussions with patients and families. With regard to bereavement, all respondents were proponents of incorporating greater bereavement support into patient care at TMC. Most believed that palliative care providers are well-suited to play a leading role in that process and continue to provide an avenue for families to communicate with the care team after the death of a loved one.

As a testament to the important role palliative care played in support of families during the pandemic, we would like to share this note from an 89-year-old woman whose brother died at TMC, whereas his relatives were in Atlanta and Arizona.

I was so deeply touched by the write up you gave to the BlueCross BlueShield reporter about my brother and my family and your effort to ease the distance between us. Thank you so very much for that beautiful tribute to my family and especially to my brother.

Your calls to M [his nephew] and me were very precious in that you were so calming and caring. That meant so much and added to the comfort of making our decisions. Both M and I feel as if we made the right call and hope that B [my brother] is, at last, at peace.

With love,

—E [B's sister]

SUMMARY

The Codes of Ethics published by the American Medical Association, American Nursing Association, and American Society of Health-Systems Pharmacists each, respectively, addresses the long-standing responsibility of physicians, nurses, and pharmacists in protecting and promoting the health of the public.[19–21] Although these perspectives are a small sampling of the experiences of pediatric providers in meeting that call, our hope is that through these stories we have shared some unique viewpoints and innovations, and we have provided a window into the contributions of pediatric teams to our communities. It was not only our responsibility to do so, but an honor to be a cornerstone of care delivery during the pandemic.

CLINICS CARE POINTS

- Redeployment of pedatric providers was essential for many hospitals to deliver adequate care during the SARS-CoV-2 pandemic.
- With proper education, supervision and interdisciplinary support, scope of practice for pediatric providers can be expanded to deliver effective and safe care.

REFERENCES

1. Chomton M, Marsac L, Deho A, et al, Robert-Debré University Hospital Study Group. Transforming a paediatric ICU to an adult ICU for severe Covid-19: lessons learned. Eur J Pediatr 2021 Jul;180(7):2319–23.
2. Deep A, Knight P, Kernie SG, et al. A hybrid model of pediatric and adult critical care during the Coronavirus disease 2019 surge: the experience of two tertiary hospitals in London and New York. Pediatr Crit Care Med 2021 Feb 1;22(2): e125–34. https://doi.org/10.1097/PCC.0000000000002584. PMID: 33027239.
3. Gist RE, Pinto R, Kissoon N, et al. Repurposing a PICU for adult care in a state Mandated COVID-19 only hospital: outcome comparison to the MICU Cohort to Determine safety and Effectiveness. Front Pediatr 2021;9:665350.
4. Joyce CL, Howell JD, Toal M, et al. Critical care for Coronavirus disease 2019: perspectives from the PICU to the medical ICU. Crit Care Med 2020;48(11): 1553–5.
5. Kneyber MCJ, Engels B, van der Voort PHJ. Paediatric and adult critical care medicine: joining forces against Covid-19. Crit Care 2020;24(1):350.
6. Levin AB, Bernier ML, Riggs BJ, et al. Transforming a PICU into an adult ICU during the Coronavirus disease 2019 pandemic: meeting multiple needs. Crit Care Explor 2020;2(9):e0201.
7. Sinha R, Aramburo A, Deep A, et al. Caring for critically ill adults in paediatric intensive care units in England during the COVID-19 pandemic: planning, implementation and lessons for the future. Arch Dis Child 2021;106(6):548–57.
8. Yager PH, Whalen KA, Cummings BM. Repurposing a pediatric ICU for adults. N Engl J Med 2020;382(22):e80. https://doi.org/10.1056/NEJMc2014819. Epub 2020 May 15. PMID: 32412712.
9. Bhatt-Mehta V, Buck ML, Chung AM, et al. Recommendations for meeting the pediatric patient's need for a clinical pharmacist: a joint opinion of the pediatrics practice and research network of the American College of clinical pharmacy and the pediatric pharmacy advocacy group. Pharmacotherapy 2013;33(2): 243–51.
10. Lat I, Paciullo C, Daley MJ, et al. Position Paper on critical care pharmacy services: 2020 update. Crit Care Med 2020;48(9):e813–34. https://doi.org/10.1097/ CCM.0000000000004437. PMID: 32826496.
11. Damari E, Fargel A, Berger I, et al. Pediatric residents' perception of medical education, general Wellness and patient care Following the Shortening of shifts during the COVID-19 pandemic. Isr Med Assoc J 2021;23(4):214–8. PMID: 33899352.
12. Kazmerski TM, Friehling E, Sharp EA, et al. Pediatric faculty and trainee Attitudes toward the COVID-19 pandemic. Hosp Pediatr 2021;11(2):198–207. https://doi. org/10.1542/hpeds.2020-001990. Epub 2021 Jan 11. PMID: 33431427.

13. Siva N, Knight P, Deep A. COVID-19: trainee perspectives from unprecedented changes on the Paediatric Intensive Care Unit (PICU). Pediatr Res 2022; 91(1):70–1.

14. Macy ML, Leslie LK, Turner A, et al. Growth and changes in the pediatric medical subspecialty workforce pipeline. Pediatr Res 2021;89(5):1297–303.

15. Horak RV, Marino BS, Werho DK, et al. Assessment of physician training and prediction of workforce needs in paediatric cardiac intensive care in the United States. Cardiol Young 2021;1–6. https://doi.org/10.1017/S1047951121004893. Epub ahead of print. PMID: 34924098.

16. LaRovere KL, Murphy SA, Horak R, et al. Pediatric neurocritical care: Evolution of a new clinical service in PICUs across the United States. Pediatr Crit Care Med 2018;19(11):1039–45. https://doi.org/10.1097/PCC.0000000000001708. PMID: 30134362.

17. Kramer AH, Zygun DA. Do neurocritical care units save lives? Measuring the impact of specialized ICUs. Neurocrit Care 2011;14(3):329–33.

18. Vesel T, Ernst E, Vesel L, et al. A qualitative study of the role of palliative care during the COVID-19 pandemic: perceptions and experiences among critical care clinicians, hospital leaders, and spiritual care providers. Am J Hosp Palliat Care 2021;13. https://doi.org/10.1177/10499091211055900. 104990912110559.

19. Brotherton S, Kao A, Crigger BJ. Professing the Values of medicine: the Modernized AMA *Code of medical Ethics*. JAMA 2016;316(10):1041–2. https://doi.org/10.1001/jama.2016.9752.

20. Code of Ethics for nurses with Interpretive Statements. American nurses Association. 2015. Available at: https://www.nursingworld.org/coe-view-only. Accessed June 29, 2022.

21. Code of Ethics for Pharmacists. American society of health-systems pharmacists. 1994. Available at: https://www.ashp.org/-/media/assets/policy-guidelines/docs/endorsed-documents/code-of-ethics-for-pharmacists.ashx. Accessed June 29, 2022.

Pediatric Critical Care
Outcomes: State of the Science

Mallory A. Perry-Eaddy, PhD, RN, CCRN[a,b,]*,
Leslie A. Dervan, MD, MS[c], Joseph C. Manning, PhD, RN[d,e],
R. Scott Watson, MD, MPH[c], Martha A.Q. Curley, PhD, RN[f,g,h]

KEYWORDS

- Pediatric • Critical care • Outcomes • Postintensive care syndrome • Follow-up

KEY POINTS

- Survivors of pediatric critical care are at risk of developing post-intensive care syndrome in pediatrics (PICS-p).
- PICS-p includes physical, cognitive, emotional, and social health impairments that can affect the child and/or their family and that can last for years.
- Future PICS-p research should prioritize prospective studies, data harmonization, data sharing, and creation of large multisite data repositories.
- Reframing pediatric intensive care unit (PICU) care to focus on improving survivorship and promoting resiliency may help mitigate the negative effects of PICS-p in PICU survivors and their families.

INTRODUCTION

Advances in pediatric critical care have improved the survival of critically ill infants and children worldwide.[1] Although mortality rates have decreased, survival after pediatric critical illness is often accompanied by new morbidities, leading researchers and clinicians to shift attention from child survival to family survivorship.[2] As such, pediatric

[a] University of Conneticut School of Nursing, 231 Glenbrook Road, U-4026, Storrs, CT 06269, USA; [b] Department of Pediatrics, University of Connecticut School of Medicine, 200 Academic Way, Farmington, CT 06032, USA; [c] Department of Pediatrics, Division of Pediatric Critical Care Medicine, University of Washington, Seattle Children's Hospital, M/S FA2.112, 4800 Sand Point Way NE, Seattle, WA 98105, USA; [d] Paediatric Critical Care Outreach, Nottingham Children's Hospital, Nottingham University Hospitals NHS Trust, Queens Medical Centre Campus, Derby Road, Nottingham, NG7 2UH, UK; [e] Centre for Children and Young People Health Research, School of Health Sciences, University of Nottingham, Medical School, Queen's Medical Centre, Nottingham, NG7 2HA, UK; [f] Department of Family and Community Health, University of Pennsylvania School of Nursing, 418 Curie Boulevard, Philadelphia, PA 19104, USA; [g] Children's Hospital of Philadelphia Research Institute, 3401 Civic Center Boulevard, Philadelphia, PA 19104, USA; [h] Department of Anesthesia and Critical Care, Perelman School of Medicine, University of Pennsylvania, 3400 Civic Center Boulevard, Philadelphia, PA 19104, USA
* Corresponding author.
E-mail address: mallory.perry-eaddy@uconn.edu

Crit Care Clin 39 (2023) 309–326
https://doi.org/10.1016/j.ccc.2022.09.007
0749-0704/23/© 2022 Elsevier Inc. All rights reserved.
criticalcare.theclinics.com

critical care clinicians focus on prevention of pediatric intensive care unit (PICU)-related factors that may increase an individual child's risk for new PICU morbidities after hospital discharge.

New PICU morbidities, including new or worsening problems in physical, cognitive, social, and/or emotional health that persist beyond PICU discharge, are collectively described as post-intensive care syndrome-pediatrics (PICS-p; **Fig. 1**).[3,4] Symptoms in these domains can vary and vacillate over time. Unique from adult frameworks of PICS, the PICS-p framework embeds a developmental and family perspective. Baseline status is assessed within the context of the family, including parents and siblings. Factors contributing to PICS-p include child and family characteristics, premorbid health, developmental level, critical illness trajectory including severity of illness, PICU therapies, the PICU environment itself, and family socioeconomic factors both before and after PICU admission.[5] Recovery trajectories may span days or decades—some children and families improve rapidly, others worsen, others experience peaks and valleys, whereas others remain unchanged.

Although PICU hospitalization places all children and families at risk for PICS-p, it is important to note that each child and family who develop PICS-p will have a unique experience. Early recognition and timely intervention are essential to prevent the acquisition of new morbidity in this already vulnerable pediatric population. This article will detail the current state of the science of PICS-p, outline strategies to improve recovery and make recommendations for future research priorities.

Post-Intensive Care Syndrome-Pediatrics Framework Domains

The PICS-p framework encompasses 4 distinct domains of child and family dynamics and outcomes after critical illness.[3] The following will detail each domain, precipitating factors, and example symptomatology (**Table 1**).

Physical health

Overall physical health and associated functional status are central to a child's daily activities. They encompass a child's ability to perform daily activities of living to meet their most basic needs and developmental milestones. New functional impairments are common after critical illness, with a broad range of difficulties experienced—including pain, sensation changes, impairments in mobility, self-care, feeding, and respiratory functions.[6] Precritical illness functional status varies, with an increasing effect on the PICU population due to the increase in medically complex children admitted to PICUs.[7] As such, determining baseline functional status is critical to understanding the recovery trajectory after critical illness. Validated functional status scales in the PICU include the widely used pediatric overall performance category (POPC) and pediatric cerebral performance category,[8] the Functional Status Scale,[9] and the Stein Jessop Functional Status II-R for children with developmental disability.[10]

A scoping review of 25 studies including 72,780 critically ill children found that up to 36% of children experienced newly acquired functional status decline essential to their daily routines at PICU discharge, with 26% and 13% showing improvement at 6 months and 1 year, respectively.[6] A recent study found that at 6 months after PICU discharge, approximately two-thirds of critically ill children who survived had signs of recovery of functional impairment.[11] A substantial population of children who survive critical illness experience new functional impairments and may benefit from increased efforts to support functional recovery. Recent studies using long-term follow-up after PICU discharge have found new functional impairments may persist in children who survive critical illness, with an improvement during 1 to 2 years.[6,12,13] Studies beyond 2 years post-PICU discharge are limited but needed.[6,14]

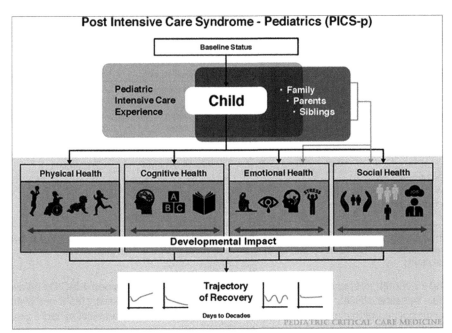

Fig. 1. Conceptualizing PICS-p in children. (*From* Manning, Joseph C.; Pinto, Neethi P.; Rennick, Janet E.; Colville, Gillian; Curley, Martha A. Q. Conceptualizing Post Intensive Care Syndrome In Children – The PICS-P Framework. PCCM. 19(4):298-300, April 2018. https://doi.org/10.1097/PCC.0000000000001476; with permission.)

In a scoping review by Ong and colleagues, of 25 PICU follow-up studies included, only 5 evaluated functional outcomes beyond 2 years after PICU discharge.[15–19] These studies included not only POPC but also the PedsQL,[20] Modified Glasgow Outcome Scale,[21] and the Health Utilization Index.[22]

A recent scoping review synthesized the existing literature on post-PICU physical function. A total of 68 studies were identified with 23,967 children. Within these studies, up to 52% of children experienced impaired physical function after PICU hospitalization. Moderate-to-severe difficulty in physical function was associated with prolonged hospital stay and preexisting comorbidities.[23] Yet, there is a discrepancy in the evaluation of baseline preexisting comorbidities, especially regarding baseline physical function. In a recent scoping review of 102 studies evaluating post-PICU physical function, only 7% of studies included an assessment of baseline physical function.[24] Recognizing the association of moderate-to-severe difficulty in physical function after PICU with preexisting comorbidities is important. Especially given that the PICU population includes an increasing number of children with special healthcare needs, medical complexity, and chronic critical illnesses.[25] Children in these special populations frequently experience prolonged admission, which may further increase their risk of post-PICU physical dysfunction. Although medical comorbidity is a significant risk factor for new physical dysfunction, children without preexisting conditions are not immune. Within the Life After Pediatric Sepsis Evaluation (*LAPSE*) Study cohort, many children without complex chronic conditions did not recover to their baseline health-related quality of life (HRQL).[26] Specifically, 56%, 41%, 32%, and 38% remained at least 1 mean clinically important difference (MCID) below their baseline HRQL as assessed by the PedsQL at 1-month, 3-month, 6-month,

Table 1
Postintensive care syndrome in pediatrics domain examples

PICS-p Domain Examples			
Physical Health	**Cognitive Health**	**Emotional Health**	**Social Health**
• Decline in functional status • Pain (acute/chronic) • Fatigue • Feeding difficulties • Mobility issues • Delayed growth • Poor sleep hygiene	• Poor school performance • Memory issues • Attention difficulties • Aphasia	• Mood lability • PTSSs • Depressive symptoms • Anxiety • Regression (developmental)	• Withdrawn from usual activities • School absenteeism • Social anxiety • Identity issues (dependency)

Although this table is not all-inclusive, these are some key examples of physical, cognitive, emotional, and social health examples of PICS-p, which may affect a child and its family after critical illness.

and 12-month, respectively, and 50%, 16% 15%, and 17% remained 4 MCIDs below their baseline HRQL.[26,27] Notably, older children (aged >2 years) and those with abnormal neurologic examination and/or injury during their PICU admission had worse physical HRQL at 1-year after discharge.[26]

Children also frequently experience pain and altered sleep after PICU discharge.[28] A recent study showed that severe pain episodes during PICU stays were independently associated with lower postdischarge HRQL after controlling for potential confounding factors such as age, baseline cognitive function, and illness severity.[29] Considering the number of painful procedures children experience in the PICU (averaging >10 per child per day),[30–32] pain is a common, and potentially modifiable, risk factor for poor outcomes even if a single painful episode is experienced. Sleep is important to multiple aspects of health and is also often interrupted in the PICU. Studies have consistently demonstrated the importance of restorative sleep for healing during critical illness.[14,33–35] Sleep interruption in PICU is multifaceted, with environmental, pharmacologic, and physical causes, and likely has short-term and long-term implications for the child including, but not limited to, cognitive decline, immune dysfunction, increased inflammation, respiratory compromise, catabolism, impaired glucose metabolism, and delayed healing,[28,33,36] all of which are important in critically ill children. In adult intensive care unit (ICU) survivors, sleep impairments are one of the most frequently reported problems after discharge.[37] Unfortunately, studies evaluating sleep in children after PICU discharge are limited. One study conducted a median of 5 months after PICU discharge found that up to 80% of children who survived critical illness were at risk for sleep disturbance.[38]

Cognitive health
The National Institutes of Health (NIH) National Institute on Aging defines cognitive health as, "the ability to clearly think, learn, and remember –[it] is an important component of performing everyday activities."[39] In the context of critical illness, children who survive are at risk for deficits in attention, memory, communication, and/or processing speed.[40,41] In a retrospective analysis of 29,352 admissions in the Virtual PICU System (VPS) Database, the overall prevalence of newly acquired cognitive disability was 3.4% from January 1, 2009 to December 31, 2010 in children aged 1 month to 18 years, who survived to discharge.[42] Children with increased severity of illness,

receipt of invasive mechanical ventilation, longer PICU stay, cardiopulmonary resuscitation, renal replacement therapy, and extracorporeal membrane oxygenation were associated with greater risk of newly acquired cognitive disability.[42] Additional risk factors for poor cognitive outcomes after pediatric critical illness include young age during illness, older age at follow-up, lower socioeconomic status, oxygen requirements during PICU admission, and the receipt of opioids while in the PICU.[43,44] The notion that younger age during critical illness and older age at follow-up are independently associated with poor cognitive function is consistent with the developmental neurology concept of "growing into deficits."[45] This phenomenon posits that early brain damage and/or injury during key stages of brain development are cumulative as a child matures, and an increasing number of deficits may surface as the child ages chronologically and executive functions are expected to mature.[46,47]

Cognitive and neurodevelopmental outcomes have been specifically evaluated among critically ill children who require sedation to facilitate safe PICU care. Polypharmacy and administration of opioids and sedatives, particularly benzodiazepines, during critical illness are consistently associated with the likelihood of developing ICU delirium.[48,49] Although ICU delirium is associated with decreased postdischarge cognitive function in adults, the impact of these medications and ICU delirium on long-term neurocognition in children is not well understood.[50–52] A recent study by Watson and colleagues[41] examined the role of critical illness—acute respiratory failure requiring mechanical ventilation—and its association with neurocognitive outcomes. Children without a prior history of cognitive dysfunction who survived critical illness without severe cognitive dysfunction at PICU discharge and matched biological siblings underwent neurocognitive evaluation of intelligence quotient (IQ) memory, visuospatial, skills, motor skills, language, and executive function 3 to 8 years after critical illness. The critical illness survivors had significantly lower estimated IQ scores compared with their otherwise healthy siblings, with the greatest difference among children hospitalized at the youngest ages. Although the differences were significant, the authors cautioned that the absolute differences were small, and their clinical significance requires further investigation.

These findings concur with an earlier study evaluating intellectual function, memory, attention, and teacher assessment of children after critical illness in 88 children with meningoencephalitis, sepsis, or other critical illness (respiratory, surgical—elective and emergency, metabolic, cardiac failure).[53] Survivors performed worse on neuropsychological testing compared with healthy controls, and teachers perceived these children as emotionally labile and having difficulty with schoolwork, executive functioning, and attention. Dysfunction was more prevalent in younger children, those of lower socioeconomic status, and if the child experienced a seizure during the PICU admission. Finally, dysfunction was worse in children with severe infection, specifically sepsis and meningoencephalitis.[53]

Similar associations have also been observed in a cohort of children diagnosed with bacterial meningitis specifically. In a meta-analysis of 39 studies including 2015 children with IQ data and 12 studies on developmental delay with 382 subjects, children with bacterial meningitis frequently experience significant decline in IQ of approximately 5 points less compared with healthy controls. Survivors are also 5 times more likely to have intellectual impairment.[54] As such, children who survive severe infections should be considered at particular risk and should be assessed and treated for cognitive deficits beyond the immediate PICU period. Although follow-up after PICU may not be feasible or beneficial in all children, special emphasis for those at greatest risk of neurocognitive decline after PICU, including those of younger age, of seizure history, and of lower socioeconomic status, should be considered.

Emotional health

A facet of mental health, emotional health refers to one's ability to cope with negative and positive stressors, adapt to change, and have overall awareness of one's own emotions.[55] A review by Nelson and Gold found that at least a quarter of children who survive critical illness developed posttraumatic stress disorder (PTSD), and up to 62% of children will demonstrate posttraumatic stress symptoms (PTSS).[56] Studies of illness-specific PICU cohorts have identified sepsis as an independent predictor of PTSS.[38,57] In addition to PTSD and PTSS, other psychopathologies affecting one's health such as anxiety and depression after PICU discharge are prevalent in children who survive critical illness, although the reporting of their prevalence is variable. In a review of 17 studies examining psychiatric symptoms and disorders after PICU, the point prevalence of clinically significant depressive symptoms ranged from 7% to 13%, with a median point prevalence of 10% (2 studies, n = 51). Major depression diagnosed via diagnostic interview occurred in 0% to 6% of children, with a median prevalence of 3% (3 studies, n = 128).[58] Although prevalence is variable, pre-PICU psychosocial characteristics are risk factors for post-PICU distress in children who survived critical illness. In a small single-center study, 51% of survivors reported pre-PICU adverse childhood events and nearly all (96%) reported posttraumatic stress. There was a strong association with acute stress, PTSD, and impaired HRQL before the current PICU admission,[57] indicating baseline psychosocial factors are important indices and predictors for emotional health after discharge from the PICU, although the authors acknowledged that baseline HRQL may have been impacted by potential recall bias and should be considered in interpretations of the findings.

The emotional influence of pediatric critical illness spans beyond the child into the family unit. Parents, guardians, and caregivers are particularly susceptible to the emotional effects of their child's critical illness as well. These effects are variable, ranging from PTSS, depression-like symptoms, a sense of powerlessness, loss of work, and financial hardship.[59,60] This is not a comprehensive list, and these effects are influenced by baseline factors such as social support and social determinants of health, which may impact many facets of post-PICU wellness, including quality of life and emotional health in both the child and their family.[61–63] Parents of children who survive critical illness frequently experience PTSD and PTSS, up to 21% and 84%, respectively.[56] PTSD and PTSS experienced in parents of survivors may contribute to family dysfunction, which may substantially affect the child's overall well-being. A pilot randomized controlled trial of 31 parents of children who survived critical illness was conducted in the United Kingdom. Parents were randomized to usual treatment or a post-PICU psychoeducational tool administered by a telephone call. Those parents who received the intervention reported lower PTSS, as well as fewer emotional and behavioral health problems with their child.[63] Although underpowered, this study demonstrated feasibility. A larger trial is necessary to understand if such an intervention improves parent outcomes in a broader context.

Critical illness and ICU admission are associated with PTSD and/or PTSS; however, positive aspects of survival and posttraumatic growth have also been reported.[64] Posttraumatic growth is well studied in survivors of traumatic events (eg, abuse, disaster)[65,66] and adolescent cancer survivorship[67]; it is less well studied in ICU populations. It is defined as positive psychological change and improvement that can result from processing trauma.[68] In the case of children who survive critical illness, and their families, the traumatic event is the critical illness and the PICU environment itself. Colville and Cream surveyed parents of critically ill children who survived 4 months after discharge, and found that a majority (88%) experienced posttraumatic growth as a direct result of their experience in the PICU.[64] Parents of ventilated children and older children reported higher levels of posttraumatic growth after discharge. Interestingly, posttraumatic growth scores were positively correlated with PTSS scores, suggesting that these experiences do not happen in isolation. Another study of parents of children who survived critical illness also confirmed that posttraumatic growth is a common experience. More than a third of parents (37%) reported at least a medium level of posttraumatic growth 6 months after their child's PICU discharge.[69] These results suggest that parents/guardians of critically ill children demonstrate incredible resiliency in the face of adversity.

Social health

Social outcomes encompass a child's ability to participate in social activities, engage meaningfully with other people, and feel socially connected and supported by others.[70] Such social interactions are crucial to a child's development, and critical illness can deeply affect the social health of both children and their families. Children surviving critical illnesses still want to "fit in" with their friends, despite new physical changes and limitations. They can suffer from isolation and loneliness, partly related to difficulty talking about the experience,[71] as well as from experienced or anticipated social stigma.[72]

Similar to adults and work, a large proportion of life for many children is spent in school. Although not all children attend school, for many, school serves as the foundation not only for scholastic growth but also for social development, and relationship-building outside the family is crucial for overall development. In a prospective study of critically ill children in an urban PICU, 43% missed at least 7 days of school while admitted to the PICU.[73] After discharge, more than two-thirds (70%) of critically ill children who survived missed school, with a median absence of 16.9 days.[74] At 3 months after discharge from the PICU, up to 20% had not returned to school, and for those who did, a third of parents or caregivers thought that their child's school performance declined.[75] Moreover, 1 in 5 caregivers thought that their school did not do enough to support the child through services to catch up academically.[73] Even years following ICU discharge, children admitted to the PICU as infants remain at higher risk of academic impairment based on standardized testing compared with age-matched peers.[76] School absenteeism in the setting of critical illness and subsequent recovery may lead to poor scholastic performance, economic hardship, and poor health outcomes in adulthood.[74]

Family social considerations. Family social effects are wide-ranging, including community, relationship, parenting, employment, and other economic effects. Namely, missed work is common among caregivers of critically ill children; with nearly half of primary caregivers having to miss work pre-PICU and post-PICU discharge to care for their critically ill child.[74] This may lead to job loss, financial and mental health strains on the caregiver and the family unit and may last for years beyond the PICU discharge.[60] The child's post-PICU disposition, their baseline functional and health status, increased length of PICU stay, and discharge functional status are all associated with the caregiver's need to miss work.[74] Caregivers and families of critically ill children must be assessed at individual levels to ensure that aside from the burden of the actual critical illness, they are not burdened by outside factors such as financial strain that may be associated with medical bills, lost wages, and hospital-associated costs such as meals, lodging, and transportation costs.[77–79]

In addition to economic hardship, parental relationships are often strained. In a qualitative study of 10 parents conducted 2 years after PICU admission, parents cited persistent strain in their interpersonal relationships due to the theme of "losing manageability."[60] Parents struggled with feelings of isolation, leading to loss of friendships, and difficulty with parental attachment to their critically ill child. Despite these difficulties, some parents described strengthened relationships because they were able to handle hardships together.[60] This is a unique finding because it has long been hypothesized that parents of seriously and/or chronically ill children experience disproportionately higher divorce rates yet evidence for this is not supported in the literature.[80]

Another unique consideration is the role the siblings may play in the critically ill child's life and vice versa.[81] Similar to parents, siblings of critically ill children are not shielded from the negative effects of critical illness.[82] Unlike parents, they are often excluded from the PICU environment for various reasons including concerns of increased risk of infection, perceived psychological trauma, and effects on the child.[83] Although literature exploring sibling response to chronic illnesses such as cancer are abundant,[84,85] there are limited studies in pediatric critical care.[86] In a recent qualitative study of siblings of critically ill children, several themes were found to be experienced by siblings: pre-illness stressors, the PICU environment, their sibling's appearance, uncertainty, and their parent's stress.[81] None of these stressors occurred in isolation. Presence in the PICU for some siblings was quite therapeutic, whereas it was distressing and anxiety-inducing for others. Much of this variation was age-dependent and varied by pre-illness factors such as social support, sibling-patient interactions, and sibling relationship. Sibling wellness (physical, social, emotional, and spiritual) is likely affected by the experience of having a critically ill sibling, and changes to the sibling relationship may also affect the critically ill child once discharged.

Future Directions

Within the last decade, research evaluating pediatric critical care and postdischarge outcomes have dramatically increased.[24,40] There is an increasing need to understand the rapidly evolving population of children who survive critical illness, including their own unique needs and priorities. The following section will outline the process of creating the PICU Core Outcome Set (COS) and Core Outcome Measurement Set (COMS), to support more systematic assessment of long-term function and morbidity in children who survive critical illness. Both efforts may be useful from a data harmonization perspective in order to better answer clinical questions regarding post-PICU care. Additionally, we will discuss the emergence of PICU follow-up clinics to support the child and family's recovery after PICU discharge and discuss mitigation strategies to reduce PICS-p and optimize recovery in the post-PICU period.

PICU core outcome set

Reliably assessing PICS-p across studies has been challenging due to the sheer breadth of measurement tools used in PICU outcomes studies. Each measurement tool assesses unique domains of PICS-p, and not all tools are equally robust. The Pediatric Outcomes STudies after PICU Investigators of the Pediatric Acute Lung Injury and Sepsis Investigators (PALISI) Network and the Eunice Kennedy Shriver National Institute of Child Health and Human Development (NICHD)-funded Collaborative Pediatric Critical Care Research Network (CPCCRN) recently put forth recommendations for a COS for pediatric critical care. As defined by the Core Outcomes Measurements in Effectiveness Trials initiative, a COS is an "agreed upon standardized set of outcomes that should be measured and reported, as a minimum, in all clinical trials in specific areas of health or healthcare."[87,88] Using an in-depth multinational modified Delphi consensus process, 333 key stakeholders were surveyed, including researchers, clinicians, and family/advocates. After 2 rounds, stakeholders agreed on the inclusion of 4 global domains (physical, cognitive, emotional, and overall health) and 4 specific outcome domains (survival, child HRQL, pain, and communication). In addition to the COS, an extended COS (PICU COS-Extended) was generated because 21 additional domains were identified as important by families but were not included in the COS. Identifying a PICU-specific COS for pediatric critical care research may enhance research harmonization across studies. In addition, future studies with similar outcome metrics, will be available for data-sharing across studies, which may help to better understand and answer clinical questions related to PICU survivorship.

Following the development of the COS is the development of a PICU COMS.[89] Using a similar standardized approach of key stakeholders, the COMS is a robust recommendation of instruments and measurement tools for clinicians and researchers to assess pediatric critical care outcomes. Development of the PICU COMS is an important step in harmonizing data across pediatric critical care outcomes research.

Surveillance, large research networks, and data sharing

With the use of electronic medical records and the generation of data repositories, the potential for data sharing is greatly increasing. The VPS is the largest collaborative database for quality improvement based on severity of illness-adjusted comparisons specifically in pediatric critical research.[90,91] VPS has more than 200 enrolled PICUs who opt to share data, with more than 1.5 million patient admission records. Variables for analysis include severity of illness scores, basic laboratories, and vital signs. Although VPS is a robust research tool, it is a voluntary registry limited to the acute inpatient PICU stay and the data include very little information on social determinants of health. Although quite different, other pediatric-specific databases may capture some of this data, such as the Kids' Inpatient Database (KID), a large population-based administrative database provided by the US government-funded Agency for Healthcare Research and Quality.[92] The KID database includes all pediatric inpatient admissions, including those to the PICU but many pediatric critical care-specific variables are not collected (eg, PICU-specific severity of illness scores) because it is compiled from billing records. However, some patient-level socioeconomic variables are recorded, as well as discharge location and readmissions to units other than the PICU. This makes the KID database a useful tool to explore social determinants of health because the data may pertain to the entire hospital course and discharge, although there are no outcomes after discharge. A noteworthy model worth mentioning for its robust nature is the Paediatric Intensive Care Audit Network (PICANet) for the UK Network.[93] Established in 2002, PICANet is a United Kingdom-funded audit database that records all National Health Service-funded PICU patient encounters and now includes 2 Dublin PICUs as well. This data is available in aggregate and de-identified patient-level on a by-request basis to researchers with the proper ethics approvals.

In addition to these large databases of pediatric inpatient clinical data, an additional potential source is the NIH, which commits to data sharing from NIH-funded studies. The NIH does not fund or support other databases. Funded Principal Investigators are required to upload their relevant data to NIH repositories such as the NICHD Data and Specimen Hub (DASH—https://dash.nichd.nih.gov/) and the National Heart, Lung, and Blood Institute Biological Specimen and Data Repository Information Coordinating Center (BioLINCC—https://biolincc.nhlbi.nih.gov/home/). Although there are several other NIH-funded data and biospecimen repositories, an exemplar study submitted and available through the DASH biorepository is the aforementioned, *LAPSE* observational Study. *LAPSE* includes the clinical data of 389 critically ill children with severe sepsis and/or septic shock, including biospecimens and robust follow-up data. In addition to clinical data, biological specimens may be requested by qualified researchers. Such datasets need to be used to draw conclusions on large populations of children who survive critical illness.

Although large repositories such as DASH and BioLINCC are useful in making data readily available to pediatric critical researchers who may not otherwise have the resources, these datasets are limited to the primary research questions. In the example of *LAPSE*, collected clinical variables are related to sepsis, and all included children had sepsis or septic shock. To answer questions outside of a specific population, more representative datasets are required. The integration of electronic health records (EHRs) and data sharing has made data accessible to researchers and clinicians alike. An example of an NIH repository integrating EHR is the National Coronavirus disease (COVID) Cohort Collaborative (N3C) Enclave an initiative by the National Center for Accelerating Translational Sciences (NCATS) and the Center for Data to Health (CD2H). N3C is unique because it incorporates more than 50 health systems, including pediatric inpatient units/hospitals, collecting COVID-specific clinical and outcomes data. Any scientist interested in asking COVID-specific questions is invited to request data from the Enclave to answer specific questions. Although the N3C is population-specific (COVID-19–positive children and adults), the creation of similar collaboratives to share EHR data could provide a powerful tool for critical care research. Members of the PALISI subgroup Pediatric Data Science and Analytics are in the process of creating a PICU Data Collaborative (http://vpicu.net/). The PICU Data Collaborative will allow members to contribute and share anonymized EHR data. This, along with improving outcome standardization across new research studies by using the COMS, may help support data aggregation, and algorithm development to improve long-term post-PICU outcomes.

Strategies to Optimize Recovery After Pediatric Intensive Care Unit Discharge

Post-PICU follow-up clinics

Increased survival, awareness of PICS-p, and increased interest in long-term outcomes after PICU have spurred an exploration into the utility of PICU follow-up clinics worldwide. Post-ICU follow-up clinics have become potentially feasible solutions for adult ICU survivors to improve outcomes,[94] especially in the time of the COVID-19 pandemic.[95,96] However, their overall feasibility for general ICU patients remains questionable. The optimal patient eligibility, timing, method of delivery, and cost-effectiveness of Post-ICU follow-up clinics are not well understood.[94,97] Initiatives such as the Society of Critical Care Medicine's THRIVE collaborative aim to establish a multinational effort of multidisciplinary post-ICU follow-up clinics and peer support to facilitate post-ICU growth and recovery.[98,99] However, such clinics and their feasibility and utility in critically ill children and their families have been minimally evaluated. A cross-sectional web-based study conducted in the entire United Kingdom and the Republic of Ireland assessed the prevalence of post-PICU follow-up. Data collection included responses from 22/28 PICUs. Of the 22 PICUs providing data, only 4 PICUs provided postdischarge PICU follow-up, using telephone (n = 2), follow-up clinic consultation (n = 1), or home visit (n = 1) methods.[100]

In a single, large academic PICU, Fitzgerald and colleagues[101] implemented a nurse-led follow-up system for pediatric sepsis survivors embedded within an existing health-care system. A multidisciplinary approach was taken, including therapists (occupational, physical, speech), teachers, neuropsychology, and coordinators from existing survivorship programs—neonatology, stroke, and oncology. The program included predischarge education and referrals, with postdischarge follow-up at 2 to 3 months to screen for new physical and/or psychosocial morbidity for referral purposes. This method of care coordination was found to be cost-effective and feasible to screen for potential new morbidity while making formal diagnoses and referrals within an existing system. A survey of active PICU follow-up clinics was conducted by Williams and colleagues. Results yielded responses from 17 active clinics, with significant variation among each regarding services provided. Of the respondents, more than 80% agreed that post-PICU follow-up clinics were beneficial to children and supported knowledge advancement. However, clinics are limited by "lack of support," citing funding constraints, including reimbursement, and lack of clinical space to lead successful follow-up programs.[102]

ICU liberation bundles

Adult ICUs have focused on attempts to reduce ICU-associated morbidity through implementing ABCDEF care bundle elements, including Assess, prevent, and manage pain; Both spontaneous awakening and breathing trials; Choice of analgesia and sedation; Delirium—assess, prevent, and manage; Early mobility; and Family engagement.[103] Implementation of this care bundle improves post-ICU outcomes, including reducing the development of PICS by reducing deep sedation and prolonged immobilization.[104]

Although PICUs globally are implementing some of these bundle elements, they are implemented inconsistently. In the Prevalence of Acute Rehabilitation for Kids in PICU study (PARK-PICU), less than 10% of the 161 international PICUs (18 countries) incorporated all 6 components of the ABCDEF bundle into routine clinical practice.[105] The most common component was standardized pain assessment (91%), followed by family engagement (88%) and routine sedation assessment (84%).[105] Within PARK-PICU, early mobility was the least commonly implemented component (26%). Despite poor adoption of early mobilization in PICUs, quality improvement initiatives, such as PICU Up!,[106] demonstrate early mobilization programs in critically ill children are generally feasible and safe.[106] The Society of Critical Care Medicine is committed to increasing access and knowledge of the ABCDEF bundles in PICUs to promote ICU liberation and limit ICU morbidity.[107]

SUMMARY

Advances in pediatric critical care have led to increased survival for critically ill children. Shifting attention from an exclusive focus on saving lives to PICU survivorship in children who survive critical illness, with emphasis on PICS-p, has increased in the past decade. Using the PICS-p Framework as a guide to clinical practice and research is necessary to optimize recovery for critically ill children and their families. Understanding the ever-changing epidemiologic landscape of children who survive critical illness is vital. Standardized post-PICU assessment, data harmonization, and data sharing to create large datasets may help optimize research efforts in this area. Additionally, strategies such as effective post-PICU clinics, ICU Liberation bundle implementation, and resiliency interventions to promote posttraumatic growth may help offset the negative effects of critical illness and PICU-related therapies, promoting recovery among children who survive critical illness.

CLINICS CARE POINTS

- Post-Intensive Care Syndrome in pediatrics (PICS-p) is now acknowledged as a phenomenon commonly experienced by children who survive critical illness and their families.

- Symptoms of PICS-p should be assessed in survivors of pediatric critical illness. Though uncertainties exist in which PICU patients may benefit most, when assessments should occur, and what interventions should be considered for support.
- Assessments should consider both a biopsychosocial and developmental approaches as described within the PICS-p framework, including elements of physical, cognitive, emotional and social well-being of the child and family, parents, and siblings.
- Core outcomes, evaluated systematically following PICU discharge, may allow for early detection and intervention in high-risk patients. However, the selection and implementation of specific instruments evaluating these outcomes will depend on access, resources, and context.
- Interventions within the PICU, including incorporation of ICU liberation and chronotherapeutic bundles, may aid in promoting resilience and recovery in children who survive critical illness.

DISCLOSURE

The authors declare no conflicts of interest. Dr. M.A. Perry-Eaddy is funded by an NIH, United States/NIGMS MOSAIC K99/R00 (4R00GM145411) and American Association of Critical Care Nurses Impact Grant Award. Dr. J.C. Manning is funded by an NIHR, United KingdomICA Clinical Lectureship (ICA-CL-2018–04-ST2-009). Dr. M.A.Q. Curley is currently funded by NIH/NHLBI (5UH3HL141736); and both Drs M.A.Q. Curley and R.S. Watson are MPIs funded by the NIH/NICHD (1R01HD098269).

REFERENCES

1. Epstein D, Brill JE. A history of pediatric critical care medicine. Pediatr Res 2005;58(5):987–96.
2. Heneghan JA, Pollack MM. Morbidity: changing the outcome paradigm for pediatric critical care. Pediatr Clin North Am 2017;64(5):1147–65.
3. Manning JC, Pinto NP, Rennick JE, et al. Conceptualizing post intensive care syndrome in children-the PICS-p framework. Pediatr Crit Care Med 2018. https://doi.org/10.1097/pcc.0000000000001476.
4. Needham DM, Davidson J, Cohen H, et al. Improving long-term outcomes after discharge from intensive care unit: report from a stakeholders' conference. Crit Care Med 2012;40(2):502–9.
5. Long DA, Fink EL. Transitions from short to long-term outcomes in pediatric critical care: considerations for clinical practice. Transl Pediatr 2021;10(10): 2858–74.
6. Ong C, Lee JH, Leow MK, et al. Functional outcomes and physical impairments in pediatric critical care survivors: a scoping review. Pediatr Crit Care Med 2016; 17(5):e247–59.
7. Shapiro MC, Henderson CM, Hutton N, et al. Defining pediatric chronic critical illness for clinical care, research, and policy. Hosp Pediatr 2017;7(4):236–44.
8. Fiser DH. Assessing the outcome of pediatric intensive care. J Pediatr 1992; 121(1):68–74.
9. Pollack MM, Holubkov R, Glass P, et al. Functional Status Scale: new pediatric outcome measure. Pediatrics 2009;124(1):e18–28.
10. Stein RE, Jessop DJ. Functional status II(R). A measure of child health status. Med Care 1990;28(11):1041–55.
11. Choong K, Fraser D, Al-Harbi S, et al. Functional recovery in critically ill children, the "WeeCover" multicenter study. Pediatr Crit Care Med 2018;19(2):145–54.

12. Sankar J, Moodu S, Kumar K, et al. Functional outcomes at 1 year after PICU discharge in critically ill children with severe sepsis. Pediatr Crit Care Med 2021;22(1):40–9.
13. Polic B, Mestrovic J, Markic J, et al. Long-term quality of life of patients treated in paediatric intensive care unit. Eur J Pediatr 2013;172(1):85–90.
14. Herrup EA, Wieczorek B, Kudchadkar SR. Characteristics of postintensive care syndrome in survivors of pediatric critical illness: a systematic review. World J Crit Care Med 2017;6(2):124–34.
15. van der Heide P, Hassing MB, Gemke RJ. Characteristics and outcome of long-stay patients in a paediatric intensive care unit: a case-control study. Acta Paediatr 2004;93(8):1070–4.
16. Butt W, Shann F, Tibballs J, et al. Long-term outcome of children after intensive care. Crit Care Med 1990;18(9):961–5.
17. Taylor A, Butt W, Ciardulli M. The functional outcome and quality of life of children after admission to an intensive care unit. Intensive Care Med 2003;29(5):795–800.
18. Namachivayam P, Taylor A, Montague T, et al. Long-stay children in intensive care: long-term functional outcome and quality of life from a 20-yr institutional study. Pediatr Crit Care Med 2012;13(5):520–8.
19. Conlon NP, Breatnach C, O'Hare BP, et al. Health-related quality of life after prolonged pediatric intensive care unit stay. Pediatr Crit Care Med 2009;10(1):41–4.
20. Varni JW, Seid M, Kurtin PS. PedsQL 4.0: reliability and validity of the Pediatric Quality of Life Inventory version 4.0 generic core scales in healthy and patient populations. Med Care 2001;39(8):800–12.
21. Jennett B, Bond M. Assessment of outcome after severe brain damage. Lancet 1975;1(7905):480–4.
22. Feeny DH, Torrance GW, Furlong WJ. Health utilities index. In: Spilker B, editor. Qual life pharmacoeconomics in clin trials26, 2nd edition. Philadelphia, PA: Lippincott-Raven Press; 1996. p. 239–52.
23. Bossen D, de Boer RM, Knoester H, et al. Physical functioning after admission to the PICU: a scoping review. Crit Care Explor 2021;3(6):e0462.
24. Maddux AB, Pinto N, Fink EL, et al. Postdischarge Outcome domains in pediatric critical care and the instruments used to evaluate them: a scoping review. Crit Care Med 2020;48(12):e1313–21.
25. Murphy Salem S, Graham RJ. Chronic illness in pediatric critical care. Front Pediatr 2021;9:686206.
26. Meert KL, Reeder R, Maddux AB, et al. Trajectories and risk factors for altered physical and psychosocial health-related quality of life after pediatric community-acquired septic shock. Pediatr Crit Care Med 2020;21(10):869–78.
27. Zimmerman JJ, Banks R, Berg RA, et al. Trajectory of mortality and health-related quality of life morbidity following community-acquired pediatric septic shock. Crit Care Med 2020;48(3):329–37.
28. Hartman ME, Williams CN, Hall TA, et al. Post-Intensive-Care Syndrome for the pediatric neurologist. Pediatr Neurol 2020;108:47–53.
29. Smith MB, Killien EY, Dervan LA, et al. The association of severe pain experienced in the pediatric intensive care unit and postdischarge health-related quality of life: a retrospective cohort study. Paediatr Anaesth 2022. https://doi.org/10.1111/pan.14460.
30. Stevens BJ, Abbott LK, Yamada J, et al. Epidemiology and management of painful procedures in children in Canadian hospitals. CMAJ 2011;183(7):E403–10.

31. Baarslag MA, Jhingoer S, Ista E, et al. How often do we perform painful and stressful procedures in the paediatric intensive care unit? A prospective observational study. Aust Crit Care 2019;32(1):4–10.

32. LaFond CM, Hanrahan KS, Pierce NL, et al. Pain in the pediatric intensive care unit: how and what are we doing? Am J Crit Care 2019;28(4):265–73.

33. Kudchadkar SR, Aljohani OA, Punjabi NM. Sleep of critically ill children in the pediatric intensive care unit: a systematic review. Sleep Med Rev 2014;18(2):103–10.

34. Berger J, Zaidi M, Halferty I, et al. Sleep in the hospitalized child: a contemporary review. Chest 2021. https://doi.org/10.1016/j.chest.2021.04.024.

35. Barnes SS, Kudchadkar SR. Sedative choice and ventilator-associated patient outcomes: don't sleep on delirium. Ann Transl Med 2016;4(2):34.

36. Dervan LA, Wrede JE, Watson RS. Sleep architecture in mechanically ventilated pediatric ICU patients receiving goal-directed, dexmedetomidine- and opioid-based sedation. J Pediatr Intensive Care 2022;11(1):32–40.

37. Freedman NS, Gazendam J, Levan L, et al. Abnormal sleep/wake cycles and the effect of environmental noise on sleep disruption in the intensive care unit. Am J Respir Crit Care Med 2001;163(2):451–7.

38. Als LC, Picouto MD, Hau SM, et al. Mental and physical well-being following admission to pediatric intensive care. Pediatr Crit Care Med 2015;16(5):e141–9.

39. National Institute of Aging. Cognitive health and older adults. 2022. Available at: https://www.nia.nih.gov/health/cognitive-health-and-older-adults#:~:text=Cognitive%20health%20%E2%80%94%20the%20ability%20to,aspect%20of%20overall%20brain%20health. Accessed June 6, 2022.

40. Woodruff AG, Choong K. Long-term outcomes and the post-intensive care syndrome in critically ill children: a North American perspective. Child (Basel) 2021;8(4). https://doi.org/10.3390/children8040254.

41. Watson RS, Beers SR, Asaro LA, et al. Association of acute respiratory failure in early childhood with long-term neurocognitive outcomes. JAMA 2022;327(9):836–45.

42. Bone MF, Feinglass JM, Goodman DM. Risk factors for acquiring functional and cognitive disabilities during admission to a PICU. Pediatr Crit Care Med 2014;15(7):640–8.

43. Madurski C, Treble-Barna A, Fink EL. Cognitive impairment following pediatric critical illness: time to pay attention. Pediatr Crit Care Med 2018;19(3):277–8.

44. Kachmar AG, Irving SY, Connolly CA, et al. A systematic review of risk factors associated with cognitive impairment after pediatric critical illness. Pediatr Crit Care Med 2018;19(3):e164–71.

45. Baron IS, Weiss BA, Litman FR, et al. Latent mean differences in executive function in at-risk preterm children: the delay-deficit dilemma. Neuropsychol 2014;28(4):541–51.

46. Aarsen FK, Paquier PF, Reddingius RE, et al. Functional outcome after low-grade astrocytoma treatment in childhood. Cancer 2006;106(2):396–402.

47. van Houdt CA, Oosterlaan J, van Wassenaer-Leemhuis AG, et al. Executive function deficits in children born preterm or at low birthweight: a meta-analysis. Dev Med Child Neurol 2019;61:1015–24.

48. Block RI, Thomas JJ, Bayman EO, et al. Are anesthesia and surgery during infancy associated with altered academic performance during childhood? Anesthesiology 2012;117(3):494–503.

49. Mody K, Kaur S, Mauer EA, et al. Benzodiazepines and development of delirium in critically ill children: estimating the causal effect. Crit Care Med 2018;46(9): 1486–91.

50. Girard TD, Jackson JC, Pandharipande PP, et al. Delirium as a predictor of long-term cognitive impairment in survivors of critical illness. Crit Care Med 2010; 38(7):1513–20.

51. Mart MF, Williams Roberson S, Salas B, et al. Prevention and management of delirium in the intensive care unit. Semin Respir Crit Care Med 2021;42(1): 112–26.

52. Pandharipande PP, Girard TD, Jackson JC, et al. Long-term cognitive impairment after critical illness. N Engl J Med 2013;369(14):1306–16.

53. Als LC, Nadel S, Cooper M, et al. Neuropsychologic function three to six months following admission to the PICU with meningoencephalitis, sepsis, and other disorders: a prospective study of school-aged children. Crit Care Med 2013; 41(4):1094–103.

54. Christie D, Rashid H, El-Bashir H, et al. Impact of meningitis on intelligence and development: a systematic review and meta-analysis. PLoS One 2017;12(8): e0175024.

55. National Institutes of Health. Emotional wellness toolkit. NIH. 2022. Available at: https://www.nih.gov/health-information/emotional-wellness-toolkit. Accessed June 7, 2022.

56. Nelson LP, Gold JI. Posttraumatic stress disorder in children and their parents following admission to the pediatric intensive care unit: a review. Pediatr Crit Care Med 2012;13(3):338–47.

57. Nelson LP, Lachman SE, Goodman K, et al. Admission psychosocial characteristics of critically ill children and acute stress. Pediatr Crit Care Med 2021;22(2): 194–203.

58. Davydow DS, Richardson LP, Zatzick DF, et al. Psychiatric morbidity in pediatric critical illness survivors: a comprehensive review of the literature. Arch Pediatr Adolesc Med 2010;164(4):377–85.

59. O'Meara A, Akande M, Yagiela L, et al. Family outcomes after the pediatric intensive care unit: a scoping review. J Intensive Care Med 2021. 8850666211056603.

60. Terp K, Sjöström-Strand A. Parents' experiences and the effect on the family two years after their child was admitted to a PICU-An interview study. Intensive Crit Care Nurs 2017;43:143–8.

61. Epstein D, Reibel M, Unger JB, et al. The effect of neighborhood and individual characteristics on pediatric critical illness. J Community Health 2014;39(4): 753–9.

62. Kachmar AG, Watson RS, Wypij D, et al, the RESTORE Investigative Team. Association of socioeconomic status with postdischarge pediatric resource use and quality of life. Crit Care Med 2022;50(2):e117–28.

63. Als LC, Nadel S, Cooper M, et al. A supported psychoeducational intervention to improve family mental health following discharge from paediatric intensive care: feasibility and pilot randomised controlled trial. BMJ Open 2015;5(12): e009581.

64. Coville G, Cream P. Post-traumatic growth in parents after a child's admission to intensive care: maybe Nietzsche was right? Intensive Care Med 2009;35(5): 919–23.

65. Cobb AR, Tedeschi RG, Calhoun LG, et al. Correlates of posttraumatic growth in survivors of intimate partner violence. J Trauma Stress 2006;19(6):895–903.

66. Cryder CH, Kilmer RP, Tedeschi RG, et al. An exploratory study of posttraumatic growth in children following a natural disaster. Am J Orthopsychiatry 2006; 76(1):65–9.

67. Zamora ER, Yi J, Akter J, et al. Having cancer was awful but also something good came out': post-traumatic growth among adult survivors of pediatric and adolescent cancer. Eur J Oncol Nurs 2017;28:21–7.

68. Tedeschi RG, Calhoun LG. The Posttraumatic Growth Inventory: measuring the positive legacy of trauma. J Trauma Stress 1996;9(3):455–71.

69. Rodríguez-Rey R, Alonso-Tapia J. Predicting posttraumatic growth in mothers and fathers of critically ill children: a longitudinal study. J Clin Psychol Med Settings 2019;26(3):372–81.

70. Daughtrey H, Slain KN, Derrington S, et al. Measuring social health following pediatric critical illness: a scoping review and conceptual framework. J Intensive Care Med 2022;22. 8850666221102815.

71. Rennick JE, McHarg LF, Dell'Api M, et al. Developing the Children's Critical Illness Impact Scale: capturing stories from children, parents, and staff. Pediatr Crit Care Med 2008;9(3):252–60.

72. Manning JC, Hemingway P, Redsell SA. Stories of survival: children's narratives of psychosocial well-being following paediatric critical illness or injury. J Child Health Care 2017;21(3):236–52.

73. Kastner K, Pinto N, Msall ME, et al. PICU follow-up: the impact of missed school in a cohort of children following PICU admission. Crit Care Explor 2019;1(8): e0033.

74. Carlton EF, Donnelly JP, Prescott HC, et al. School and work absences after critical care hospitalization for pediatric acute respiratory failure: a secondary analysis of a cluster randomized trial. JAMA Netw Open 2021;4(12):e2140732.

75. Colville GA, Pierce CM. Children's self-reported quality of life after intensive care treatment. Pediatr Crit Care Med 2013;14(2):e85–92.

76. Tomaszewski W, Ablaza C, Straney L, et al. Educational outcomes of childhood survivors of critical illness-a population-based linkage study. Crit Care Med 2022;50(6):901–12.

77. Clark ME, Cummings BM, Kuhlthau K, et al. Impact of Pediatric intensive care unit admission on family financial status and productivity: a pilot study. J Intensive Care Med 2019;34(11–12):973–7.

78. Ducharme-Crevier L, La KA, Francois T, et al. PICU follow-up clinic: patient and family outcomes 2 months after discharge. Pediatr Crit Care Med 2021;22(11): 935–43.

79. Grandjean C, Ullmann P, Marston M, et al. Sources of stress, family functioning, and needs of families with a chronic critically ill child: a qualitative study. Front Pediatr 2021;9:740598.

80. Brown RT, Wiener L, Kupst MJ, et al. Single parents of children with chronic illness: an understudied phenomenon. J Pediatr Psychol 2008;33(4):408–21.

81. Abela KM, Casarez RL, Kaplow J, et al. Siblings' experience during pediatric intensive care hospitalization. J Pediatr Nurs 2022;64:111–8.

82. Abela KM, Wardell D, Rozmus C, et al. Impact of pediatric critical illness and injury on families: an updated systematic review. J Pediatr Nurs 2020;51:21–31.

83. Rozdilsky JR. Enhancing sibling presence in pediatric ICU. Crit Care Nurs Clin North Am 2005;17(4):451–461, xii.

84. Deavin A, Greasley P, Dixon C. Children's perspectives on living with a sibling with a chronic illness. Pediatrics 2018;142(2). https://doi.org/10.1542/peds. 2017-4151.

85. Havill N, Fleming LK, Knafl K. Well siblings of children with chronic illness: a synthesis research study. Res Nurs Health 2019;42(5):334–48.
86. Manning JC, Latour JM, Curley MAQ, et al. Study protocol for a multicentre longitudinal mixed methods study to explore the Outcomes of ChildrEn and fAmilies in the first year after paediatric Intensive Care: the OCEANIC study. BMJ Open 2020;10(5):e038974.
87. Williamson PR, Altman DG, Blazeby JM, et al. Developing core outcome sets for clinical trials: issues to consider. Trials 2012;13:132.
88. Williamson PR, Altman DG, Bagley H, et al. The COMET Handbook: version 1.0. Trials 2017;18(Suppl 3):280.
89. Pinto NP, Maddux AB, Dervan LA, et al, POST-PICU Investigators of the Pediatric Acute Lung Injury and Sepsis Investigators (PALISI) Network, The Eunice Kennedy Shriver National Institute of Child Health and Human Development Collaborative Pediatric Critical Care Research Network (CPCCRN). A core outcome measurement set for pediatric critical care. Pediatr Crit Care Med 2022. https://doi.org/10.1097/PCC.0000000000003055. Epub ahead of print.
90. The virtual PICU system, LLC. 2022. Available at: https://www.myvps.org/. Accessed April 5, 2022.
91. Wetzel RC. Pediatric intensive care databases for quality improvement. J Pediatr Intensive Care 2016;5(3):81–8.
92. Kids AHRQ. Inpatient database (KID) database documentation. 2022. Available at: https://www.hcup-us.ahrq.gov/db/nation/kid/kiddbdocumentation.jsp.
93. PICANet. 2022. Available at: https://www.picanet.org.uk/. Accessed April 24, 2022.
94. Rousseau AF, Prescott HC, Brett SJ, et al. Long-term outcomes after critical illness: recent insights. Crit Care 2021;25(1):108.
95. Mayer KP, Parry SM, Kalema AG, et al. Safety and feasibility of an interdisciplinary treatment approach to optimize recovery from critical Coronavirus Disease 2019. Crit Care Explor 2021;3(8):e0516.
96. Bloom SL, Stollings JL, Kirkpatrick O, et al. Randomized clinical trial of an icu recovery pilot program for survivors of critical illness. Crit Care Med 2019; 47(10):1337–45.
97. Teixeira C, Rosa RG. Post-intensive care outpatient clinic: is it feasible and effective? A literature review. Rev Bras Ter Intensiva 2018;30(1):98–111.
98. McPeake J, Hirshberg EL, Christie LM, et al. Models of peer support to remediate post-intensive care syndrome: a report developed by the Society of Critical Care Medicine Thrive International peer support collaborative. Crit Care Med 2019;47(1):e21–7.
99. Haines KJ, Sevin CM, Hibbert E, et al. Key mechanisms by which post-ICU activities can improve in-ICU care: results of the international THRIVE collaboratives. Intensive Care Med 2019;45(7):939–47.
100. Manning JC, Scholefield BR, Popejoy E, et al. Paediatric intensive care follow-up provision in the United Kingdom and Republic of Ireland. Nurs Crit Care 2021; 26(2):128–34.
101. Fitzgerald JC, Kelly NA, Hickey C, et al. Implementation of a follow-up system for pediatric sepsis survivors in a large academic Pediatric Intensive Care Unit. Front Pediatr 2021;9:691692.
102. Williams CN, Hall TA, Francoeur C, et al. Continuing care for critically ill children beyond hospital discharge: current state of follow-up. Hosp Pediatr 2022;12(4): 359–93.

103. Marra A, Ely EW, Pandharipande PP, et al. The ABCDEF Bundle in critical care. Crit Care Clin 2017;33(2):225–43.
104. Lee Y, Kim K, Lim C, et al. Effects of the ABCDE bundle on the prevention of post-intensive care syndrome: a retrospective study. J Adv Nurs 2020;76(2): 588–99.
105. Ista E, Redivo J, Kananur P, et al. ABCDEF bundle practices for critically ill children: an international survey of 161 PICUs in 18 countries. Crit Care Med 2022; 50(1):114–25.
106. Wieczorek B, Ascenzi J, Kim Y, et al. PICU Up!: impact of a quality improvement intervention to promote early mobilization in critically ill children. Pediatr Crit Care Med 2016;17(12):e559–66.
107. Choong K, Abu-Sultaneh S. Applying the ICU liberation bundle to critically ill children. 2021. Available at: https://www.sccm.org/Communications/Critical-Connections/Archives/2020/Applying-the-ICU-Liberation-Bundle-to-Critically-I. Accessed August 11, 2021.

The Current State of Workforce Diversity and Inclusion in Pediatric Critical Care

Yuen Lie Tjoeng, MD, MS[a],*, Carlie Myers, MD, MS[b],
Sharon Y. Irving, PhD, CRNP[c,d], Ivie Esangbedo, MD[a],
Derek Wheeler, MD, MMM, MBA[e], Ndidiamaka Musa, MD[a]

KEYWORDS

- Pediatric critical care workforce • Workforce diversity • Diversity and inclusion
- Underrepresented in medicine • Race and ethnicity
- LGBTQIA+ (lesbian, gay, bisexual, transgender, intersex, asexual) • Gender
- Differences in physical ability

KEY POINTS

- The true landscape of diversity and inclusion of the pediatric critical care (PCC) workforce is not well documented.
- Increasing workforce diversity and inclusion is important to foster safe working environments and improving health care disparities in PCC.
- Avenues to improve workforce disparities in PCC include collecting additional data to understand the extent of disparity, increasing recruitment/mentorship/sponsorship for underrepresented groups, and recurring equity, diversity, and inclusion education for the existing workforce.

INTRODUCTION

The health-care workforce has been under enormous strain during the past several years. Current events surrounding social injustices and lack of minority representation in health-care providers have prioritized the need for workforce equity, diversity, and

[a] Division of Pediatric Critical Care, Seattle Children's Hospital, University of Washington School of Medicine, 4800 Sand Point Way Northeast M/S RC.2.820, Seattle, WA 98105, USA;
[b] Division of Critical Care Medicine, Cincinnati Children's Hospital Medical Center, University of Cincinnati, 3333 Burnet Avenue, Location G, Cincinnati, OH 45229, USA; [c] Department of Family and Community Health, Children's Hospital of Philadelphia, University of Pennsylvania School of Nursing, 418 Curie Boulevard, Office 415, Philadelphia, PA 19104, USA; [d] Department of Nursing and Clinical Services, Critical Care, Philadelphia, PA, USA; [e] Division of Critical Care, Ann & Robert H. Lurie Children's Hospital of Chicago, Northwestern University Feinberg School of Medicine, 225 East Chicago Avenue, Box 1, Chicago, IL 60611, USA
* Corresponding author.
E-mail address: Lie.Tjoeng@seattlechildrens.org

Crit Care Clin 39 (2023) 327–340
https://doi.org/10.1016/j.ccc.2022.09.008
0749-0704/23/© 2022 Elsevier Inc. All rights reserved.
criticalcare.theclinics.com

inclusion (EDI) across all disciplines. The coronavirus disease (COVID-19) pandemic has further emphasized disparities particular to health-care providers and the persistence of racism and discrimination in the United States. The COVID-19 pandemic has disproportionately affected non-White people in terms of exposure, infection rates, illness severity, and mortality.[1,2] Several studies have demonstrated that the COVID-19 pandemic has also had a disproportionate influence on women in the workforce in a variety of industries, particularly in health care.[3–5] Additionally, anti-Asian sentiment related to COVID-19 has resulted in overt discrimination towards and assault on members of the Asian community.[6] The multiple killings of Black individuals in the United States have highlighted the prevalence of institutional racism in society, including the health-care system. Similarly, despite the nationwide legalization of same-sex marriage in 2015, the lesbian, gay, bisexual, transgender, intersex, asexual (LGBTQIA+) community continues to face increasing levels of discrimination, including the criminalization and limitation of gender-affirming medical care.[7] Additionally, a proportion of individuals have or develop a disability during their lifetime, and differences in ability should be considered part of a diverse and inclusive workforce.[8] Collectively, these issues have brought renewed awareness for the need of a diverse health-care workforce to care for patients across the lifespan.

Significant disparities exist among critically ill children admitted to the pediatric intensive care unit (PICU).[9–13] Negative health care outcomes have been linked to structural racism and implicit bias but may be ameliorated by health-care workforce diversity.[14] Patients treated by racially, ethnically, or gender concordant providers have better outcomes.[15] Patients and families are more likely to choose a provider of the same gender, race, or ethnicity as they are, and are reportedly more satisfied with their care when they are able.[15] Additionally, a recent study of 1.5 million Medicare patients found that hospital mortality and readmission rates were lower for patients treated by female physicians compared with male physicians.[16] These studies support the assertion that workforce diversity is necessary to advance health equity. Herein, we review the current literature on diversity and inclusion in the pediatric critical care (PCC) workforce.

Race and Ethnicity Workforce Demographics Within Pediatric Critical Care

Recent efforts have been made to increase the racial and ethnic makeup of providers underrepresented in medicine (URiM), which include "racial and ethnic populations underrepresented in medicine relative to their numbers in the population" (eg, African American/Black, Hispanic/Latinx, American Indian/Alaska Native, Native Hawaiian/Pacific Islander). However, little is known about the racial or ethnic profile of the PCC workforce. A recent publication by Horak and colleagues[17] in 2021 surveyed pediatric cardiac critical care medical directors and faculty members who reported to the Society of Thoracic Surgeons Congenital Heart Surgery Database. Of the 294 faculty respondents, only 3% identified as African American/Black and 6% identified as Hispanic/Latinx, with 70% of respondents identifying as White.[17] These data reassert the disparity within the medical provider base for pediatric cardiac care.

Although data specific to race and ethnicity in the PCC attending physician workforce remains limited, exploring the pipeline into PCC across disciplines is crucial. The Association of American Medical Colleges (AAMC) reports race and ethnicity data for medical school applicants, matriculants, and graduates. Although medical school matriculants are becoming more diverse, the increase in URiM applicants, matriculants, and graduates has not kept pace with the changing US Census.[18–20] When compared with 2014, medical school enrollee race/ethnicity for multiple URiM groups increased in 2020, with 8.9% African American/Black, 11.3% Hispanic, and 0.5%

Native Hawaiian/Pacific Islander.[18] Matriculation of Black medical students increased by an unprecedented 21% in the 2021 to 2022 academic year,[18] although it is unclear what led to this increase, compared with stagnant enrollment in 1978 and 2010 of 3.1% to 2.9%, respectively.[21]

Critical care medical training programs have also failed to keep pace with the rapidly changing racial and ethnic composition of the US population.[22] According to a longitudinal analysis published by Montez and colleagues,[23] racial and ethnic diversity in pediatric subspecialty fellowships has decreased since 2007. URiM PCC fellows represent 11.5% of the fellow cohort, a decrease from 13.2% during a 12-year period, despite a stagnant proportion (16%) of URiM pediatric resident trainees.[23] With fewer URiM trainees entering PCC, the lack of racial and ethnic diversity among faculty and PCC leadership will persist.

Comparative data specific to nursing is challenging to ascertain. The 2020 National Nursing Workforce survey reported more than 80% identify as White/Caucasian, with the next largest group being Asian, accounting for more than 7%.[24] Registered nurses (RNs) identifying as African American/Black were 6.7%, and 5.6% reported a Hispanic or Latinx ethnicity.[24] This report revealed 13% of actively working RNs are in acute/critical care, with 4.2% in pediatrics.[24] Although not specific to PCC, these numbers give a general overview of the US RN workforce.

In assessing the Advanced Practice Nurse Practitioner (APRN) role, the numbers are similar to physician colleagues. Health Resources and Services Administration (HRSA) data from 2021 identify more 210,000 APRNs in the United States, not including Clinical Nurse Specialists.[25] Of this number, nearly 80% identify as White/Caucasian, approximately 7% as African American/Black, and 6% Asian. Native Hawaiian, American Indian/Alaska Native, and others make up less than 1% representation each in the general APRN workforce.[25] In their 2022 fact sheet, the American Association of Nurse Practitioners identified 0.7% of all NPs hold certification in Pediatric Acute Care.[26] The American Association of Critical Care Nurses (AACN) report just under 5% of their total membership to be pediatric providers (e-mail communication with Dr Amanda Bettencourt, AACN President, July 18, 2022). Of these, approximately 76% identify as White, 3.2% African American/Black, and 7% Asian, with Native American and Pacific Islander less than 1% of the membership. Additionally, 7.2% of the pediatric members identify as Hispanic. The lack of racially/ethnically diverse representation is also present in nursing providers.

Many URiM medical trainees attribute their decision to pursue academic pediatrics to mentorship and URiM representation.[27] The current paucity of racially and ethnically diverse faculty could deter URiM trainees from pursuing PCC subspecialty training. These proximal threats to the diversity of the PCC workforce are preceded by the societal barriers individuals from underrepresented backgrounds face, including primary/secondary school education and resource disparities, inequities and deficits in college-level counseling and mentorship, racial/ethnic biases in medical school admissions/grading/accolades, and the financial and social burden associated with the pursuit of medicine.[28] In addition to these barriers, once in the training environment, URiM trainees are subject to increased professional scrutiny[29] and are subject to daily pressure to assimilate to cisgender, white, male professional culture, microaggressions, and discrimination from patients.[29,30] Furthermore, despite making up only 5% of residents, African American/Black residents account for 20% of dismissals, according to (William McDade, unpublished, 2015) Accreditation Council for Graduate Medical Education (ACGME) analysis.[31] The cumulative effect of these stressors experienced by URiM physicians leads to burnout or burnout with attrition, which compounds existing disparities.[32]

There have been calls for attention to diversity from the AAMC, Liaison Committee on Medical Education, ACGME, the Institute of Medicine, and the American Board of Pediatrics (ABP), among others. However, despite these calls and currently available data, large gaps exist in PCC race/ethnicity workforce demographics. As of July 2022, the ABP does not publish race/ethnicity data. Interventions to increase racial/ethnic diversity in the PCC workforce have also not yet been published.

Similar challenges exist in educating and employing diverse nurse providers. Nursing organizations, nurse educators, and nurse leaders all acknowledge the need for more diversity in nursing. Enrollment in nursing schools at both the graduate and undergraduate level is not on par to align with the current and growing population diversity in the United States. Literature addressing diversity in nursing describe multiple barriers that hinder the inclusivity of underrepresented persons in the profession, these include unsuccessful entry into nursing school, financial challenges, computer literacy, lack of inclusive and supportive environments, decreased exposure to successful minority faculty and professional socialization.[33]

Understanding the Gender Gap

According to the 2021 physician report from the ABP, more men than women have been board-certified in PCC, making up 55% of 3166 total diplomates since the first certification in 1987.[34] There is also a higher proportion of men than women who are aged older than 50 years; however, this disparity does not exist in the younger age bracket. There are now more female than male board-certified pediatric intensivists among those aged younger than 45 years.[34,35] This trend toward a higher proportion of female intensivists in the younger generation is consistent with a workforce survey of practicing pediatric cardiac intensivists in the United States, with only 25% of respondents aged older than 60 years identifying as woman versus 58% in the younger age bracket.[17]

Despite the increasing number of female board-certified pediatric intensivists, there continues to be a gender pay-gap. Using 2016 data on earnings from the American Academy of Pediatrics Pediatrician Life and Career Experience Study, Frintner and colleagues[36] found that early to midcareer female pediatricians earned less money than male pediatricians. This gap persisted after adjustment for subspecialty, work characteristics, and work–family characteristics. Women earned US$51,000 less than their male counterparts before adjustment, which decreased to US$8000 after adjustment for labor force, physician-specific job, and work–family characteristics.[36] Notably, respondents who indicated making decisions about work–life balance for their children made significantly lower salaries than those who did not.[36] Female pediatricians continue to have more household and childcare responsibilities compared with their male colleagues.[37] These differences in responsibilities, along with the gender pay gap, contribute to dissatisfaction with work–life balance as well as the gender pay gap.

Men in the nursing workforce have increased more than 1% during the last several years, with current numbers approximating 9% of the total nursing workforce according to the National Council of State Boards of Nursing (NCSBN).[38] Similar to physician colleagues, one study demonstrated that men earned on average 10% more than their female counterparts in a predominately female profession.[39] The granularity of gender distribution by specialty is not accurately or easily attainable in nursing. AACN reports approximately 9% of their total membership to be men.[38] It is acknowledged that the presence of men adds to the diversity necessary to better serve the patient population.

Burnout has been studied within the PCC workforce for several years using the validated Maslach Burnout Inventory.[40] Multiple studies have demonstrated that female physicians experience higher rates of burnout,[41–43] including PCC trainees.[43] The phenomenon of burnout also exists within nursing, particularly in the critical care environment where bedside care can be the most demanding and challenging. Studies have demonstrated that women are more likely to experience burnout due to experiences such as sexual harrassment,[30] microaggressions,[29,30] and imposter syndrome.[44] Exposure to persistent microaggressions has been shown to lead to imposter syndrome, which has been associated with reduced workplace engagement and work productivity, subsequently limiting career advancement.[44] Unidentified and unaddressed, burnout by physicians and nurses can result in poor morale, decreased quality of care delivery, increased staff turnover, and altered patient and family communication with decreased satisfaction.[44,45]

There is no reliable data on the proportion of female intensivists who choose to go into academic medicine or who are involved in research in PCC. Data addressing the rates of or time to academic promotion and salaries among PCC faculty by gender has not been reported nationally, although these data may be available at the institutional level. Finally, reliable data on attrition rates and part-time careers by gender have not been reported.

Sexual and Gender Minorities Within Pediatric Critical Care

Sexual and gender minority (SGM) individuals include those who identify as LGBTQIA+, those who identify as nonbinary, and individuals whose sexual orientation or gender identity varies. There are no data on the number of physicians in PCC who identify as SGM, although there is a growing body of evidence that people who identify as an SGM experience stigma-related stress, which can lead to anxiety and stress associated with identity concealment.[46]

Multiple survey-based studies demonstrate that people in medicine who identify as SGM experience higher risks of anxiety and depression, microaggressions, and harassment at work.[47–50] In one survey of SGM, Madrigal and colleagues[49] found higher frequencies of bullying and contemplating suicide than those who do not identify as SGM. Overt and covert discrimination related to sexual and gender identity has also been reported in students pursuing other health sciences, including nursing.[51] Inclusive communities have been shown to influence specialty, job selection, and disclosure for SGM.[46,48–52] A majority of SGM medical student survey respondents rated their campus as noninclusive of SGM.[48] Students who identified as SGM were more likely to choose a specialty or career that was perceived as welcoming to the LGBTQIA + community.[46,49]

The ABP does not currently collect demographic data beyond age and gender. There are no studies that have determined the composition of the PCC workforce with regards to sexual orientation or gender identity. Therefore, the extent of workplace discrimination experienced by people who identify as SGMs has not been adequately examined.

DISABILITY AND THE DIVERSITY FRAMEWORK

With the increasing focus on diversity, equity, and inclusion because they pertain to race, ethnicity, and gender, there has also been a shift to include disability within the diversity framework. Defined by the Americans with Disability Act, disability represents a physical or mental impairment (including physical, sensory, learning, psychological, and chronic health conditions) that substantially limits one or more major life activities, as compared with others without impairment.[53] In a recent study examining medical students' self-reported disabilities, 2.7% (1,547) had a disability they disclosed to their institutions.[54] However, the percentage of undergraduate students with disabilities is higher than that seen in medical school students.[55,56] It is unknown whether this difference is due to individuals with a disability forgoing medicine as a career, whether they are not accepted into medical school, or whether they choose not to disclose their disability.

To highlight the needs of medical trainees and faculty that identify as having a disability, the University of California at San Francisco and the AAMC designed the Lived Experience Project, an examination of the culture, climate, and structure of medical institutions and training programs from the first-person perspectives of trainees.[57] Similar to other marginalized groups, people with disabilities reported that the greatest barriers to equity were related to the difficulty of removing stereotypes and stigmas from the culture of the institution.[57] Structural components included policies (or lack thereof), assistive technology, meaningful accommodation, and knowledgeable providers.[57] Nurses with physical and/or sensory disabilities reported hiding their disability if possible. Nurses with disabilities similarly noted that accommodations were suboptimal for safe and successful job performance.[58] There is a paucity of literature exploring disability within the pediatric health-care workforce, and no data specific to PCC.

Leadership and Professional Societies

The current leadership in PCC predominantly consists of white male physicians and white female nurses. In a cross-sectional study examining academic PCC centers accredited by the ACGME, Maxwell and colleagues[59] demonstrated that as of 2019, 32% of PCC division directors were women, which was not statistically different from the female proportion of the PCC workforce overall (40%; $P = .14$). Among fellowship program directors, there were more women than men, and the proportion of female fellowship program directors was higher than proportion of female intensivists ($P = .03$).[59] Although PCC medical directors were not included in this study due to missing data, Horak and colleagues[17] demonstrated that in the pediatric cardiac intensive care units, 76% of medical directors in the 2021 cardiac intensivist workforce survey were men.

Although not specific to PCC, the AAMC has published data describing percentages of medical school deans of URiM and non-URiM backgrounds during 30+ years. During this time period, 12% of Deans are from URiM backgrounds, whereas 88% are not.[60] Describing gender and racial profiles of tenure-track pediatric faculty across the United States from 2007 to 2020, Saboor and colleagues[61] found that White, non-Hispanic male academic pediatricians were the majority in all tenure-track categories across the country, with 1% African American/Black race and 1% Hispanic ethnicity. In reference to academic rank during the 14-year study period, African American/Black and Hispanic academic pediatricians increased at all ranks.[61] For chairperson positions, the number of African American/Black faculty decreased, whereas the number of Hispanic faculty increased.[61] These findings demonstrate that racial disparities in promotion persist despite an increase in the total number of academic pediatricians over the past decade.[61] Data specific to URiM in leadership positions in PCC are not currently available.

In a review of nursing, nursing leadership, and nursing education, Ihedure-Anderson reported a 2015 study from the American Hospital Association demonstrating 14% of 6000 chief executive officers to be minority.[62] Currently, there are no guidelines from the NCSBN related to minority students being enrolled in state-level board of nursing programs, hindering the creation of pathways for minorities into the profession.[62] To date, the nursing education approval and accreditation processes do not have any regulations related to the inclusion and treatment of minority nursing students or faculty.[62] Furthermore, among nurses in the highest earning bracket, more than 90% are Caucasian, in contrast to 4% of African American/Black nurses, and 2% of Hispanic or Asian nurses.[63]

Within critical care society board leadership, gender and racial inequities persist. Ravioli and colleagues[64] described critical care medicine board leadership as one of the lowest representations of women compared with other medical specialties. The Society of Critical Care Medicine, the largest medical organization dedicated to critical care medicine, has had only 10 female presidents out of 51 since its inception in 1971.[65] The percentage of women seated on the board of intensive care societies varies between 7% and 50% internationally, with the highest percentage of women on the board of Society of Critical Care Medicine.[66] The AACN Board of Directors currently consists of 13 women and 2 men, with women serving as immediate past, current, and next presidents.[67] In a recent Journal of the American Medical Association (JAMA) report, Pinho-Gomes investigated the gender distribution of 444 editors-in-chief of 410 leading medical journals and found the mean proportion of women as editors-in-chief was 21% (94 of 444) with critical care medicine having the lowest representation (1 of 10).[68]

Data on the demographics of invited speakers at PCC conferences is unknown. However, Mehta and colleagues[69] examined 5 critical care conferences during 7 years, and found that women represented 5% to 31% of speakers. Female physicians made up 5% to 26% of speakers, a larger gender gap than was found for all other allied health professionals.[69] More than 50% of allied health professional speakers were women, with nursing and allied professional accounting for 0% to 25% of speakers.[69] There is no information regarding URiM and SGM invited speakers.

The majority of data on women and URiM faculty in leadership and professional societies has been obtained by self-reported survey data, which depend on voluntary responses and are not validated. There are no data on people who identify as SGM in leadership positions and that of URiM faculty is incomplete.

Diversity and Inclusion of Additional Pediatric Critical Care Disciplines

Given the multidisciplinary team approach, diversity of the entire PCC team is important across disciplines, including nurses, pharmacists, respiratory therapists, and advanced practice providers, among other groups. Although we did not find data specific to PCC, limited data suggest that a lack of diversity and inclusion may extend to other disciplines as well. For example, although the racial and ethnic makeup of respiratory therapists is similar to the breakdown of the US Census, the gender pay gap persists.[70] Additionally, only 4.9% of all licensed pharmacists in 2019 were African American/Black race.[71] Further studies are needed to evaluate the diversity of multidisciplinary teams specific to PCC.

DISCUSSION

We seek to describe the current state of workforce diversity in PCC. We found that, although women make up an equal proportion of the PCC workforce, diversity across race/ethnicity in the field is lacking and leadership positions continue to be held predominantly by men. Additionally, there are gaps in the literature that address representation of health-care providers who identify as LGBTQIA+ or have differences in physical ability. Much of the literature that we found was not specific to the PCC workforce. However, data across the board for nursing and Advanced Practice Nurses is similar to that of physicians. The lack of diversity persists for race/ethnicity and gender, but a pay gap is ever present even in a female-dominated profession such as nursing.

Opportunity exists for improvement in workforce diversity in the PCC workforce. White non-Hispanic people make up 57.8% of the US population, with a growing number of non-White and Hispanic people.[72] However, the proportion of African American/Black and Hispanic health-care providers has not kept pace with the corresponding population growth in the United States. Furthermore, men continue to be disproportionately represented in leadership positions, despite 45% of board-certified PCC physicians being women.[34,35] Additionally, there is incomplete literature describing the diversity of other historically marginalized groups, such as URiM, LGBTQIA+, and persons with differences in physical ability.

Multiple associations have published statements calling for the increase in diversity of the health-care workforce, including the American Academy of Pediatrics (AAP),[73] the AAMC,[19] the NCSBN,[62] and the National Council on Nurse Education and Practice.[38] Despite these resources, the onus remains on the voluntary commitment of institutions to prioritize diversity and inclusion for their workforce. This article serves as a call to action to our PCC colleagues across disciplines to improve workforce diversity and inclusion through 3 avenues to improve care delivery and patient outcomes: research and data collection; focused recruitment and mentorship/sponsorship to increase diversity and inclusion; and ongoing EDI education for the existing workforce.

The extent of disparities in workforce diversity cannot be adequately assessed without complete and transparent demographic information. However, as we discovered through our review of current data, our understanding of diversity and inclusion in PCC is incomplete and not easily accessible. The ABP has demographic data relating to specialty, geography, and gender but does not include race/ethnicity in their publicly available workforce statistics. The AAMC has information regarding race/ethnicity but lacks sufficient granularity to evaluate pediatric subspecialties by race/ethnicity. The AACN data for nursing equally lacks granularity for those in PCC. Data from HRSA is not granular to the specifics of disciplines across PCC. As of 2018, SCCM reported knowing ethnicity for only 30.3% and gender for 38.8% of its members.[74]

Additionally, other factors that are important in workforce diversity (eg, first language, religion, and sexual orientation) are not included in workforce data. Many of these factors are not collected due to confidentiality concerns, and we support the protection of personal information. However, acknowledging that members of marginalized groups are often subject to discrimination and harassment in the workplace, it is recommended that routinely collected demographic data, including race/ethnicity and gender, be reported, as interventions aimed at improving the experience for one group may also benefit other underrepresented groups. We also recommend developing the capabilities to filter by more than one group, such as African American/Black women in health care, to facilitate understanding the intersectionality of identifying with multiple marginalized groups.

Despite the gaps in data and literature, it is likely that underrepresentation in the PCC workforce exists to varying degrees across pediatric subspecialties and at all levels of experience. Efforts must be made at an early stage to enhance exposure to health-care fields and provide resources for preparation and successful application into institutions of higher education to increase matriculation and retention of members of underrepresented groups.[19] Structural racism and implicit bias preclude many students from entering the pathway to medicine, nursing, and other health-care professions, contributing to underrepresentation among applicants, matriculants, and graduates. Efforts to increase diversity must begin well before the hiring process in PCC and include more people of color and underrepresented groups in programming, curriculum, and decision-making. Promoting diversity of race/ethnicity, SGM, and gender is as important as diversity of thought and approach to research, care delivery and policy.

In addition to supporting programs that lead to an increase in applicants, higher education health professional institutions, training programs, and hospitals must commit to addressing the lack of diversity among matriculants.[75] Traditional measures of academic achievement can introduce bias, including board scores, academic pedigree, and letters of recommendation, which can negatively impact underrepresented applicants.[76–79] Instead, personal statements and life experience can promote a more holistic applicant review.[75] These efforts and practices should not stop with compositional diversity but must extend into the career of the faculty, with mentorship and sponsorship opportunities such that there are pathways to leadership for underrepresented individuals. Programs that focus on women and minority faculty leadership development have made some strides but these programs have limited capacity. There is a need for similar programs at the institutional, regional, and national levels with strategic planning aimed at program stability and growth, and financial strength directed specifically toward recruitment, retention, and promotion of underrepresented individuals at all levels and disciplines across institutions. Additionally, professional societies have an obligation to review the composition of their boards, committees, and invited speakers, to ensure a diverse representation of people and perspectives.

Efforts must also be made to make the working environment hospitable, safe, and inclusive for underrepresented groups. Multiple studies demonstrate that URiM groups, women, those who identify as LGBTQIA+, and other marginalized groups experience consistent microaggressions, higher levels of imposter syndrome, harassment, and burnout.[29,30,41,48,50] Improving inclusivity and guaranteeing psychological safety at work leads to improved retention, engagement, and productivity,[80–82] particularly for women and non-White people,[83,84] which may be key in preventing burnout and attrition. Bias-reduction training programs are currently being studied and bias reporting systems may be beneficial in outlining the extent of the problem.

We acknowledge that demographic data for the PCC workforce is lacking. However, based on the current evidence, disparities in representation across multiple groups likely exist within PCC. The above recommendations for furthering diversity and inclusion in the workforce should not be precluded based on the lack of data or transparency. We also acknowledge that we are unable to consider all underrepresented groups and perspectives in this article, and that there are viewpoints absent from our analysis. We encourage further discussion surrounding workplace diversity, culture, and interventions to promote a diverse and inclusive PCC environment across disciplines for all our patients and colleagues.

SUMMARY

There is a paucity of data surrounding the demographics of the PCC workforce. Further studies are needed to better delineate the landscape of the PCC workforce. However, several areas have demonstrated that there are a number of underrepresented groups in health care, and efforts should be made to increase their visibility, entrance and presence, inclusion, and retention to better serve our patient population and enhance the PCC working environment.

CLINICS CARE POINTS

- Significant disparities exist in outcomes among critically ill children.
- There continue to be gaps in data related to the makeup of the PCC workforce. However, based on current data, it is likely that underrepresentation of multiple groups exists to varying degrees in PCC.

- Increasing workforce diversity and inclusion may improve health outcomes for critically ill pediatric patients in addition to reducing burnout for the PCC workforce.

ACKNOWLEDGMENTS

The authors would like to acknowledge current AACN President, Amanda Bettencourt, PhD, APRN, CCRN-K, ACCNS-P and her team, Natasha S. Varn-Davis, PhD (Community Impact Director), and Monica Simmerman (AACN Community Operations Insight Analyst) for providing current AACN data.

DISCLOSURE

The authors declare that they have no relevant or material financial interests that relate to the research described in this article.

REFERENCES

1. Cucinotta D, Vanelli M. WHO declares COVID-19 a pandemic. Acta Biomed 2020;91(1):157–60.
2. Tai DBG, Shah A, Doubeni CA, et al. The disproportionate Impact of COVID-19 on racial and ethnic minorities in the United States. Clin Infect Dis 2021;72(4):703–6.
3. Bateman N, Ross M. Why has COVID-19 been especially harmful for working women?. In: Brookings. 2020. Available at: https://www.brookings.edu/essay/why-has-covid-19-been-especially-harmful-for-working-women/. Accessed July 20, 2022.
4. Rabinowitz LG, Rabinowitz DG. Women on the frontline: a changed workforce and the fight against COVID-19. Acad Med 2021;96(6):808–12.
5. Woitowich NC, Jain S, Arora VM, et al. COVID-19 Threatens progress toward gender equity within academic medicine. Acad Med 2021;96(6):813–6.
6. Shang Z, Kim JY, Cheng SO. Discrimination experienced by Asian Canadian and Asian American health care workers during the COVID-19 pandemic: a qualitative study. CMAJ Open 2021;9(4):E998–1004.
7. Martin S, Sandberg ES, Shumer DE. Criminalization of gender-affirming care - interfering with essential treatment for transgender children and adolescents. N Engl J Med 2021;385(7):579–81.
8. Waliany S. Health professionals with disabilities: motivating inclusiveness and representation. AMA J Ethics 2016;18(10):971–4.
9. Epstein D, Reibel M, Unger JB, et al. The effect of neighborhood and individual characteristics on pediatric critical illness. J Community Health 2014;39(4):753–9.
10. Andrist E, Riley CL, Brokamp C, et al. Neighborhood poverty and pediatric intensive care use. Pediatrics 2019;144(6):e20190748.
11. Stockwell DC, Landrigan CP, Toomey SL, et al, GAPPS Study Group. Racial, ethnic, and socioeconomic disparities in patient safety events for hospitalized children. Hosp Pediatr 2019;9(1):1–5.
12. Brown LE, França UL, McManus ML. Socioeconomic disadvantage and distance to pediatric critical care. Pediatr Crit Care Med 2021;22(12):1033–41.
13. Slain KN, Wurtz MA, Rose JA. US children of minority race are less likely to be admitted to the pediatric intensive care unit after traumatic injury, a retrospective analysis of a single pediatric trauma center. Inj Epidemiol 2021;8(1):14.
14. Institute of Medicine (US). Committee on understanding and eliminating racial and ethnic disparities in health care. In: Smedley BD, Stith AY, Nelson AR, editors.

Unequal treatment: confronting racial and ethnic disparities in health care. Washington, DC: National Academies Press (US); 2003. p. 1–2.

15. Silver JK, Bean AC, Slocum C, et al. Physician workforce disparities and patient care: a narrative review. Health Equity 2019;3(1):360–77.

16. Tsugawa Y, Jena AB, Figueroa JF, et al. Comparison of hospital mortality and re-admission rates for medicare patients treated by male vs female physicians. JAMA Intern Med 2017;177(2):206–13.

17. Horak RV, Bai S, Marino BS, et al. Workforce demographics and unit structure in paediatric cardiac critical care in the United States. Cardiol Young 2021;1–5. https://doi.org/10.1017/S1047951121004753, published online ahead of print, 2021 Dec 3.

18. Association of American Medical Colleges. 2021 AAMC Fall applicant, matriculant, and enrollment data 2021. 2021. Available at: https://www.aamc.org/media/57761/download?attachment. Accessed 18 July, 2022.

19. Morrison E, Cort DA. An analysis of the medical school pipeline: a high school aspirant to applicant and enrollment view. AAMC Anal Brief 2014;14(3). Available at: https://www.aamc.org/media/7556/download?attachment.

20. Morris DB, Gruppuso PA, McGee HA, et al. Diversity of the national medical student body - four decades of inequities. N Engl J Med 2021;384(17):1661–8.

21. Association of American medical colleges. Altering the course: Black males in medicine. Association of American medical colleges. 2015. Available at: https://store.aamc.org/downloadable/download/sample/sample_id/84/.   Accessed 20 July, 22.

22. Lane-Fall MB, Miano TA, Aysola J, et al. Diversity in the emerging critical care workforce: analysis of demographic trends in critical care fellows from 2004 to 2014. Crit Care Med 2017;45(5):822–7.

23. Montez K, Omoruyi EA, McNeal-Trice K, et al. Trends in race/ethnicity of pediatric residents and fellows: 2007-2019. Pediatrics 2021;148(1). e2020026666.

24. Smiley RA, Rittinger C, Oliveira CM, et al. The 2020 national nursing workforce survey. J Nurs Regul 2021;12(Suppl):S1–96.

25. Health Resources and Services Administration. Area health resource files. 2021. Available at: https://data.hrsa.gov/topics/health-workforce/ahrf#top. Accessed 8 July, 2022.

26. American Association of Nurse Practitioners. NP fact sheet. April 2022. Available at: https://www.aanp.org/about/all-about-nps/np-fact-sheet. Accessed 10 July, 2022.

27. Dixon G, Kind T, Wright J, et al. Factors that influence underrepresented in medicine (UIM) medical students to pursue a career in academic pediatrics. J Natl Med Assoc 2021;113(1):95–101.

28. Nivet MA. Commentary: diversity 3.0: a necessary systems upgrade. Acad Med 2011;86(12):1487–9.

29. Alexis DA, Kearney MD, Williams JC, et al. Assessment of perceptions of professionalism among faculty, trainees, staff, and students in a large university-based health system. JAMA Netw Open 2020;3(11):e2021452.

30. de Bourmont SS, Burra A, Nouri SS, et al. Resident physician experiences with and responses to biased patients. JAMA Netw Open 2020;3(11):e2021769.

31. McDade W. Diversity and inclusion in graduate medical education. Accreditation council for graduate medical education.. 2019. Available at: https://southernhospitalmedicine.org/wp-content/uploads/2019/10/McDade-ACGME-SHM-Presentation-McDade-Final.pdf. Accessed 19 August, 2022.

32. Dander VM, Grigsby RK, Bunton SA. Burnout among U.S medical school faculty. AAMC Anal Brief 2019;19(1). Available at: https://www.aamc.org/data-reports/analysis-brief/report/burnout-among-us-medical-school-faculty.

33. Phillips JM, Malone B. Increasing racial/ethnic diversity in nursing to reduce health disparities and achieve health equity. Public Health Rep 2014;129(Suppl 2):45–50.

34. American Board of Pediatrics. Pediatric workforce: data from the american board of pediatrics. 2021. Available at: https://www.abp.org/content/pediatric-subspecialists-ever-certified. Accessed June 2022.

35. American Board of Pediatrics. Pediatric subspecialists age/gender distribution and summary. 2021. Available at: https://www.abp.org/content/pediatric-subspecialists-agegender-distribution-and-summary. Accessed June 2022.

36. Frintner MP, Sisk B, Byrne BJ, et al. Gender differences in earnings of early- and midcareer pediatricians. Pediatrics 2019;144(4):e20183955.

37. Starmer AJ, Frintner MP, Matos K, et al. Gender discrepancies related to pediatrician work-life balance and household responsibilities. Pediatrics 2019;144(4):e20182926.

38. American association of colleges of nursing. Enhancing diversity in the workforce. 2019. Available at. https://www.aacnnursing.org/News-Information/Fact-Sheets/Enhancing-Diversity. Accessed 10 July, 2022.

39. Wilson BL, Butler MJ, Butler RJ, et al. Nursing gender pay differentials in the new millennium. J Nurs Scholarsh 2018;50(1):102–8.

40. Schaufeli WB, Bakker AB, Hoogdui K, et al. On the clinical validity of the maslach burnout inventory and the burnout measure. Psychol Health 2001;16:565–82.

41. Fields AI, Cuerdon TT, Brasseux CO, et al. Physician burnout in pediatric critical care medicine. Crit Care Med 1995;23(8):1425–9.

42. Shenoi AN, Kalyanaraman M, Pillai A, et al. Burnout and psychological distress among pediatric critical care physicians in the United States. Crit Care Med 2018;46(1):116–22.

43. Suttle ML, Chase MA, Sasser WC 3rd, et al. Burnout in pediatric critical care medicine fellows. Crit Care Med 2020;48(6):872–80.

44. Acholonu RG, Oyeku SO. Addressing microaggressions in the health care workforce-a path toward achieving equity and inclusion. JAMA Netw Open 2020;3(11):e2021770.

45. Browning SG. Burnout in critical care nurses. Crit Care Nurs Clin North Am 2019;31(4):527–36.

46. Sitkin NA, Pachankis JE. Specialty choice among sexual and gender minorities in medicine: the role of specialty prestige, perceived inclusion, and medical school climate. LGBT Health 2016;3(6):451–60.

47. Lee KP, Kelz RR, Dubé B, et al. Attitude and perceptions of the other underrepresented minority in surgery. J Surg Educ 2014;71(6):e47–52.

48. Lapinski J, Sexton P. Still in the closet: the invisible minority in medical education. BMC Med Educ 2014;14:171.

49. Madrigal J, Rudasill S, Tran Z, et al. Sexual and gender minority identity in undergraduate medical education: impact on experience and career trajectory. PLoS One 2021;16(11):e0260387.

50. Przedworski JM, Dovidio JF, Hardeman RR, et al. A comparison of the mental health and well-being of sexual minority and heterosexual first-year medical students: a report from the medical student change study. Acad Med 2015;90(5):652–9.

51. Holloway IW, Miyashita Ochoa A, Wu ESC, et al. Perspectives on academic mentorship from sexual and gender minority students pursuing careers in the health sciences. Am J Orthopsychiatry 2019;89(3):343–53.

52. Merchant RC, Jongco AM 3rd, Woodward L. Disclosure of sexual orientation by medical students and residency applicants. Acad Med 2005;80(8):786.
53. U.S. Department of Justice, Civil Rights Division. Public access section. The americans with disabilities act : title II technical assistance manual : covering state and local government programs and services. Washington, D.C.: U.S. Dept. of Justice, Civil Rights Division, Public Access Section; 2005.
54. Meeks LM, Herzer KR. Prevalence of self-disclosed disability among medical students in US allopathic medical schools. JAMA 2016;316(21):2271–2.
55. National center for education statistics. Fast facts: students with disabilities. 2022. Available at: https://nces.ed.gov/fastfacts/display.asp?id=60#:~:text=Response%3A,20%20percent%20for%20female%20students. Accessed 20 July, 2022.
56. U.S. Department of Education. Profile of students in graduate and first-professional students: 2007–08. NCES. 2010. Available at: https://nces.ed.gov/pubs2010/2010177.pdf. Accessed 19 July, 2022.
57. Meeks LM, Jain MS. Accessibility, inclusion, and action in medical education: lived experiences of learners and physicians with disabilities. AAMC.. 2018. Available at: https://sds.ucsf.edu/sites/g/files/tkssra2986/f/aamc-ucsf-disability-special-report-accessible.pdf. Accessed 19 July, 2022.
58. Neal-Boylan L, Miller M. How inclusive are we, really? Teach Learn Nurs 2020; 15(4):237–40.
59. Maxwell AR, Riley CL, Stalets EL, et al. State of the unit: physician gender diversity in pediatric critical care medicine leadership. Pediatr Crit Care Med 2019; 20(7):e362–5.
60. American Association of Medical Colleges. U.S. medical school deans by dean type and race/ethnicity (URiM vs. non-URiM) 2021. 2022. Available at: https://www.aamc.org/data-reports/faculty-institutions/interactive-data/us-medical-school-deans-trends-type-and-race-ethnicity. Accessed 19 July, 2022.
61. Saboor S, Naveed S, Chaudhary AM, et al. Gender and racial profile of the academic pediatric faculty workforce in the United States. Cureus 2022;14(2): e22518.
62. Iheduru-Anderson KC, Wahi MM. Rejecting the myth of equal opportunity: an agenda to eliminate racism in nursing education in the United States. BMC Nurs 2021;20(1):30.
63. Hader R. Nurse leaders: a closer look. Nurs Manage 2010;41(1):25–9.
64. Ravioli S, Moser N, Ryser B, et al. Gender distribution in boards of intensive care medicine societies. J Crit Care 2022;68:157–62.
65. Society of critical care medicine. Past presidents. SCCM. 2022. Available at: https://www.sccm.org/About-SCCM/Past-Presidents. Accessed July 2022.
66. Venkatesh B, Mehta S, Angus DC, et al. Women in Intensive Care study: a preliminary assessment of international data on female representation in the ICU physician workforce, leadership and academic positions. Crit Care 2018; 22(1):211.
67. American association of critical-care nurses. AACN boards. 2022. Available at: https://www.aacn.org/about-aacn/board?tab=Board%20of%20Directors. Accessed 19 August, 2022.
68. Pinho-Gomes AC, Vassallo A, Thompson K, et al. Representation of women among editors in chief of leading medical journals. JAMA Netw Open 2021; 4(9):e2123026.
69. Mehta S, Rose L, Cook D, et al. The speaker gender gap at critical care conferences. Crit Care Med 2018;46(6):991–6.

70. Data USA. Respiratory therapists. 2022. Available at: https://datausa.io/profile/ soc/respiratory-therapists#:~:text=Race%20%26%20Ethnicity&text=67.7% 25%20of%20Respiratory%20therapists%20are,or%20ethnicity%20in%20this% 20occupation. Accessed 8 July, 2022.

71. Doucette W, Gaither C, Mott D, et al. 2019 National pharmacist workforce study final report. Pharmacy Workforce Center. 2020. https://www.aacp.org/sites/ default/files/2020-03/2019_NPWS_Final_Report.pdf. [Accessed 19 August 2022].

72. Jenson E, Jones N, Rabe M, et al. 2020 U.S population more racially an ethnically diverse than in measured in 2010. 2021. Available at: https://www.census.gov/ library/stories/2021/08/2020-united-states-population-more-racially-ethnically- diverse-than-2010.html. Accessed 19 July, 2022.

73. Committee on Pediatric Workforce, Pletcher BA, Rimsza ME, et al. Enhancing pe- diatric workforce diversity and providing culturally effective pediatric care: impli- cations for practice, education, and policy making. Pediatrics 2013;132(4): e1105–16.

74. Gerlach AT, Kerr GE, Hydo LJ. Working together to advance diversity and inclu- sion. society of critical care medicine critical connections blog. 2019. Available at: https://www.sccm.org/Blog/May-2019/Working-Together-to-Advance- Diversity-and-Inclusio. Accessed 18 July, 2022.

75. Berman L, Renaud E, Pace D, et al. Inclusion and representation in the pediatric surgery workforce: strategies to mitigate bias in the fellowship application pro- cess. J Pediatr Surg 2022. https://doi.org/10.1016/j.jpedsurg.2021.12.023. S0022-3468(22)00002-1.

76. Grimm LJ, Redmond RA, Campbell JC, et al. Gender and racial bias in radiology residency letters of recommendation. J Am Coll Radiol 2020;17(1 Pt A):64–71.

77. Polanco-Santana JC, Storino A, Souza-Mota L, et al. Ethnic/racial bias in medical school performance evaluation of general surgery residency applicants. J Surg Educ 2021;78(5):1524–34.

78. Powers A, Gerull KM, Rothman R, et al. Race- and gender-based differences in descriptions of applicants in the letters of recommendation for orthopaedic sur- gery residency. JB JS Open Access 2020;5(3):e20.00023.

79. Yeo HL, Dolan PT, Mao J, et al. Association of demographic and program factors with american board of surgery qualifying and certifying examinations pass rates. JAMA Surg 2020;155(1):22.

80. Rosser VJ. Faculty members' intentions to leave: a national study on their worklife and satisfaction. Res Higher Educ 2004;45:285–309.

81. Sheridan J, Savoy JN, Kaatz A, et al. Write more articles, get more grants: the impact of department climate on faculty research productivity. J Womens Health (Larchmt) 2017;26(5):587–96.

82. Trower CA. Success on the tenure track: five keys to faculty job satisfaction. Bal- timore: Johns Hopkins University Press; 2014.

83. Callister RR. The impact of gender and department climate on job satisfaction and intentions to quit for faculty in science and engineering fields. J Technology Transfer 2006;31:367–75.

84. Pololi LH, Evans AT, Gibbs BK, et al. The experience of minority faculty who are underrepresented in medicine, at 26 representative U.S. medical schools. Acad Med 2013;88(9):1308–14.

Screening for Social Determinants of Health in the Pediatric Intensive Care Unit
Recommendations for Clinicians

Manzilat Akande, MD, MPH[a],*, Erin T. Paquette, MD[b],
Paula Magee, MD, MPH[b], Mallory A. Perry-Eaddy, PhD, RN, CCRN[c,d],
Ericka L. Fink, MD, MS[e], Katherine N. Slain, DO[f,g]

KEYWORDS

- Health status disparities • Intensive care unit • Pediatric
- Social determinants of health

KEY POINTS

- SDoH impact children along the continuum of critical illness, making screening an important first step in improving clinical care delivery through quality improvement and research initiatives.
- A child's admission to a PICU offers a unique opportunity for social screening. High staff to patient ratios, parent presence, and availability of social workers at tertiary centers can make screening feasible.
- Widespread implementation of SDoH screening across PICUs has the potential to increase our understanding of mechanisms that potentiate health disparities, facilitate linkage of vulnerable families to social resources, and enable development of public health interventions.

Funding Source: No funding was secured for this study.
Financial Disclosure: The authors have no financial relationships relevant to this article to disclose.
[a] Section of Critical Care, Department of Pediatrics, Oklahoma University Health Sciences Center, OU Children's Physicians Building, 1200 Children's Avenue, Oklahoma City, OK 73104, USA; [b] Division of Critical Care Medicine, Ann & Robert H. Lurie Children's Hospital of Chicago, 225 East, Chicago Avenue, Box 73, Chicago, IL 60611, USA; [c] University of Connecticut School of Nursing, 231 Glenbrook Rd, U-4026, Storrs, CT 06269, USA; [d] Department of Pediatrics, University of Connecticut School of Medicine, 200 Academic Way, Farmington, CT 06032, USA; [e] Department of Critical Care Medicine, UPMC Children's Hospital of Pittsburgh, 4401 Penn Avenue, Faculty Pavilion, 2nd floor, Pittsburgh, PA 15206, USA; [f] Division of Pediatric Critical Care Medicine, University Hospitals Rainbow Babies & Children's Hospital, 11100 Euclid Avenue, RBC 6010 Cleveland, OH 44106, USA; [g] Department of Pediatrics, Case Western Reserve University School of Medicine, 9501 Euclid Avenue, Cleveland, OH 44106, USA
* Corresponding author.
E-mail address: manzi-akande@ouhsc.edu

Crit Care Clin 39 (2023) 341–355
https://doi.org/10.1016/j.ccc.2022.09.009
0749-0704/23/© 2022 Elsevier Inc. All rights reserved.

INTRODUCTION

In the United States (US), more than 100,000 deaths annually are linked with adverse social determinants of health (SDoH), many of which are preventable with access to supportive resources.[1] SDoH are the economic, political, and environmental systems that affect a person's capacity to live a healthy life.[2] Key SDoH include socioeconomic status, education, neighborhood and physical environment, employment, social support networks, and access to health care. Differences in individual, family, and neighborhood SDoH are primary drivers of health disparities among US children and are exacerbated by inequitable distribution of societal resources, and discriminatory and exclusionary public policies.[3–5] Racial and ethnic minority groups have been especially affected by these inequities. Black children have higher death rates than White children across all age groups; in fact, all minority US children, including Black, Latino, Asian, Pacific Islander, American Indian, have worse health indices compared with their White peers.[5–7] With racial and ethnic diversity among US children growing, identifying, understanding, and eliminating differential health outcomes becomes increasingly important.[8]

In the next 10 years, an estimated 1 million US children will require critical care services.[9] Given the emerging evidence that SDoH negatively affect children across the continuum of critical illness, placing them at risk for higher illness severity, higher hospital utilization, and challenges in posthospital recovery, it is imperative that we understand and address the equity gaps in pediatric critical care and outcomes.[10] To meet the standards of health care quality set forth by the National Academies of Medicine and adopted by the Agency for Healthcare Quality, the pediatric critical care community must ensure that care we deliver is equitable.[11] In this article, we provide a rationale for universal SDoH screening and resource provision in the pediatric intensive care unit (PICU) as a key first step to the implementation of a clinical and research agenda to understand and mitigate health disparities affecting critically ill children. Our objectives therefore are 2-fold: (1) summarize SDoH impact on pediatric critical illness and outcomes to provide justification for routine screening and resource provision and (2) highlight important practical aspects of social screening that should be considered before implementation in the PICU setting.

IMPACT OF SOCIAL DETERMINANTS OF HEALTH ON PEDIATRIC CRITICAL ILLNESS

SDoH affect people throughout the life course through varied, complex, and interrelated mechanisms, and their influence on health make routine screening in both the outpatient and inpatient settings imperative. Multicenter PICU database studies show that Hispanic, Black, publicly insured, and low-income children have higher illness severity, rates of PICU admission, in-hospital mortality, readmission rates, and poorer functional outcomes than children who are White, commercially insured, or come from higher-income families.[10,12–17] Routine screening and associated data collection can contribute to our mechanistic understanding of how SDoH influence pediatric critical illness. SDoH are categorized by the Centers for Disease Control and Prevention into 5 domains: economic stability, community and built environment, education access and quality, health care access and quality, and social and community context (**Fig. 1**).[18] Below is a brief summary of what is currently known about the relationship between these SDoH domains and pediatric critical illness and injury.

Health Care Access and Quality

This domain includes factors that influence a person's access to health care, an individual's health literacy, and existence of differential health-care quality based on social

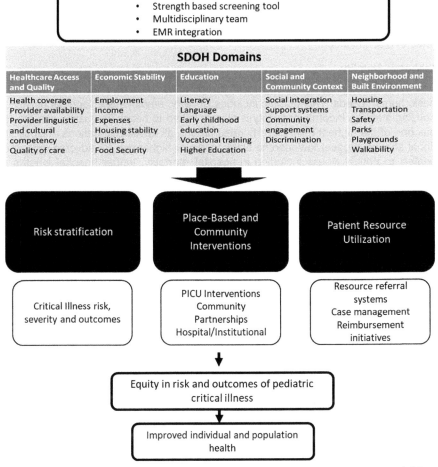

Fig. 1. Impact of universal social screening on risk and outcomes of critical illness in children. (SDOH Domains adapted from Artiga S and Hinton E. Beyond Health Care: The Role of Social Determinants in Promoting Health and Health Equity. Kaiser Family Foundation via https://www.kff.org/racial-equity-and-health-policy/issue-brief/beyond-health-care-the-role-of-social-determinants-in-promoting-health-and-health-equity/. Accessed November 2015; with permission.)

factors, including race or ethnicity. The evidence for inequality in the American health-care system is overwhelming and sobering. Among high-income countries, the US ranks among the lowest in objective measures of health-care access.[19] Low health literacy, defined as difficulties in understanding and navigating the health-care system, may affect half of all US adults.[20] The National Academies of Medicine landmark publication *Unequal Treatment* describes pervasive differences in health-care quality between White and minority race populations.[21] Socioeconomic and racial differences in rates of health insurance and access to preventive care, subspecialty care (including critical care), and pharmacy resources may place children, especially those with chronic health-care needs, at higher risk for critical illness and associated high hospital utilization.[22–25] Disturbingly, race-based differences in in-hospital and surgical-related mortality exist.[26–28] Single-center PICU studies suggest that publicly insured families and families of minority race or ethnicity experience differential care compared with White and privately insured families. This includes more instances of failed communication, higher rate of conflicts with the health care team, and higher rates of discrimination.[29–32]

Economic Stability

Economic stability has a profound influence on health due to its direct relationship with basic human needs. This domain includes poverty, employment, food security, and housing stability. Income inequality is closely linked to health inequality, and the US has one of the highest child poverty rates among all developed nations.[33] Observational studies suggest low-income children are at higher risk for adverse outcomes related to critical illness including in-hospital mortality, longer hospital lengths of stay, and more frequent hospital readmissions.[12,34] All poverty-related SDoH can be considered adverse childhood exposures, which predisposes a child to toxic stress. The eco-bio-developmental model of childhood health posits that repeated exposures to toxic stress can alter immune/inflammatory responses, providing a potential mechanistic explanation for the unfavorable hospital outcomes frequently observed in low-income children.[35] Household poverty is also associated with substandard living conditions and lower use of preventative care, which may predispose children to higher risk of critical disease and higher severity of illness on presentation.[12,14] Low-income families are also overburdened by out-of-pocket expenses related to their child's hospitalization and required follow-up care.[36] In addition, children and their families may also experience financial effects after critical illness, including inability of caregivers to return to work, which could hinder recovery and potentiate post-PICU morbidity.[37]

Community and Built Environment

There is increasing evidence that where one lives affects health status, quality of life, and even life expectancy.[38] In addition to child-level and family-level SDoH, the neighborhood context also contributes to disparities in a child's risk of illness, hospital course, and recovery. Availability of public transportation, pharmacies and doctors, employment and educational opportunities, healthy foods, green space, and exposure to violence, crime, and pollutants are neighborhood factors potentially placing children at risk for higher severity of illness and need for intensive care services.[39,40] Disadvantaged neighborhoods may lack resources needed to make the physical and built environment conducive for optimal health. This situation leaves families underequipped to support children recovering from critical illness or children with chronic health issues, thus increasing their risk for acute exacerbations and acute care use. Furthermore, neighborhood measures of relative socioeconomic disadvantage have been linked to worse PICU outcomes, such as longer length of stay, increased need for mechanical ventilation, and increased mortality.[12,34,41] Higher PICU admission rates and severity of illness scores have been observed in neighborhoods with higher rates of persons living in poverty.[14] Children residing in lower socioeconomic areas seem to be at higher risk of critical illness and traumatic injury, and Black children residing in these areas have lower rates of bystander out-of-hospital resuscitation for cardiac arrests, compared with children living in more socioeconomically advantaged areas.[10,42] Neighborhoods with high rates of PICU readmissions for asthma have high social vulnerability, and higher exposure to environmental toxins such as industrial pollutants, airborne microparticles, and higher ozone concentrations.[43] Understanding the resources and limitations of the child's neighborhood may inform discharge planning to reduce the risk of adverse outcomes and readmission following an episode of critical illness.

Education Access and Quality

This domain includes access to early childhood education, overall educational attainment, and literacy.[18] There is strong evidence linking education and health; increasing educational attainment is associated with healthier behaviors, longer life expectancy, and overall well-being throughout the life course.[44,45] In resource-limited countries, higher maternal education is linked to lower child mortality but the association between parental education and risk of severe illness and death, outside the neonatal period, among US children is not well described.[46–48] Additionally, a severe illness or injury during childhood may have a profound influence on cognitive outcomes and school performance, and this relationship may be exacerbated by SDoH.[49] As educational attainment is linked to long-term health outcomes, income stability, and wealth generation, preventing and responding to disparities in educational outcomes is crucially important for child survivors of critical illness.[50]

Social and Community Context

Studies routinely demonstrate a protective effect of social support, social cohesion, and community engagement on overall health and well-being.[51,52] Accordingly, increasing community and social support is a major objective of the Healthy People 2030 initiative.[53] There are limited studies on the relationship between community and social context and the risk and outcomes of critical illness in children, in part due to challenges in operationalizing the definition of "social outcome."[54]

SOCIAL DETERMINANTS OF HEALTH SCREENING IN THE PEDIATRIC INTENSIVE CARE UNIT

To date, there are no studies directly linking routine social risk screening to improved health outcomes in hospitalized children. In the outpatient setting, 2 randomized studies conducted in primary care clinics associated implementation of social risk screening with improved child health, operationalized as a decrease in documented medical abuse and neglect in one study, and an improvement in parent-reported child health in another study.[55,56] Despite lack of empiric evidence, routine screening is universally endorsed by professional societies and federal agencies, and the Centers for Medicare and Medicaid Services recently issued guidance to state Medicaid directors to encourage universal screening as part of an overall shift from fee-for-service reimbursement models to value-based care.[57] These organizations recognize that investment in social health has the potential to improve individual and population-level health and lead to significant cost savings to the health care sector.[58] We believe that routine, standardized screening for the SDoH is imperative for identification and mitigation of health disparities among children admitted to the PICU. We think that social screening, as part of a larger effort to achieve pediatric health equity, has the potential to improve the health of individuals and populations, and is required if we are to successfully provide just, ethical, and equitable care for critically ill children.

Screening for Social Determinants of Health May Improve the Health of Individuals

There are several potential benefits to families if routine social risk screening is implemented in an intensive care setting. First, family-centered care requires effective patient–provider communication, cultural humility and competence, acknowledgment of implicit biases, knowledge of health literacy, and an understanding of a family's lived experiences, cultural and religious beliefs, and goals of care—all of which can be facilitated by routine screening for SDoH.[59,60] Second, understanding if families struggle with food security, housing stability, adequate health-care access, and fragile support systems can allow PICU providers to contextualize a family's ability to navigate their child's hospitalization.[61] Third, for families with identified needs, social resources that may be available within the health-care system can be mobilized.[62] Fourth, the PICU encounter offers an opportunity to identify social needs in children previously not screened by their primary care providers. Although most pediatricians acknowledge its importance, few screen.[63] Finally, screening can identify family and community factors that could help or hinder recovery after critical illness. Up to 70% of children develop a new morbidity following the PICU stay, and it is increasingly recognized that the development of postintensive care syndrome is related to both illness factors and the social milieu, including SDoH.[64,65] In-depth assessments of family social needs during the acute phase of critical illness are necessary for provision of optimal anticipatory guidance to families in preparation for recovery after critical illness.

Screening for Social Determinants of Health May Improve the Health of Populations

Section 4302 (*Understanding Health Disparities: Data Collection and Analysis*) of the Affordable Care Act outlines minimum data-collection standards for race, ethnicity, sex, language, and disabilities for all Department of Health and Human Services programs and surveys.[66] The Institute for Healthcare Improvement and the Agency for Healthcare Research and Quality have independently stated systematic collection of the aforementioned demographic data, as well as universal screening for SDoH, is necessary for identification, understanding, and elimination of the root causes of health disparities.[67–69] As part of local and multicenter collaborative patient safety initiatives, PICUs routinely perform quality improvement projects that rely on accurate data collection for stratification and dissemination of quality performance. Examples of improvement targets include health-care–acquired conditions, patient handoffs, antibiotic and blood culture stewardship, and pediatric severe sepsis.[70–73] To date, there are no large-scale databases with SDoH data for critically ill children, which could inform health equity projects.[74] The Virtual Pediatric Systems (VPS, LLC http://www.myvps.org/) database includes more than 1 million PICU admissions from more than 130 centers and was developed to improve PICU care delivery through quality improvement and research initiatives.[75] The Pediatric Health Information System (Children's Hospital Association, Lenexa, KS) is an administrative database including resource utilization data from more than 45 tertiary centers associated with the Children's Hospital Association. Both datasets were designed, in part, to drive health care improvement through benchmarking, quality improvement, and research initiatives, although arguably they currently lack the data necessary to fully identify inequitable health-care delivery.[75,76] For example, race and ethnicity was not a "mandatory" data field in VPS until 2021, and neither registry collects data on family-level social determinants.

Collection of demographic and social determinant data should be standardized, and when possible, captured in institutional electronic health records (EHRs) and multiinstitutional research and administrative databases. This would allow PICUs to stratify outcome data, including mortality, length of stay, hospital-acquired conditions, and readmissions-a necessary first step in the effort to achieve health equity. Social screening can promote better understanding of the unique needs of the PICU patient population, and spur hospital-wide initiatives aimed to improve population health, such as financial navigation programs[77] for medical-related financial stress, hospital-based food pantries,[62] and housing interventions[78] for food and housing insecurity. Finally, adding a social risk "score" alongside an index of mortality or illness severity score (eg, pediatric logistic organ dysfunction-2 [PELOD-2] score) could highlight those patients who may have a more difficult PICU course, or those who will be at higher risk for mortality or require intensive post-PICU follow-up to optimize chances for good health outcomes. Furthermore, there is a critical need for empirical research on SDoH screening in the PICU, and implemented interventions aimed at reducing identified inequalities or disparities. Any research program, however, must collect and report on race and ethnicity, recognizing these labels as social constructs. Data must be collected with adequate rigor to allow sufficient evaluation of race and ethnicity as contributors to the research outcomes of interest, within a racial equity framework.[79]

As evidence builds for place-based disparities in risk of pediatric critical illness, collecting neighborhood-level data can facilitate identification of "hot spots" amenable to public health interventions collaboratively developed by health systems, communities, and governments.[80] The influence of neighborhood on child health is complex, with research revealing multiple, distinct, but overlapping relationships between a child's environment and its health. For example, unfavorable asthma outcomes have independently been linked to poor housing quality, high levels of air pollution, challenges in access to preventative care and pharmacies, and lack of transportation.[81] Identifying communities conferring high levels of risk with composite markers of neighborhood health, such as the publicly available Child Opportunity Index, could allow researchers to measure associations between multidimensional, interrelated neighborhood characteristics and health outcomes.[82] The *Breathe Easy at Home* program in Boston and the *Collaboration to Lessen Environmental Asthma Risks* at Cincinnati Children's Hospital are examples of neighborhood-based programs through which disparities in asthma outcomes were identified and mitigated through health system-community collaborations.[83,84] Furthermore, incorporating composite neighborhood risk scores into the EHR could facilitate a deeper understanding of disease risk and challenges with recovery, allowing clinicians the opportunity to tailor their anticipatory guidance and therapeutic choices for individual patients, and support the development of relationships with community partnerships to affect population health outcomes.[81]

Screening in an Acute Care Setting

In the last decade, the American Academy of Pediatrics (AAP) has recognized the importance of poverty and related social determinants to child health and well-being by releasing 4 policy statements.[85–88] Although most pediatricians think that routine screening for social needs is important, few think that implementation is feasible.[89] In outpatient clinics, time constraints, lack of staff and referral resources, workflow disruptions, and inadequate reimbursement policies contribute to overall low rates of screening.[90] Subspecialty pediatricians and hospital-based pediatricians report similar barriers to screening.[90,91] Although the AAP makes no specific recommendations surrounding SDoH screening in the acute care setting, in developing an interdisciplinary approach to mitigating social risk, the Academy emphasizes the benefits of the medical home, medical-legal partnerships, health system-community partnerships, and care coordination, all of which can—and should—be facilitated by hospital-based care teams.[85] A PICU admission offers a unique opportunity for SDoH screening; however, to our knowledge, no implementation framework or validated tool exists for SDoH screening in the PICU.[92] High staff-to-patient ratios, parent and guardian presence, and the availability of social workers and case workers at many tertiary care PICUs make screening for SDoH and resource referral potentially feasible. When planning the implementation of SDoH screening and data collection, the following should be considered:

1. *Educate providers on the impact of SDoH and the relevance of screening.* All staff members involved in the direct care of PICU patients should be educated on influences SDoH have on the continuum of critical illness and the influence of screening, with the goal of improving their understanding of the structures, practices, policies and processes that contribute to health inequities, and the importance of addressing unmet social needs of patients and their families.
2. *All families should undergo screening.* Universal screening, as part of the intake process, will minimize a family from feeling targeted, identify needs in families who may otherwise not ask for help if not screened, allows staff members to gain expertise in screening through repetition, and provides an accurate population-based picture of the social needs of the PICU population.
3. *Employ a strength-based approach.* Each family has unique strengths, and most thrive despite adversity. These strengths should be recognized and celebrated through strength-based screening, which provides families with opportunities and experiences to build their protective factors, such as parental resilience and social support.[93] This approach will improve participation and engagement of patients and families.[94] Providers should avoid screening approaches that may create a sense of shame, or that place blame for structural socio-economic conditions outside of families' control.[93,94]
4. *Staff should be trained to screen.* Families may be reticent to answer sensitive questions, and those who conduct social needs screening with families must be trained and/or have experience in the core competencies of trauma-informed and culturally effective care.[93]
5. *SDoH needs identified from screening should be paired with appropriate referrals and resources.* SDoH screening followed by linkage to appropriate resources within the hospital and/or community has been associated with improved child health outcomes.[55] Hospitals have successfully partnered with community organizations to establish food pantries, offer transportation resources, and provide housing vouchers to families in need. A compendium of local and national resources, such as the United Way's national 2-1-1[95] program, can be created and made readily available to share with families in need.
6. *Build upon existing systems.* To successfully implement widespread screening and intervention processes across PICUs, it will be important to leverage existing systems and ensure collaboration occur across multidisciplinary teams, both within and across institutions. Integrating SDoH screening tools into the EHR available to different care providers at transition points in a patient's care will facilitate resource provision and rapid analysis of social risk as a factor that may directly or indirectly affect the patient's critical care trajectory and can also prevent families from undergoing repeated screening within the same institution.[95] Consideration should be made for EHR documentation of identified social needs, using the International Classification of Diseases, 10th revision "miscellaneous Z codes" for the purposes of case management and follow-up, risk-adjustment modeling, and for inclusion in future reimbursement initiatives.[96–98]
7. *Develop valid and reliable screening tools.* Few screening tools currently used in pediatric practice have undergone validity and reliability testing.[99] Ensuring the tools are accurate and inform care for intended patient populations should be a priority area of research in this area.

Screening for the Social Determinants of Health is Required for Just and Equitable Health Care

As a group, critical care clinicians provide ethically sound care and are well-versed in maximizing patient good (beneficence) and minimizing patient harm (nonmaleficence). Ethical health-care delivery must also incorporate principles of justice that affect individual-level and population-level care. As a core principle of biomedical ethics, achieving justice in health care requires that (1) individuals have an equal right to basic needs and liberties and (2) when resources are limited, decisions related to resource distribution ensure those individuals with the greatest need are benefited, and all individuals have equal opportunity to obtain resources.[100] Addressing health-related social risks through SDoH screening can ensure that basic health needs are met, whereas assessing for and responding to structural barriers or systemic inequities will promote justice.

Identification of structural barriers to health may uncover social needs that we are unable to provide immediate resources for thus creating moral dilemma for both health-care providers and patients. However, building a narrative for resources or policy changes to address these concerns is critical to ultimately reducing their impact. Collaborating with medical legal partnerships can be an effective mechanism both to address individual and systemic level social risks through advocacy-recent research suggests that this collaborative approach can lead to improved health outcomes.[101]

SUMMARY

Disparities in the risk, care, and outcomes of critical illness in children are prevalent and unacceptable. Widespread implementation of SDoH screening in our PICUs is an important first step in addressing the causes of these disparities. Beyond increasing our understanding of the mechanisms that potentiate disparities, SDoH screening will facilitate identification of vulnerable families and children likely to benefit from linkage to resources within the hospital and community. Furthermore, information gathered through screening will enable the development of effective interventions and policies aimed at ensuring distribution of resources to those with the greatest need—a core element of just and equitable health care.

CLINICS CARE POINTS

- Multicenter cohort studies have demonstrated the existence of disparities in illness severity, rates of PICU admission, in-hospital mortality, readmission rates, and long-term functional outcomes based on race, ethnicity, insurance status, and socioeconomic status.
- Implementation of universal SDoH screening in a PICU should include appropriate staff training, employ a strengths-based approach, and be paired with appropriate hospital-based and community-based resource referral.
- Development of a valid and reliable screening tools for use in the PICU setting should be a priority of future research.

ACKNOWLEDGEMENT

Dr. Talati Paquette's work is supported by the Eunice Kennedy Shriver National Institute of Child Health and Human Development (1K23HD098289)

REFERENCES

1. Galea S, Tracy M, Hoggatt KJ, et al. Estimated deaths attributable to social factors in the United States. Am J Public Health 2011;101(8):1456–65.
2. Social determinants of health. 2018. Available at: http://www.who.int/social_determinants/en/. Accessed May 30, 2022.
3. Braveman P, Egerter S, Williams DR. The social determinants of health: coming of age. Annu Rev Public Health 2011;32:381–98.
4. Braveman P, Gottlieb L. The social determinants of health: it's time to consider the causes of the causes. Public Health Rep 2014;129(Suppl 2):19–31.
5. Flores G, Committee On Pediatric R. Technical report–racial and ethnic disparities in the health and health care of children. Pediatrics 2010;125(4):e979–1020.
6. Howell E, Decker S, Hogan S, et al. Declining child mortality and continuing racial disparities in the era of the Medicaid and SCHIP insurance coverage expansions. Am J Public Health 2010;100(12):2500–6.
7. Oberg C, Colianni S, King-Schultz L. Child health disparities in the 21st century. Curr Probl Pediatr Adolesc Health Care 2016;46(9):291–312.
8. U.S. child population decreasing, becoming more diverse. [press release]. November 1, 2021. Available at: https://publications.aap.org/aapnews/news/17443. Accessed June 13th, 2022.
9. Garber N, Watson RS, Linde-Zwirble WT. The size and scope of intensive care for children in the US. Crit Care Med 2003;31(Suppl):A78.
10. Mitchell HK, Reddy A, Perry MA, et al. Racial, ethnic, and socioeconomic disparities in paediatric critical care in the USA. Lancet Child Adolesc Health 2021;5(10):739–50.
11. Records CotRSaBDaMfEH. Capturing social and behavioral domains and measures in electronic health records: phase 2. Washington, DC: Institute of Medicine; Board on Population Health and Public Health Practice; 2014.
12. Andrist E, Riley CL, Brokamp C, et al. Neighborhood poverty and pediatric intensive care use. Pediatrics 2019;144(6):e20190748.
13. Czaja AS, Zimmerman JJ, Nathens AB. Readmission and late mortality after pediatric severe sepsis. Pediatrics 2009;123(3):849–57.
14. Epstein D, Reibel M, Unger JB, et al. The effect of neighborhood and individual characteristics on pediatric critical illness. J Community Health 2014;39(4):753–9.
15. Turner D, Simpson P, Li SH, et al. Racial disparities in pediatric intensive care unit admissions. Southampt Med J 2011;104(9):640–6.
16. Lopez AM, Tilford JM, Anand KJ, et al. Variation in pediatric intensive care therapies and outcomes by race, gender, and insurance status. Pediatr Crit Care Med 2006;7(1):2–6.
17. Epstein D, Wong CF, Khemani RG, et al. Race/Ethnicity is not associated with mortality in the PICU. Pediatrics 2011;127(3):e588–97.
18. Prevention CfDCa. About social determinants of health. Available at: https://www.cdc.gov/socialdeterminants/about.html. Accessed June 6, 2022.
19. Weaver MR, Nandakumar V, Joffe J, et al. Variation in health care access and quality among US states and high-income countries with universal health insurance coverage. JAMA Netw Open 2021;4(6):e2114730.
20. Institute of Medicine (US) Committee on Health Literacy. Health Literacy. In: Nielsen-Bohlman L, Panzer AM, Kindig DA, editors. A Prescription to End

Confusion. Washington, DC: National Academies Press; 2004. Available at: https://pubmed.ncbi.nlm.nih.gov/25009856/.

21. Institute of Medicine (US) Committee on Understanding and Eliminating Racial and Ethnic Disparities in Health Care. Unequal Treatment: Confronting Racial and Ethnic Disparities. In: Smedley BD, Stith AY, Nelson AR, editors. Health Care. Washington, DC: National Academies Press; 2003.

22. Brown LE, Franca UL, McManus ML. Socioeconomic disadvantage and distance to pediatric critical care. Pediatr Crit Care Med 2021;22(12):1033–41.

23. Guagliardo MF, Ronzio CR, Cheung I, et al. Physician accessibility: an urban case study of pediatric providers. Health Place 2004;10(3):273–83.

24. Shi L, Stevens GD. Disparities in access to care and satisfaction among U.S. children: the roles of race/ethnicity and poverty status. Public Health Rep 2005;120(4):431–41.

25. Flores G, Tomany-Korman SC. Racial and ethnic disparities in medical and dental health, access to care, and use of services in US children. Pediatrics 2008;121(2):e286–98.

26. Castellanos MI, Dongarwar D, Wanser R, et al. In-hospital mortality and racial disparity in children and adolescents with acute myeloid leukemia: a population-based study. J Pediatr Hematol Oncol 2022;44(1):e114–22.

27. Mitchell HK, Reddy A, Montoya-Williams D, et al. Hospital outcomes for children with severe sepsis in the USA by race or ethnicity and insurance status: a population-based, retrospective cohort study. Lancet Child Adolesc Health 2021;5(2):103–12.

28. Willer BL, Mpody C, Tobias JD, et al. Association of race and family socioeconomic status with pediatric postoperative mortality. JAMA Netw Open 2022; 5(3):e222989.

29. DeLemos D, Chen M, Romer A, et al. Building trust through communication in the intensive care unit: HICCC. Pediatr Crit Care Med 2010;11(3):378–84.

30. Studdert DM, Burns JP, Mello MM, et al. Nature of conflict in the care of pediatric intensive care patients with prolonged stay. Pediatrics 2003;112(3 Pt 1):553–8.

31. Zurca AD, Wang J, Cheng YI, et al. Racial minority families' preferences for communication in pediatric intensive care often overlooked. J Natl Med Assoc 2020;112(1):74–81.

32. Epstein D, Unger JB, Ornelas B, et al. Satisfaction with care and decision making among parents/caregivers in the pediatric intensive care unit: a comparison between English-speaking whites and Latinos. J Crit Care 2015;30(2):236–41.

33. Bor J, Cohen GH, Galea S. Population health in an era of rising income inequality: USA, 1980-2015. Lancet 2017;389(10077):1475–90.

34. Slain KN, Shein SL, Stormorken AG, et al. Outcomes of children with critical bronchiolitis living in poor communities. Clin Pediatr (Phila) 2018;57(9):1027–32.

35. Shonkoff JP, Garner AS, Committee on Psychosocial Aspects of C, et al. The life-long effects of early childhood adversity and toxic stress. Pediatrics 2012; 129(1):e232–46.

36. Clark ME, Cummings BM, Kuhlthau K, et al. Impact of pediatric intensive care unit admission on family financial status and productivity: a pilot study. J Intensive Care Med 2019;34(11–12):973–7.

37. Kamdar BB, Sepulveda KA, Chong A, et al. Return to work and lost earnings after acute respiratory distress syndrome: a 5-year prospective, longitudinal study of long-term survivors. Thorax 2018;73(2):125–33.

38. Prochaska JD, Jupiter DC, Horel S, et al. Rural-urban differences in estimated life expectancy associated with neighborhood-level cumulative social and environmental determinants. Prev Med 2020;139:106214.

39. Kirby JB, Kaneda T. Neighborhood socioeconomic disadvantage and access to health care. J Health Soc Behav 2005;46(1):15–31.

40. Wooldridge G, Murthy S. Pediatric critical care and the climate emergency: our responsibilities and a call for change. Front Pediatr 2020;8:472.

41. Colvin JD, Zaniletti I, Fieldston ES, et al. Socioeconomic status and in-hospital pediatric mortality. Pediatrics 2013;131(1):e182–90.

42. Naim MY, Griffis HM, Burke RV, et al. Race/ethnicity and neighborhood characteristics are associated with bystander cardiopulmonary resuscitation in pediatric out-of-hospital cardiac arrest in the United States: a study from CARES. J Am Heart Assoc 2019;8(14):e012637.

43. Grunwell JR, Opolka C, Mason C, et al. Geospatial analysis of social determinants of health identifies neighborhood hot spots associated with pediatric intensive care use for life-threatening asthma. J Allergy Clin Immunol Pract 2022;10(4):981–991 e981.

44. The Lancet Public H. Education: a neglected social determinant of health. Lancet Public Health 2020;5(7):e361.

45. Assari S, Caldwell CH, Bazargan M. Association between parental educational attainment and youth outcomes and role of race/ethnicity. JAMA Netw Open 2019;2(11):e1916018.

46. Makate M, Makate C. The causal effect of increased primary schooling on child mortality in Malawi: universal primary education as a natural experiment. Soc Sci Med 2016;168:72–83.

47. Andriano L, Monden CWS. The causal effect of maternal education on child mortality: evidence from a quasi-experiment in Malawi and Uganda. Demography 2019;56(5):1765–90.

48. Gage TB, Fang F, O'Neill E, et al. Maternal education, birth weight, and infant mortality in the United States. Demography 2013;50(2):615–35.

49. Tomaszewski W, Ablaza C, Straney L, et al. Educational outcomes of childhood survivors of critical illness-A population-based linkage study. Crit Care Med 2022;50(6):901–12.

50. Hahn RA, Truman BI. Education improves public health and promotes health equity. Int J Health Serv 2015;45(4):657–78.

51. Reblin M, Uchino BN. Social and emotional support and its implication for health. Curr Opin Psychiatry 2008;21(2):201–5.

52. Singh R, Javed Z, Yahya T, et al. Community and social context: an important social determinant of cardiovascular disease. Methodist Debakey Cardiovasc J 2021;17(4):15–27.

53. Healthy People 2030: Social Determinants of Health. U.S. Department of Health and Human Services. https://health.gov/healthypeople/priority-areas/social-determinants-health. Accessed June 17th, 2022.

54. Daughtrey H, Slain KN, Derrington S, et al, POST-PICU and PICU-COS Investigators of the Pediatric Acute Lung Injury and Sepsis Investigators (PALISI) and the Eunice Kennedy Shriver National Institute of Child Health and Human Development Collaborative Pediatric Critical Care Research Networks (CPCCRN). Measuring social health following pediatric critical illness: a scoping review and conceptual framework. J Intensive Care Med 2022. https://doi.org/10.1177/08850666221102815.

55. Gottlieb LM, Hessler D, Long D, et al. Effects of social needs screening and in-person service navigation on child health: a randomized clinical trial. JAMA Pediatr 2016;170(11):e162521.
56. Dubowitz H, Feigelman S, Lane W, et al. Pediatric primary care to help prevent child maltreatment: the Safe Environment for Every Kid (SEEK) Model. Pediatrics 2009;123(3):858–64.
57. Centers for Medicaid and Medicare Services. State Health Official # 21-001. (2021). RE: Opportunities in medicaid and CHIP to address social determinants of health (SDOH). https://www.medicaid.gov/federal-policy-guidance/downloads/sho21001.pdf. Accessed June 12, 2022.
58. Lipson DJ. Medicaid's Role in improving the social determinants of health: opportunities for states, 14, 2017. Available at: https://www.nasi.org/wp-content/uploads/2017/06/Opportunities-for-States_web.pdf. Accessed June 8, 2022.
59. Perez-Stable EJ, El-Toukhy S. Communicating with diverse patients: how patient and clinician factors affect disparities. Patient Educ Couns 2018;101(12):2186–94.
60. Greene-Moton E, Minkler M. Cultural competence or cultural humility? Moving beyond the debate. Health Promot Pract 2020;21(1):142–5.
61. Kangovi S, Barg FK, Carter T, et al. Challenges faced by patients with low socio-economic status during the post-hospital transition. J Gen Intern Med 2014;29(2):283–9.
62. Gany F, Lee T, Loeb R, et al. Use of hospital-based food pantries among low-income urban cancer patients. J Community Health 2015;40(6):1193–200.
63. Fleegler EW, Lieu TA, Wise PH, et al. Families' health-related social problems and missed referral opportunities. Pediatrics 2007;119(6):e1332–41.
64. Watson RS, Choong K, Colville G, et al. Life after critical illness in children-toward an understanding of pediatric post-intensive care syndrome. J Pediatr 2018;198:16–24.
65. Kachmar AG, Watson RS, Wypij D, et al. Randomized evaluation of sedation titration for respiratory failure investigative T. Association of socioeconomic status with postdischarge pediatric resource use and quality of life. Crit Care Med 2022;50(2):e117–28.
66. Dorsey R, Graham G, Glied S, et al. Implementing health reform: improved data collection and the monitoring of health disparities. Annu Rev Public Health 2014;35:123–38.
67. Wyatt RLM, Botwinick L, Mate K, et al. Achieving health equity: a guide for health care organizations. Cambridge, Massachusetts: Institute for Healthcare Improvement; 2016.
68. Forum NQ. A roadmap for promoting health equity and eliminating disparities. Washington (DC): The Four I's for Health Equity; 2017.
69. O'Kane M ea. An equity agenda for the field of health care quality improvement. Washington, DC: National Academy of Medicine; 2021.
70. Miller MR, Niedner MF, Huskins WC, et al. Reducing PICU central line-associated bloodstream infections: 3-year results. Pediatrics 2011;128(5):e1077–83.
71. Malenka EC, Nett ST, Fussell M, et al. Improving handoffs between operating room and pediatric intensive care teams: before and after study. Pediatr Qual Saf 2018;3(5):e101.
72. Larsen GY, Brilli R, Macias CG, et al. Development of a quality improvement learning collaborative to improve pediatric sepsis outcomes. Pediatrics 2021;147(1):e20201434.

73. Woods-Hill CZ, Colantuoni EA, Koontz DW, et al. Association of diagnostic stewardship for blood cultures in critically ill children with culture rates, antibiotic use, and patient outcomes: results of the bright STAR collaborative. JAMA Pediatr 2022;176(7):690–8.

74. Riley C, Maxwell A, Parsons A, et al. Disease prevention & health promotion: what's critical care got to do with it? Transl Pediatr 2018;7(4):262–6.

75. Wetzel RC. Pediatric intensive care databases for quality improvement. J Pediatr Intensive Care 2016;5(3):81–8.

76. Kittle K, Currier K, Dyk L, et al. Using a pediatric database to drive quality improvement. Semin Pediatr Surg 2002;11(1):60–3.

77. Watabayashi K, Steelquist J, Overstreet KA, et al. A pilot study of a comprehensive financial navigation program in patients with cancer and caregivers. J Natl Compr Canc Netw 2020;18(10):1366–73.

78. Kelly A, Fazio D, Padgett D, et al. Patient views on emergency department screening and interventions related to housing. Acad Emerg Med 2022;29(5):589–97.

79. Zurca AD, Suttle ML, October TW. An antiracism approach to conducting, reporting, and evaluating pediatric critical care research. Pediatr Crit Care Med 2022;23(2):129–32.

80. Beck AF, Anderson KL, Rich K, et al. Cooling the hot spots where child hospitalization rates are high: a neighborhood approach to population health. Health Aff (Millwood) 2019;38(9):1433–41.

81. Beck AF, Sandel MT, Ryan PH, et al. Mapping neighborhood health geomarkers to clinical care decisions to promote equity in child health. Health Aff (Millwood) 2017;36(6):999–1005.

82. Krager MK, Puls HT, Bettenhausen JL, et al. The child opportunity index 2.0 and hospitalizations for ambulatory care sensitive conditions. Pediatrics 2021;148(2).

83. Beck AF, Simmons JM, Sauers HS, et al. Connecting at-risk inpatient asthmatics to a community-based program to reduce home environmental risks: care system redesign using quality improvement methods. Hosp Pediatr 2013;3(4):326–34.

84. Rosofsky A, Reid M, Sandel M, et al. Breathe easy at home: a qualitative evaluation of a pediatric asthma intervention. Glob Qual Nurs Res 2016;3. 2333393616676154.

85. COUNCIL ON COMMUNITY PEDIATRICS. Poverty and child health in the United States. Pediatrics 2016;137(4):e20160339.

86. Pascoe JM, Wood DL, Duffee JH, et al, COMMITTEE ON PSYCHOSOCIAL ASPECTS OF CHILD AND FAMILY HEALTH, COUNCIL ON COMMUNITY PEDIATRICS.. Mediators and adverse effects of child poverty in the United States. Pediatrics 2016;137(4):e20160340.

87. COUNCIL ON COMMUNITY PEDIATRICS, COMMITTEE ON NUTRITION.. Promoting food security for all children. Pediatrics 2015;136(5):e1431–8.

88. COUNCIL ON COMMUNITY PEDIATRICS. Providing care for children and adolescents facing homelessness and housing insecurity. Pediatrics 2013;131(6):1206–10.

89. Garg A, Cull W, Olson L, et al. Screening and referral for low-income families' social determinants of health by US pediatricians. Acad Pediatr 2019;19(8):875–83.

90. Schwartz B, Herrmann LE, Librizzi J, et al. Screening for social determinants of health in hospitalized children. Hosp Pediatr 2020;10(1):29–36.

91. Lax Y, Bathory E, Braganza S. Pediatric primary care and subspecialist providers' comfort, attitudes and practices screening and referring for social determinants of health. BMC Health Serv Res 2021;21(1):956.

92. La Count S, McClusky C, Morrow SE, et al. Food insecurity in families with critically ill children: a single-center observational study in pittsburgh. Pediatr Crit Care Med 2021;22(4):e275-7.

93. Flacks J. and Boynton-Jarrett R.F., A Strengths-based Approaches to Screening Families for Health-Related Social Needs in the Healthcare Setting. The Center for the Study of Social Policy. Washington, DC, 2018. https://www.ctc-ri.org/sites/default/files/uploads/A-strengths-based-approach-to-screening.pdf. Accessed May 23, 2022.

94. Frankowski BL, Leader IC, Duncan PM. Strength-based interviewing. Adolesc Med State Art Rev 2009;20(1):22-40, vii-viii.

95. Lindau ST. CommunityRx, an E-prescribing system connecting people to community resources. Am J Public Health 2019;109(4):546-7.

96. Clark MA, Gurewich D. Integrating measures of social determinants of health into health care encounters: opportunities and challenges. Med Care 2017;55(9):807-9.

97. Torres JM, Lawlor J, Colvin JD, et al. ICD social codes: an underutilized resource for tracking social needs. Med Care 2017;55(9):810-6.

98. Weeks WB, Cao SY, Lester CM, et al. Use of Z-codes to record social determinants of health among fee-for-service medicare beneficiaries in 2017. J Gen Intern Med 2020;35(3):952-5.

99. Sokol R, Austin A, Chandler C, et al. Screening children for social determinants of health: a systematic review. Pediatrics 2019;144(4):e20191622.

100. Political JR. Liberalism. New York, NY: Columbia University Press; 1993.

101. Beck AF, Henize AW, Qiu T, et al. Reductions in hospitalizations among children referred to a primary care-based medical-legal partnership. Health Aff (Millwood) 2022;41(3):341-9.

Youth Firearm Injury
A Review for Pediatric Critical Care Clinicians

Elinore J. Kaufman, MD, MSHP[a], Therese S. Richmond, PhD, RN[b],*,
Katelin Hoskins, PhD, MBE, CRNP[c]

KEYWORDS

- Firearm injury • Public health • Injury prevention • Youth

KEY POINTS

- Firearms are now the leading cause of death for youth in the United States. The most common cause of youth firearm death is homicide. Boys account for 90% of deaths, and youth of color are affected disproportionately.
- The presence of firearms in the home increases youth risk of homicide, suicide, and unintentional injury, particularly when firearms are stored loaded or unlocked.
- Families are open to counseling on firearm storage from clinicians, and counseling can reduce risk of injury, particularly when combined with the distribution of secure storage devices.
- Trauma informed approaches, including dedicated support for recovering youth, can improve outcomes after firearm injury.

INTRODUCTION

Firearms are the leading cause of death among children and adolescents (youth) in the United States, ending more lives than cancer, congenital anomalies, or chronic respiratory disease.[1] The SARS-CoV-2 pandemic has ushered in escalating risks for youth and families. Rising community gun violence has impacted youth disproportionately[2] and youth suicides have risen,[3] particularly among Black youth.[4] Moreover, 2.9% of US adults became firearm owners for the first time during the pandemic, exposing more than 5 million youth to the risks of firearms in the home.[5–7] The escalation in firearm-related death for youth is particularly disturbing because of how preventable these deaths are.

[a] Division of Traumatology, Surgical Critical Care, and Emergency Surgery, University of Pennsylvania Perelman School of Medicine, Penn Presbyterian Medical Center, MOB Suite 120, 51 North 39th Street, Philadelphia, PA 19104, USA; [b] University of Pennsylvania School of Nursing, Fagin Hall 330, 418 Curie Boulevard, Philadelphia, PA 19104, USA; [c] University of Pennsylvania School of Nursing, Fagin Hall 312, 418 Curie Boulevard, Philadelphia, PA 19104, USA
* Corresponding author.
E-mail address: terryr@nursing.upenn.edu

Crit Care Clin 39 (2023) 357–371
https://doi.org/10.1016/j.ccc.2022.09.010   criticalcare.theclinics.com
0749-0704/23/© 2022 Elsevier Inc. All rights reserved.

Pediatric critical care clinicians are highly skilled at providing life-saving care to injured youth. While organized systems of trauma care and sophisticated critical care units are essential elements of treating the disease of firearm injury, they are not sufficient. Clinicians have an ethical obligation to address firearm violence as they would any other health problem.[8] Therefore, we must move upstream to prevent firearm-related harm before it brings children to our intensive care units, and we must think beyond the unit to focus on healing the scars of youth, families, and communities.[9]

The reasons for the escalation of firearm injury and death among youth are complex and crosssocietal sectors from social policy to education to health care and beyond. The complexity of the issue is challenging but also opens up a wealth of potential points of intervention that can be designed, implemented, and evaluated. In this paper, we seek to equip pediatric critical care clinicians with necessary information about the epidemiology of firearm-related harm and related costs, risk and protective factors, the impact of firearm violence on youth, and public health approaches to prevent firearm-related harm to inform actions that pediatric critical care clinicians can take.

EPIDEMIOLOGY OF FIREARM INJURY AMONG YOUTH

Youth accounted for almost 12% of firearm deaths in 2020, with a death rate of 6.32 per 100,000 for youth below age 21.[10] While suicide is the leading intent of firearm death in the general population, in youth, homicides account for the majority of deaths (**Fig. 1**). The proportion of youth homicides that are firearm-related increased significantly from 1980 to 2016.[11]

The public health epidemic of firearm-related death is dominated by boys, with 4710 boys dying as compared with 704 girls in 2020. Firearm-related deaths are not evenly distributed across race/ethnicity (**Fig. 2**). Including all intents of injury, Black boys have the highest death rate per 100,000 (35.05) followed by American Indian/Alaska Native (18.58), Latino (7.54), White (6.13), and Asian/Pacific Islander boys (2.49).[10] The pattern changes for firearm suicide, with American Indian/Native Alaskan boys dominating followed by White and Black boys. Among girls, Black girls bear a disproportionate burden of firearm homicide. This disparity extends to firearm-related deaths due to legal intervention (shootings carried out by law enforcement officers in the course of their duties). Between 2003 and 2018, Black and Hispanic adolescents between 12 and 17 years of age had higher risks of firearm-related deaths due to legal intervention than their non-Hispanic White peers (RR 6.01 and 2.78, respectively).[12]

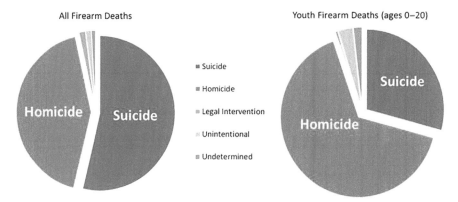

Fig. 1. Firearm deaths according to the intention of injury 2020 firearm deaths. Firearm deaths for all ages n = 45,222. Youth firearm deaths (ages 0–20) n = 5414. *Data from* WISQARS. https://www.cdc.gov/injury/wisqars/index.htm.

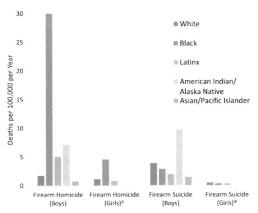

Fig. 2. Firearm Homicide and Suicide by Race and Ethnicity for Boys and Girls. [a]Rates for American Indian/Alaska Native and Asian/Pacific Islander girls unstable and not reported.

There is no comprehensive data source for nonfatal firearm injuries. Limited data on emergency department (ED) visits and hospitalizations suggest that more than 4 times as many youth survive firearm injuries than die.[13] This case fatality ratio is lower for youth than for adults, largely because youth incur more unintentional injuries, which rarely lead to death. More than 4 in 5 nonfatal firearm injuries are in adolescents, and more than 4 in 5 injured youth are boys. Assaults account for 71% of nonfatal firearm injuries in youth, but unintentional injuries are more common in rural areas.[14,15] Racial disparities mirror those present in homicides,[15–17] and a disproportionate share of injuries occur in low income neighborhoods,[17] and in the South.[18]

RISK AND PROTECTIVE FACTORS

A public health approach to youth firearm injury prevention focuses on boosting protective factors and reducing risk factors at the individual, family, community, environmental, and societal levels. This understanding can aid the development, implementation, and scale-up of tailored interventions. A recent scoping review from the Firearm safety Among Children and Teens (FACTS) Consortium highlights that much of youth firearm violence literature has focused on individual-level risk factors (ie, beliefs, attitudes, behaviors).[19] Substance use, truancy, low academic achievement, delinquency, and firearm carriage are all notable risk factors for interpersonal firearm violence victimization. Specific to firearm suicide, study results are inconsistent as to whether mental health diagnosis, treatment, and prior attempts affect youth's risk for firearm suicide.[19] Peer-related factors also influence the risk of firearm injury for adolescents, who are more likely to carry a firearm if their peers do, or if they expect to encounter other youth who are carrying.[19,20]

At the household level, a well-established body of literature highlights the risks associated with the presence of firearms in the home for youth firearm unintentional injury, homicide, and suicide.[19–22] These risks are amplified when firearms are stored unlocked or loaded. Approximately 30 million children live in US households with firearms, with 4.6 million youth living in households with loaded and unlocked firearms.[23] Updated estimates suggest that adolescents' risk of dying by suicide is at least three times higher living in a home with a firearm versus without.[5,24] Moreover, an examination of National Violent Death Reporting System data across five US states found that for 77% of youth who died by firearm suicide, the firearms used mostly came from parents, but also grandparents, brothers, and parents' intimate partners.[6] Though older children are at higher risk for injury, households with only older children are more likely to store at least one firearm loaded and unlocked compared with households with younger children.[25]

Youth from communities with high levels of socioeconomic disadvantage are at the highest risk for firearm injuries.[17] Black youth disproportionately live in historically racialized spaces with increased exposure to living conditions shaping violence and contributing to high rates of firearm homicide.[26] Multiple neighborhood-level factors fuel violence inequities, including limited economic opportunities, alcohol outlets, narcotic sales, and high concentrations of firearms.[17,19,27] Recent findings indicate that higher county poverty concentration is associated with youth firearm-related deaths across all intents.[28] Youth living in rural counties are at higher risk for firearm-related suicides and unintentional deaths, but lower risk for homicide; differences may be attributable to lethal means access, social isolation, or limited access to mental health services.[28] The causal pathways by which poverty and structural racism lead to injury are complex, and interventions to disrupt this trajectory are sorely needed.[29]

Surprisingly little is known about protective factors for youth firearm outcomes.[19] Parental monitoring and involvement,[30] future orientation,[31] higher levels of school attachment, exposure to school-based drug and violence prevention programs, and stricter state-level firearm policies are associated with decreased propensity to carry firearms in cross-sectional studies.[20]

COSTS OF YOUTH FIREARM INJURY

As the incidence of firearm injury rises in youth, so do the economic costs to individuals, families, and the health care system. The Government Accountability Office estimates the total annual costs of acute care for firearm injuries in the US for all intents and age groups is approximately $1 billion annually, with Medicaid accounting for approximately half of these costs.[32]

Direct health care costs include acute care in the ED for most injuries, but care and accompanying costs vary widely by anatomic injury. Even simple fractures may require physical therapy, prescription drugs, or durable medical equipment such as crutches, scooters, or wheelchairs. Injuries to the organs of the chest and abdomen can require complex surgical management and prolonged inpatient hospitalizations, as well as subsequent rehabilitation. Injuries to the head or spinal cord can require prolonged recovery or result in permanent disability. The mental health impacts of firearm injury can lead to the need for mental and behavioral health care which may extend beyond the individual to victims of secondary trauma stemming from the firearm injury itself: family, friends, and community.[32]

For 2016 to 2017, the average cost of an ED visit for firearm injury was $1478 and the average cost of an inpatient hospitalization was $34,791. Taken together, total acute care costs for youth were $1,153,186,636. Readmissions are common after firearm injury, and affect 4.5% of youth,[33] with an average cost of $8311.[34]

There are limited data on long-term costs for youth who survive firearm injury. Costs are difficult to track, as individuals frequently change insurance carriers. It is difficult to link services to the initial injury, particularly when it comes to behavioral health.[32] Song and colleagues found that in the year after a nonfatal firearm injury, medical spending increased more than 400% among survivors, and also increased 4.2% among family members of survivors, speaking to the wider burden of these injuries and care.[35] Pulcini and colleagues used data from Medicaid and the Children's Health Insurance Program to track health care spending for youth ages 0 to 17 who survived firearm injuries, identifying an increase of $9,084 in health care costs per patient in the year following injury. The greatest increases were seen in self-inflicted injuries.[36]

Costs of youth firearm injury extend beyond direct medical care. Including legal costs, the price tag rises to $270,399 for each death and $52,585 for each nonfatal injury,[37] but little information exists on the impact of lost work for caregivers, or the economic consequences of missed school and disrupted health. The broader costs of firearm violence include not only the need to maintain emergency care systems to treat injured individuals and legal costs, but also lost value of housing and business in neighborhoods impacted by violence. For example, research from The Urban Institute estimated that for every 10 fewer incidents of gun fire, one new business could open, one fewer businesses would close, 20 more jobs could be created, and more than a million dollars of sales could accrue.[38]

CONTEXTUAL IMPACT OF FIREARM INJURY AND EXPOSURE TO VIOLENCE ON YOUTH

Exposure to firearm violence has long-term effects for those who are injured, but also for their peers, families, and communities. Indeed, social network analysis reveals that almost everyone (99.85%) will know a firearm violence victim over the course of a lifetime.[39] For youth of color living in communities marginalized by structural racism, these impacts are greatly magnified, making firearm violence both a cause and a consequence of racial disparities in health and well-being. Both direct and indirect exposures can have profound effects on health and well-being over the short- and long-term. Here we examine firearm-related harm on youth within the broader context of firearm violence in homes, communities, and schools.

There is ample evidence of adverse mental health impacts on youth who have been shot, including depression, posttraumatic stress disorder (PTSD), anxiety, and substance use.[40] One in four youth who survive a firearm injury are diagnosed with a new mental health disorder within a year.[41] It is essential that care provided to youth from the moment of the shooting to long-term follow-up embrace a holistic, trauma-informed approach, and to provide the support necessary for holistic recovery.

Youth report high levels of exposure to community violence and to firearm violence in particular. Exposures can extend from hearing about events in neighborhoods and directly witnessing an event in addition to being victimized. In one study, 95% of 10 to 16 year olds in Philadelphia reported hearing about, 87% witnessing, and 54% being directly victimized by violence in their communities.[42]

"They was like, actually like shooting past me. One was standing down the street and the other one was standing up the street and they was actually like firing back and forth. Like it was fires shot back and forth. I was shocked. I had the trash in my hand 'cause I was putting it out, and I was just shocked. I couldn't move or nothing 'cause I couldn't believe that it was happening."

Closer proximity to a firearm violence incident and closer relationships to firearm violence victims increase the risk for posttraumatic stress.[43]

High exposure to firearm violence is associated with high rates of future injury and firearm injury,[44] and victimization during adolescence is positively associated with the likelihood of owning a handgun in the future.[45] Third graders attending schools located within higher concentration areas of gunshots score lower in standardized state tests.[46] Exposure to violence in youth in 9th grade reduces future educational expectations and increases the likelihood of subsequently carrying a firearm.[47] Youth are aware of crime in their neighborhoods, and as crime rate increases perceptions of safety decrease.[48,49] As a consequence youth develop a level of constant vigilance and make moment by moment decisions about how to safely navigate their neighborhoods.[50] In some ways, this vigilance is protective, but it can also lead to health-harming biological stress and chronic health problems.[51,52] Parents in low-resource neighborhoods where violence is common report keeping their children indoors and restricting movement through the environment.[53] This can be harmful to healthy growth and development, contribute to lack of exercise and obesity, result in missed school and work, and limit age-appropriate social connections.

Youth reside in family systems, thus firearm violence that affects a parent, sibling, or other close relatives affect youth. Consider, for example, when a youth gains access to an unsecured firearm and unintentionally wounds or kills a sibling or when intimate partner violence involves a firearm. Interpersonal firearm violence is disproportionately borne by young Black men, who are also subject to mass incarceration. Therefore, Black youth living in poverty are indirectly harmed as they often living in homes where fathers have been killed or incarcerated.[54] Black men are by far the most likely to be killed by police. In addition to this loss of life, fear of police violence drives adverse mental health, decreased care-seeking and institutional distrust in affected communities.[55–58]

The burden of firearm-related harm in society drives the allocation of resources that can negatively affect youth. For example, the potential for violence in schools drives decisions to install metal detectors and hire school safety officers drawing resources away from books and extracurricular programs. Just as firearm violence is not evenly distributed, the schools affected are more often in under-resourced, minoritized neighborhoods.

SCHOOL SHOOTINGS AND OTHER PUBLIC MASS SHOOTINGS

There have been 2,069 school shootings in the US since 1970, killing 684 and injuring another 1937.[59] These deaths account for < 1% of youth firearm fatalities, but are nonetheless far too common, and carry enormous weight in the public consciousness. School shootings are preventable. Most shooters showed warning signs; improving community response systems has the potential to save lives.[60] Most attackers used weapons obtained in their own homes, indicating that secure storage can act to reduce these shootings as well.[60] Licensing laws, magazine limits, and waiting periods may also play a role in decreasing potential shooters' access to lethal weapons.

Beyond the loss of life, school shootings contribute to posttraumatic stress in survivors and peers,[40] generate fear in students, teachers, and parents, and decrease communities' sense of safety. These shootings have also inspired schools around the country to enact lockdown and active shooter drills. Unfortunately, these drills have been shown to increase stress, with no evidence that they improve safety.[61] Likewise, increasing calls to arm staff in schools are likely to increase, rather than decrease, risk of harm.[62]

PRIMARY PREVENTION OF YOUTH FIREARM INJURY

Prevention is a key priority for promoting the overall health of youth. While pediatric critical care clinicians and other healthcare providers specialize in secondary prevention—minimizing harm and reducing adverse consequences once an injury has occurred—the lethality of firearms makes primary prevention paramount. For example, firearms have a 90% case fatality rate for suicide,[63] and opportunities for secondary prevention and second chances are scarce.

Interventions to Promote Secure Firearm Storage

Reducing opportunities for youth to access firearms in their homes and the homes of others is a key aspect of prevention for youth suicide, unintentional injury, and assault.

Engaging caregivers to increase secure storage in households with youth can prevent injuries and save lives.[64] A recent modeling study found that up to 32% of youth firearm deaths could be avoided if 20% of households with at least one firearm unlocked moved to locking all firearms.[65] Uptake of storage recommendations has the potential to yield significant reductions in both unintentional injury and suicide.

Health care settings are highly relevant intervention points. Clinician counseling on firearm safety in pediatric settings is generally acceptable to parents,[66,67] though questions remain about optimal approaches to motivating behavior change (and associated mechanisms) given the complex and socially situated reasons for both firearm ownership and storage.[65,68–70] A nonjudgmental, patient-centered approach with explicit framing around the shared goal of youth safety may enhance the acceptability and subsequent effectiveness of these conversations.[71–73] Moreover, counseling can also be tailored to specific injury risk factors, like developmental stages or mental health diagnoses.[71]

Despite recommendations from multiple leading organizations (eg, American Academy of Pediatrics) that clinicians discuss firearm safety in health care settings,[74] uptake of this guidance is low.[67,75–77] For example, in one survey of pediatric residents, most respondents indicated never providing firearm-related counseling or only doing so in 1% to 5% of well-child visits, despite agreeing that physicians have a responsibility to counsel on firearm-related risks.[77] In a survey of 54 pediatric-focused advance practice nurses, 70.3% reported asking parents about firearms in the home; advanced practice nurses with higher level of education, pediatric certification, and firearm ownership were most likely to conduct screening and teaching.[78] Identified barriers to counseling include guidance on appropriate language, correct use of locking devices, technical aspects of firearms, and time during visits, highlighting the need for implementation strategies to increase routine delivery.[75,76] Training resources are available through the AAP,[79] Zero Suicide Institute,[80] and the BulletPoints Project.[81]

Evaluations of the effectiveness of clinician counseling to reduce youth household firearm access have been limited by sample size, reliance on self-reported storage practices, and lack of measurement of injury outcomes.[82] However, several studies indicate a positive effect of clinician counseling when accompanied by free locking device provision.[68,83,84] The SAFETY study, a clustered ED-based, multisite trial, evaluated whether a brief counseling intervention reduced at-risk youths' access to lethal means.[85] Hospitals were provided with free handgun safes, cable locks, and medication lockboxes to offer families. Intervention adoption led to a twofold improvement in firearm storage after caregivers returned home from the ED; however, results for improved firearm safety did not persist.[85] One takeaway from this study was the importance of locking device features.[86] With a variety of commercially available options, further research should leverage principles of user-centered design to elicit firearm owners' preferences for locking devices to facilitate usage.[86–89]

Interventions must also be developed and implemented outside of health care settings to expand their reach to firearm owners and individuals with less access to clinical care.[88] Community-based interventions to improve firearm safety include locking device giveaways, community education programs, and firearm buyback programs.[90] Study results generally suggest improved self-reported storage following device distribution regardless of setting, with mixed results on secure storage education programs.[90] Since the 1990s, voluntary buyback programs to reduce the prevalence of firearms in communities have been deployed more broadly across US cities.[91] Though buybacks increase the number of firearms relinquished, support is mixed, with further evaluation needed for pediatric injury outcomes.[90,91]

Environmental interventions to prevent youth firearm injury

Researchers have increasingly focused on structural changes in the built environment (eg, blight reduction through the improvement of dilapidated buildings and abandoned properties) in places whereby violence occurs.[92] Residential segregation of racially and ethnically minoritized youth in settings of concentrated disadvantage necessitates multilevel interventions that target social and political determinants of firearm injury.[17,69,93] Place-based interventions addressing poverty may confer protection and demonstrate promising impact.[26,92,94] For example, a recent randomized trial demonstrated that both (1) greening and (2) mowing and trash cleanup interventions significantly reduced shootings, with no evidence of violence displacement to nearby areas.[95] Well-maintained vacant lots and the presence of parks are associated with a reduction in the odds of adolescent homicide, suggesting potential targets for future urban revitalization strategies.[96]

The role of firearm policy in preventing youth firearm injury

Youth-focused, evidence-based firearm policy is another component of firearm-related injury prevention at the population level. Child Access Prevention (CAP) laws aim to motivate secure firearm storage by imposing liability on adults who permit children to have unsupervised access to firearms. CAP law provisions vary between states, with different levels of criminal liability conferred for specific situations, such as negligent firearm storage or reckless provision of a firearm to a minor.[97] CAP laws are associated with reductions in unintentional firearm injury deaths and firearm suicides, though the magnitude of effects requires further examination.[98,99] Moreover, more evidence is needed about the features of CAP laws and their implementation that enhance effectiveness.[97]

Comprehensive background checks are a potential tool to reduce youth firearm carriage and illegal possession. Federal law mandates background checks to determine eligibility for firearm transfers from federally authorized dealers. However, the federal requirements do not extend to private firearm transfers or sales (eg, sales between individuals in person, online, or at gun shows), generating variability in firearm accessibility and availability across states.[98,100] Thirteen states have laws that mandate background checks at the point of all sales and transfers.[97] One recent study found that adolescents in states that require universal background checks at the point of sale are less likely to carry firearms, suggesting that both state and federal laws may work together to reduce adolescent firearm carriage.[100] In addition, a 5-year analysis found that states with stricter gun laws, particularly universal background checks for firearm purchases, had lower rates of firearm-related deaths in children.[101]

SECONDARY AND TERTIARY PREVENTION

Secondary prevention focuses on the prevention of mental health and behavioral sequelae after youth are exposed to firearm injury, and tertiary prevention addresses risks of recurrent firearm injury. While the occurrence of firearm injury is associated with future firearm injury and high rates of posttraumatic stress symptoms, a scoping review found little empirical research on potential secondary prevention interventions to target long-term effects.[40] However, hospital-based violence intervention programs have shown promise for improving outcomes and reducing reinjury for youth survivors. These programs use trained lay people who serve as credible messengers, often with shared backgrounds and experience to the patients they treat. Staff provide psychosocial support and case management services to patients and families to help them recover and to help them navigate the health care and social services sector to meet their needs. These programs can meet mental health needs[102] and reduce recurrent violent injury, arrests, unemployment, and aggression while improving self-efficacy.[103,104]

SUMMARY: WHAT CAN PEDIATRIC CRITICAL CARE CLINICIANS DO?

Pediatric critical care clinicians first and foremost are responsible to provide life-saving and life-affirming care to injured youth and family. Trauma-informed care should be fully integrated within the plan of care. Research has shown that providers across disciplines have positive attitudes, but would benefit from education to enhance their knowledge and competence in delivering trauma-informed care in trauma settings.[105,106] Training can be considered at the unit or institutional level using existing resources, such as those available on at the National Child Traumatic Stress Network.[107] Life-affirming care extends to planning for appropriate physical and psychological follow-up care postdischarge.

The disproportionate burden of firearm violence affects Black youth. Evidence indicates subtle negative descriptors of racialized comments are documented in electronic health records.[108] Clinicians would be well-served to self-examine the potential of stigma and judgments about the circumstances surrounding shooting events and their own implicit bias given its known association with quality of care.[109]

Primary prevention of youth firearm injury is within the purview of all clinicians and communities. Pediatric critical care clinicians should move upstream to prevent the firearm injury from occurring in the first place. For example, discussion and counseling focused on universal risk reduction regarding firearms, as well as specific safety planning in the context of risk can occur anywhere in the health care system. It does not need to be the purview of general pediatricians or psychiatrists alone.[81]

In this politicized environment of pro-firearm and anti-firearm diatribes, pediatric critical care clinicians bring an important perspective to the conversation because they deal daily with the human anguish of youth who sustain a gunshot wound. It is important to always ask "what can I do?". **Table 1** frames the mnemonic SPEAK

Table 1		
Speak up: actions that critical care providers can take to reduce firearm-related harm		
S	Separate facts from opinions	Understand the incidence and consequences of youth firearm injury
P	Partner with others such as your health system, professional societies & community organizations	Collaborate with community organizations to facilitate community-based prevention and recovery for injured youth
E	Educate yourself, your peers, your community, and your leaders	Ex: risks of firearms in the home and the benefits of secure storage
A	Advocate using current evidence to achieve the goal to create safe communities	Support evidence-based policy such as CAP laws, and programming, such as storage device distribution
K	Know how you will evaluate all interventions and programmatic initiatives	Focus on injury-related outcomes
U	Unite on common ground and be inclusive of divergent views	Center youth safety and well-being
P	Provide trauma informed care and services to help reintegrate youth into the community	Understand the impact of prior and current trauma on youth and families' reactions and interactions with the health care team

UP to provide a sample of concrete strategies and Clinics Care Points that critical care clinicians can take to reduce firearm-related harm.

DISCLOSURE

The authors have no conflicts of interest to disclose. Dr E.J. Kaufman is supported by AHRQ K12-HS026372. Dr K. Hoskins received funding from the National Institute of Mental Health Training Fellowship (T32 MH109433; Mandell/Beidas MPIs).

REFERENCES

1. Goldstick JE, Cunningham RM, Carter PM. Current causes of death in children and adolescents in the United States. N Engl J Med 2022;386(20):1955–6.
2. Afif IN, Gobaud AN, Morrison CN, et al. The changing epidemiology of interpersonal firearm violence during the COVID-19 pandemic in Philadelphia, PA. Prev Med 2022;158:107020.
3. Charpignon ML, Ontiveros J, Sundaresan S, et al. Evaluation of suicides among US adolescents during the COVID-19 pandemic. JAMA Pediatr 2022;176(7): 724–6.
4. California Department of Public Health. Suicide in California – data trends in 2020, COVID impact, and prevention strategies. Available at: https://www. psnyouth.org/wp-content/uploads/2021/08/Suicide-in-California-Data-Trends-in-2020-COVID-Impact-and-Prevention-Strategies-Slide-Deck.pdf. Accessed June 24, 2022.
5. Swanson SA, Eyllon M, Sheu YH, et al. Firearm access and adolescent suicide risk: toward a clearer understanding of effect size. Inj Prev 2020;2019:043605.
6. Barber C, Azrael D, Miller M, et al. Who owned the gun in firearm suicides of men, women, and youth in five US states? Prev Med 2022;107066. https://doi. org/10.1016/j.ypmed.2022.107066.
7. Miller M, Zhang W, Azrael D. Firearm purchasing during the COVID-19 pandemic: results from the 2021 national firearms survey. Ann Intern Med 2021. https://doi.org/10.7326/M21-3423.
8. Shultz BN, Tolchin B, Kraschel KL. The "rules of the road": ethics, firearms, and the physician's "lane. J Law Med Ethics 2020;48(4_suppl):142–5.
9. Hills-Evans K, Mitton J, Sacks CA. Stop posturing and start problem solving: a call for research to prevent gun violence. AMA J Ethics 2018;20(1). https://doi. org/10.1001/journalofethics.2018.20.1.pfor1-1801.
10. U.S. Centers for Disease Control and Prevention. Wide-ranging online data for epidemiological research. Available at: http://wonder.cdc.gov/. Accessed May 11, 2016.
11. Manley NR, Huang DD, Lewis RH, et al. Caught in the crossfire: 37 Years of firearm violence afflicting America's youth. J Trauma Acute Care Surg 2021; 90(4):623–30.
12. Badolato GM, Boyle MD, McCarter R, et al. Racial and ethnic disparities in firearm-related pediatric deaths related to legal intervention. Pediatrics 2020; 146(6). e2020015917.
13. Fowler KA, Dahlberg LL, Haileyesus T, et al. Firearm injuries in the United States. Prev Med 2015;79:5–14.
14. Kaufman EJ, Wiebe DJ, Xiong RA, et al. Epidemiologic trends in fatal and nonfatal firearm injuries in the US, 2009-2017. JAMA Intern Med 2021;181(2): 237–44.

15. Fowler KA, Dahlberg LL, Haileyesus T, et al. Childhood firearm injuries in the United States. Pediatrics 2017;140(1):e20163486.

16. Leventhal JM, Gaither JR, Sege R. Hospitalizations due to firearm injuries in children and adolescents. Pediatrics 2014;133(2):219–25.

17. Carter PM, Cook LJ, Macy ML, et al. Individual and neighborhood characteristics of children seeking emergency department care for firearm injuries within the PECARN network. Acad Emerg Med 2017;24(7):803–13.

18. Patel SJ, Goyal M, Badolato G, et al. Emergency department visits for pediatric firearm-related injury: by intent of injury. Pediatrics 2019; 144(2_MeetingAbstract):407.

19. Schmidt CJ, Rupp L, Pizarro JM, et al. Risk and protective factors related to youth firearm violence: a scoping review and directions for future research. J Behav Med 2019;42(4):706–23.

20. Oliphant SN, Mouch CA, Rowhani-Rahbar A, et al. A scoping review of patterns, motives, and risk and protective factors for adolescent firearm carriage. J Behav Med 2019;42(4):763–810.

21. Dahlberg LL, Ikeda RM, Kresnow MJ. Guns in the home and risk of a violent death in the home: findings from a national study. Am J Epidemiol 2004; 160(10):929–36.

22. Miller M, Hemenway D, Azrael D. State-level homicide victimization rates in the US in relation to survey measures of household firearm ownership, 2001–2003. Soc Sci Med 2007;64(3):656–64.

23. Miller M, Azrael D. Firearm storage in US households with children: findings from the 2021 national firearm survey. JAMA Netw Open 2022;5(2):e2148823.

24. Brent DA, Perper JA, Moritz G, et al. Psychiatric risk factors for adolescent suicide: a case-control study. J Am Acad Child Adolesc Psychiatry 1993;32(3): 521–9.

25. Azrael D, Cohen J, Salhi C, et al. Firearm storage in gun-owning households with children: results of a 2015 national survey. J Urban Health 2018;95(3):295–304.

26. Bottiani JH, Camacho DA, Lindstrom Johnson S, et al. Annual Research Review: youth firearm violence disparities in the United States and implications for prevention. J Child Psychol Psychiatr 2021;62(5):563–79.

27. Hohl BC, Wiley S, Wiebe DJ, et al. Association of drug and alcohol use with adolescent firearm homicide at individual, family, and neighborhood levels. JAMA Intern Med 2017;177(3):317.

28. Barrett JT, Lee LK, Monuteaux MC, et al. Association of county-level poverty and inequities with firearm-related mortality in US youth. JAMA Pediatr 2022;176(2): e214822.

29. Ellyson AM, Rivara FP, Rowhani-Rahbar A. Poverty and firearm-related deaths among US youth. JAMA Pediatr 2022;176(2):e214819.

30. Khetarpal SK, Szoko N, Culyba AJ, et al. Associations between parental monitoring and multiple types of youth violence victimization: a brief report. J Interpers Violence 2021;4. 8862605211035882.

31. Khetarpal SK, Szoko N, Ragavan MI, et al. Future orientation as a cross-cutting protective factor Against multiple forms of violence. J Pediatr 2021;235:288–91.

32. Office USGA. Firearm injuries: health care service needs and costs. Available at: https://www.gao.gov/products/gao-21-515. Accessed July 17, 2021.

33. Wheeler KK, Shi J, Xiang H, et al. Pediatric trauma patient unplanned 30 Day readmissions. J Pediatr Surg 2018;53(4):765–70.

34. Spitzer SA, Vail D, Tennakoon L, et al. Readmission risk and costs of firearm injuries in the United States, 2010-2015. PLoS One 2019;14(1):e0209896.

35. Song Z, Zubizarreta JR, Giuriato M, et al. Changes in health care spending, use, and clinical outcomes after nonfatal firearm injuries among survivors and family members. Ann Intern Med 2022. https://doi.org/10.7326/M21-2812.

36. Pulcini CD, Goyal MK, Hall M, et al. Mental health utilization and expenditures for children pre–post firearm injury. Am J Prev Med 2021;61(1):133–5.

37. The economic cost of gun violence. Everytown research & policy. Available at: https://everytownresearch.org/report/the-economic-cost-of-gun-violence/. Accessed December 17, 2021.

38. Is gun violence stunting business growth? Urban Institute. Available at: https://www.urban.org/features/gun-violence-stunting-business-growth. Accessed June 28, 2022.

39. Kalesan B, Weinberg J, Galea S. Gun violence in Americans' social network during their lifetime. Prev Med 2016;93:53–6.

40. Ranney M, Karb R, Ehrlich P, et al. What are the long-term consequences of youth exposure to firearm injury, and how do we prevent them? A scoping review. J Behav Med 2019;42(4):724–40.

41. Oddo ER, Maldonado L, Hink AB, et al. Increase in mental health diagnoses among youth with nonfatal firearm injuries. Acad Pediatr 2021;21(7):1203–8.

42. McDonald CC, Deatrick JA, Kassam-Adams N, et al. Community violence exposure and positive youth development in urban youth. J Community Health 2011; 36(6):925–32.

43. Montgomerie JZ, Lawrence AE, LaMotte AD, et al. The link between posttraumatic stress disorder and firearm violence: a review. Aggression Violent Behav 2015;21:39–44.

44. Tracy M, Braga AA, Papachristos AV. The transmission of gun and other weapon-involved violence within social networks. Epidemiol Rev 2016;38(1): 70–86.

45. Gresham M, Demuth S. Who owns a handgun? An analysis of the correlates of handgun ownership in young adulthood. Crime Delinq 2020;66(4):541–71.

46. Bergen-Cico D, Lane SD, Keefe RH, et al. Community gun violence as a social determinant of elementary school achievement. Soc Work Public Health 2018; 33(7–8):439–48.

47. Lee DB, Hsieh HF, Stoddard SA, et al. Longitudinal pathway from violence exposure to firearm carriage among adolescents: the role of future expectation. J Adolesc 2020;81:101–13.

48. McCray TM, Mora S. Analyzing the activity spaces of low-income teenagers: how do they perceive the spaces where activities are carried out? J Urban Aff 2011;33(5):511–28.

49. Wiebe DJ, Guo W, Allison PD, et al. Fears of violence during morning travel to school. J Adolesc Health 2013;53(1):54–61.

50. Teitelman A, McDonald CC, Wiebe DJ, et al. Youth's strategies for staying safe and coping. J Community Psychol 2010;38(7):874–85.

51. Theall KP, Shirtcliff EA, Dismukes AR, et al. Association between neighborhood violence and biological stress in children. JAMA Pediatr 2017;171(1):53–60.

52. Kapur G, Stenson AF, Chiodo LM, et al. Childhood violence exposure predicts high blood pressure in black American young adults. J Pediatr 2022; S0022-3476(22):00491–507. https://doi.org/10.1016/j.jpeds.2022.05.039.

53. Jacoby SF, Tach L, Guerra T, et al. The health status and well-being of low-resource, housing-unstable, single-parent families living in violent neighbourhoods in Philadelphia, Pennsylvania. Health Soc Care Community 2017;25(2): 578–89.

54. Race, poverty, and U.S. Children's exposure to neighborhood incarceration - alexander F. Roehrkasse. 2021. Available at: https://journals.sagepub.com/doi/full/10.1177/23780231211067871. Accessed June 21, 2022.

55. Sewell AA. The illness associations of police violence: differential relationships by ethnoracial composition. Sociological Forum 2017;32(S1):975–97.

56. Kerrison EM, Sewell AA. Negative illness feedbacks: high-frisk policing reduces civilian reliance on ED services. Health Serv Res 2020;55(S2):787–96.

57. Lett E, Asabor EN, Corbin T, et al. Racial inequity in fatal US police shootings, 2015–2020. J Epidemiol Community Health 2020;2020:215097.

58. Bor J, Venkataramani AS, Williams DR, et al. Police killings and their spillover effects on the mental health of black Americans: a population-based, quasi-experimental study. Lancet 2018;392(10144):302–10.

59. Data map. K-12 school shooting database. Available at: https://www.chds.us/ssdb/data-map/. Accessed June 25, 2022.

60. Alathari L, Drysdale D, Driscoll S, et al. PROTECTING AMERICA'S SCHOOLS A U.S. SECRET SERVICE ANALYSIS OF TARGETED SCHOOL VIOLENCE. Available at: https://www.secretservice.gov/sites/default/files/2020-04/Protecting_Americas_Schools.pdf.

61. Schonfeld DJ, Melzer-Lange M, Hashikawa AN, et al. Participation of children and adolescents in live crisis drills and exercises. Pediatrics 2020;146(3). e2020015503.

62. Arming teachers introduces new risks into schools. Everytown research & policy. Available at: https://everytownresearch.org/report/arming-teachers-introduces-new-risks-into-schools/. Accessed June 25, 2022.

63. Conner A, Azrael D, Miller M. Suicide case-fatality rates in the United States, 2007 to 2014: a nationwide population-based study. Ann Intern Med 2019; 171(2):885–95.

64. Mann JJ, Michel CA, Auerbach RP. Improving suicide prevention through evidence-based strategies: a systematic review. AJP 2021;178(7):611–24.

65. Monteaux MC, Azrael D, Miller M. Association of increased safe household firearm storage with firearm suicide and unintentional death among US youths. JAMA Pediatr 2019;173(7):657–62.

66. Knoepke C, Allen A, Ranney M, et al. Loaded questions: internet commenters' opinions on physician-patient firearm safety conversations. WestJEM 2017; 18(5):903–12.

67. Garbutt JM, Bobenhouse N, Dodd S, et al. What are parents willing to discuss with their pediatrician about firearm safety? A parental survey. J Pediatr 2016; 179:166–71.

68. Rowhani-Rahbar A, Simonetti JA, Rivara FP. Effectiveness of interventions to promote safe firearm storage. Epidemiol Rev 2016;38(1):111–24.

69. Metzl JM. What guns mean: the symbolic lives of firearms. Palgrave Commun 2019;5(1):35.

70. Betz ME, Anestis MD. Firearms, pesticides, and suicide: a look back for a way forward. Prev Med 2020;138:106144.

71. Haasz M, Boggs JM, Beidas RS, et al. Firearms, physicians, families, and kids: finding words that work. J Pediatr 2022;247:133–7.

72. Hoskins K, Johnson C, Davis M, et al. A mixed methods evaluation of parents' perspectives on the acceptability of the S.A.F.E. Firearm program. J Appl Res Child Informing Policy Child Risk 2022;12(2). Available at: https://digitalcommons.library.tmc.edu/childrenatrisk/vol12/iss2/2.

73. Fuzzell LN, Dodd S, Hu S, et al. An informed approach to the development of primary care pediatric firearm safety messages. BMC Pediatr 2022;22(1):26.

74. Council on injury, violence, and poison prevention executive committee. Firearm-related injuries affecting the pediatric population. Pediatrics 2012; 130(5):e1416–23.

75. Roszko PJD, Ameli J, Carter PM, et al. Clinician attitudes, screening practices, and interventions to reduce firearm-related injury. Epidemiol Rev 2016;38(1): 87–110.

76. Ketabchi B, Gittelman MA, Southworth H, et al. Attitudes and perceived barriers to firearm safety anticipatory guidance by pediatricians: a statewide perspective. Inj Epidemiol 2021;8(S1):21.

77. Hoops K, Crifasi C. Pediatric resident firearm-related anticipatory guidance: why are we still not talking about guns? Prev Med 2019;124:29–32.

78. Cho AN, Dowdell EB. Unintentional gun violence in the home: a survey of pediatric advanced practice nurses' preventive measures. J Pediatr Health Care 2020;34(1):23–9.

79. Safer: storing firearms prevents harm - AAP. Available at: https://shop.aap.org/safer-storing-firearms-prevents-harm/. Accessed June 23, 2022.

80. Zero suicide. Available at: https://zerosuicidetraining.edc.org/. Accessed June 23, 2022.

81. The BulletPoints Project. Available at: https://www.bulletpointsproject.org/. Accessed June 23, 2022.

82. Conner A, Azrael D, Miller M. Access to firearms and youth suicide in the US: implications for clinical interventions. In: Lee LK, Fleegler EW, editors. Pediatric firearm injuries and fatalities : the clinician's guide to policies and approaches to firearm harm prevention. Switzerland: Springer International Publishing; 2021. p. 13–29.

83. Barkin SL, Finch SA, Ip EH, et al. Is office-based counseling about media use, timeouts, and firearm storage effective? Results from a cluster-randomized, controlled trial. Pediatrics 2008;122(1):e15–25.

84. Carbone PS, Clemens CJ, Ball TM. Article. Arch Pediatr Adolesc Med 2005; 159(11):1049.

85. Miller M, Salhi C, Barber C, et al. Changes in firearm and medication storage practices in homes of youths at risk for suicide: results of the SAFETY study, a clustered, emergency department–based, multisite, stepped-wedge trial. Ann Emerg Med 2020;76(2):194–205.

86. Barber C, Azrael D, Berrigan J, et al. Selection and use of firearm and medication locking devices in a lethal means counseling intervention. Crisis 2022. https://doi.org/10.1027/0227-5910/a000855.

87. Beidas RS, Rivara F, Rowhani-Rahbar A. Safe firearm storage: a call for research informed by firearm stakeholders. Pediatrics 2020;146(5):e20200716.

88. Simonetti J, Simeona C, Gallagher C, et al. Preferences for firearm locking devices and device features among participants in a firearm safety event. West-JEM 2019;20(4):552–6.

89. Lyon AR, Bruns EJ. User-centered redesign of evidence-based psychosocial interventions to enhance implementation—hospitable soil or better seeds? JAMA Psychiatry 2019;76(1):3–4.

90. For the FACTS Consortium, Ngo QM, Sigel E, et al. State of the science: a scoping review of primary prevention of firearm injuries among children and adolescents. J Behav Med 2019;42(4):811–29.

91. Hazeltine MD, Green J, Cleary MA, et al. A review of gun buybacks. Curr Trauma Rep 2019;5(4):174–7.

92. Kondo MC, Andreyeva E, South EC, et al. Neighborhood interventions to reduce violence. Annu Rev Public Health 2018;39(1):253–71.

93. Branas CC, Reeping PM, Rudolph KE. Beyond gun laws—innovative interventions to reduce gun violence in the United States. JAMA Psychiatry 2021; 78(3):243–4.

94. Dong B, Branas CC, Richmond TS, et al. Youth's daily activities and situational triggers of gunshot assault in urban environments. J Adolesc Health 2017;61(6): 779–85.

95. Moyer R, MacDonald JM, Ridgeway G, et al. Effect of remediating blighted vacant land on shootings: a citywide cluster randomized trial. Am J Public Health 2019;109(1):140–4.

96. Culyba AJ, Jacoby SF, Richmond TS, et al. Modifiable neighborhood features associated with adolescent homicide. JAMA Pediatr 2016;170(5):473–80.

97. Capozzi Lindsay. Preventing unintentional firearm injury & death among youth: examining the evidence. Available at: https://policylab.chop.edu/evidence-action-briefs/preventing-unintentional-firearm-injury-death-among-youth-examining-evidence. Accessed June 23, 2022.

98. For the FACTS Consortium, Zeoli AM, Goldstick J, et al. The association of firearm laws with firearm outcomes among children and adolescents: a scoping review. J Behav Med 2019;42(4):741–62.

99. Miller M, Zhang W, Rowhani-Rahbar A, et al. Child access prevention laws and firearm storage: results from a national survey. Am J Prev Med 2022;62(3): 333–40.

100. Timsina LR, Qiao N, Mongalo AC, et al. National instant criminal background check and youth gun carrying. Pediatrics 2020;145(1):e20191071.

101. Goyal MK, Badolato GM, Patel SJ, et al. State gun laws and pediatric firearm-related mortality. Pediatrics 2019;144(2):e20183283.

102. Juillard C, Smith R, Anaya N, et al. Saving lives and saving money: hospital-based violence intervention is cost-effective. J Trauma Acute Care Surg 2015; 78(2):252–8.

103. Cooper C, Eslinger DM, Stolley PD. Hospital-based violence intervention programs work. J Trauma Inj Infect Crit Care 2006;61(3):534–40.

104. Cheng TL, Haynie D, Brenner R, et al. Effectiveness of a mentor-implemented, violence prevention intervention for assault-injured youths presenting to the emergency department: results of a randomized trial. Pediatrics 2008;122(5):938–46.

105. Kassam-Adams N, Rzucidlo S, Campbell M, et al. Nurses' views and current practice of trauma-informed pediatric nursing care. J Pediatr Nurs 2015;30(3): 478–84.

106. Bruce MM, Kassam-Adams N, Rogers M, et al. Trauma Providers' knowledge, views, and practice of trauma-informed care. J Trauma Nurs 2018;25(2):131–8.

107. The National Child Traumatic Stress Network. The national child traumatic stress network. https://www.nctsn.org/. Accessed June 28, 2022.

108. Sun M, Oliwa T, Peek ME, et al. Negative patient descriptors: documenting racial bias in the electronic health record. Health Aff 2022;41(2):203–11.

109. FitzGerald C, Hurst S. Implicit bias in healthcare professionals: a systematic review. BMC Med Ethics 2017;18(1):19.

Taking the Pulse of the Current State of Simulation

Anisha Kshetrapal, MD, MSEd[a,*], Mary E. McBride, MD, MEd[b],
Candace Mannarino, MD[b]

KEYWORDS

- Simulation • Medical education • Critical care • Learning theory

KEY POINTS

- Simulation is a learning technique that has a broad history both outside of and within medicine.
- Its use in medical education is supported by multiple learning theories.
- Future directions include the use of virtual reality, better understanding of teamwork in medicine, and increasing diversity.

A BRIEF OVERVIEW OF SIMULATION HISTORY

Simulation in health care has its roots in other fields, including military training and aviation, and has become the standard process for training in those fields. To understand future directions of simulation in medical education, it is helpful to review its history. This article will give readers a broad overview of the history of simulation in other fields, the trajectory of simulation-based medical education (SBME) in general and in critical care, as well as outline future directions for simulation education and research.

In the past 2 centuries, medical education has evolved from being a simple apprenticeship to incorporating scientific principles, and now to defining learner competence across the spectrum of knowledge, skills, and attitudes. Deliberate practice has been applied to medical education only recently,[1] and the introduction of simulation in the second half of the twentieth century was a major step toward developing learner competence.[1]

The first visionary in simulation training in the modern era was Edwin Link, who invented the "blue box" flight trainer.[2] He believed that there must be a safer and less expensive way to learn to fly. It was initially an amusement park ride but when

[a] Department of Pediatrics, Division of Emergency Medicine, Ann & Robert H Lurie Children's Hospital of Chicago, 225 East Chicago Avenue, Box 62, Chicago, IL 60611, USA; [b] Depatment of Pediatrics, Divisions of Cardiology and Critical Care Medicine, Ann & Robert H Lurie Children's Hospital of Chicago, 225 East Chicago Avenue, Box 62, Chicago, IL 60611, USA
* Corresponding author.
E-mail address: akshetrapal@luriechildrens.org

Crit Care Clin 39 (2023) 373–384
https://doi.org/10.1016/j.ccc.2022.09.011
0749-0704/23/© 2022 Elsevier Inc. All rights reserved.

he opened his flying school in 1930, he used it to demonstrate the value of the trainer.[3] The Army invested in Link trainers before World War II, after the deaths of pilots who could not see the ground. Realism, complexity, and technology improved during the subsequent 2 decades. In the 1970s, full flight simulation was developed by commercial airlines to teach pilots. The 1980s brought cockpit resource management (CRM, later changed to crew or crisis resource management).[3] This team training method was introduced to improve team communication by junior pilots as well as address authoritative behavior by senior pilots. In the early 1990s, CRM expanded to include the flight crew, and later in the decade, shifted its focus to error management.[2]

SIMULATION IN MEDICINE

Rudimentary clinical simulation began with anatomic models used as early as the sixteenth century[4] but modern medical simulation began in the second half of the twentieth century under the influence of the medical education reform movement,[5] the resuscitation movement, and the Institute of Medicine's "To Err is Human" report.[6]

One of the first commercially available manikins was developed by toymaker and publisher Åsmund Lærdal in concert with anesthesiologists in 1960.[7] "Resusci-Anne" was a part-task trainer used to teach mouth-to-mouth ventilation and later chest compressions.[7] The first high-fidelity simulator was developed for anesthesiologists as well and named Sim One.[8] Sim One could be ventilated, breathe on its own, had carotid and temporal pulses, and responded to various interventions.[8] This model failed to achieve acceptance, in part because of cost, and in part, because a need for education outside of apprenticeship was not yet defined.[3] Since then, the use of simulation has increased steadily.

In the 1980s, David Gaba developed the comprehensive anesthesia simulation environment (CASE)[9] and developed a taxonomy of simulation: verbal (ie, role playing), standardized patients, part-task trainers, computer patients, and electronic patients.[10] Simulation came into widespread use with the recognition of information overload in medical education, as well as the changes of increased supervision and duty hour limits in graduate education. Proponents of simulation-based education recognized that simulation could provide a safe and effective learning environment without the risk of harm to patients. It allows learners of any level to improve skills, gain knowledge, and then apply those skills. Simulation training may also facilitate the transfer of knowledge from the simulation to the clinical environment.

Theoretic Bases of Simulation Research

Although Gaba asserted that "No industry in which human lives depend on the skilled performance of responsible operators has waited for the unequivocal proof of the benefit of simulation before embracing it,"[11,12] there has been an exponential increase of simulation research in the past 2 decades. As health-care simulation research has matured, it has moved away from whether simulation works to understanding the prerequisites for learning in the simulated environment, including understanding the theoretic underpinnings of simulation education, measuring outcomes, and addressing problems in simulation education.

Multiple complementary learning theories inform simulation and simulation research in health professions education, including social cognitive, adult learning, behavioral, constructivist, and cognitive load theories.[13] Social cognitive theory posits that all learning and professional development is contextual, with an emphasis on learning in real or simulated settings and socialization of learners into communities of practice.[14] It also suggests that learners can develop self-efficacy in this way.[14,15] Its use in simulation has been underscored by the proliferation of standardized patient teaching programs. Adult learning theory assumes that learners are self-motivated and self-directed.[13] Participating in simulated patient scenarios with an effective debriefing allows adult learners opportunities to identify and reflect on performance, goals, and mastery. Behavioral learning theory includes the development of deliberate practice that supports improvement of performance.[16] It has its roots in positivist philosophy and focuses on behavior change and improvement. Practical ways in which behavioral theory has influenced simulation-based learning include reliable measurement of observable behavior and specific, measurable, actionable, and timely feedback for performance improvement. Constructivist learning theory focuses on the perceptions, interpretations, and understandings of learners that influence their actions during simulation and patient care. It also includes the idea that teachers in simulation are facilitators more than they are coaches, and the idea that learners need self-reflection to progress.[14,16] For instance, Cheung and colleagues[17] reported a randomized controlled trial that included an observational component before hands-on practice of central venous catheter insertion skills, with the observation session intended to enhance motivation and provide a mental model for the task. They found that observation greatly improved skill acquisition. Cognitive load theory is girded by the fact there is a finite working memory capacity and duration, and when the capacity or duration of working memory is surpassed, learning is impaired. For example, an experiment was performed in which the perceived cognitive load of first-year medical students after simulation training and debriefing was compared with performance outcomes. Students with "very high" reported cognitive loads performed less well on subsequent testing compared with their colleagues.[18] These and other findings should lead to careful consideration of the goals and objectives of a particular simulation.[19]

The Kirkpatrick model is a well-known outcome evaluation tool and has been used to evaluate simulation programs widely.[20] It stratifies the level of impact of education with level 4 being clinical parameters and patient outcomes, level 3 changing in the participants' behavior after training, level 2 being individual learning, and level 1 being participants' initial reactions toward training. In a parallel framework, the idea of translational outcomes (moving science from bench to bedside) has also been used in evaluating medical education.[21] In SBME, translational science can be extrapolated to show that results seen in learners in the educational setting (T1) transfer to further patient care (T2) and improved patient health (T3).[21,22]

As simulation research has evolved during the past 50 years, ways of evaluating simulation have also evolved. One example, SimZones,[23] initially developed by Roussin and Weinstock, is an organizational framework developed to organize the development of simulation programs. The problems addressed include single-loop and double-loop learning, managing training of simulation faculty, participant mix, balancing simulation environments, and organizing simulation research. Single-loop learning is about mastering known skill sets, whereas double-loop learning refers to learning how to define and solve problems de novo. In this framework, simulations are divided into 4 zones. Zone 0 simulations include autofeedback exercises with individual learners, often using virtual technology. Zone 1 simulations include instruction of basic clinical skills. Zone 2 simulations include situational instruction for acute care patient episodes, such as mock codes. Zones 0 to 2 simulations are mastery-based, whereas zone 3 simulations are exploratory in nature and involve real-life teams to facilitate addressing team and system issues. The SimZones framework can be applied as a method of competency-based assessment and provides a way to conceptualize learning for both learners and facilitators.

The Current State of Simulation in Critical Care

Simulation is used broadly in critical care training for individual skill development, formative assessment, and team performance.[24] In a survey of US fellowship program directors in pediatric critical care medicine, nearly all use SBME to train fellows, with the majority perceiving simulation as necessary training.[25] For nearly half of the programs that responded, the SBME curriculum began within the last 6 years. Challenges included variability of equipment, lack of clarity of optimal modalities, lack of consensus around its use for formative versus summative training, and lack of sufficient faculty training.[25]

In critical care, individual, learner-focused education has been shown to improve both technical skills (TS) and nontechnical skills (NTS).[24] For instance, subjective improvement in NTS was observed in a simulation-based course using standardized patients to train fellows in giving bad news.[26] Team training when beginning hospital-based employment in the form of a "boot camp" is common.[27] Focused training during orientation often uses deliberate practice[1] for procedures such as airway management, venous line placement, arterial line placement, as well as CRM for team training.[28,29]

Simulation goals around teamwork in critical care are common as patient care during acute episodes is inherently team-based. Simulation may focus on the development of interprofessional teams and their approach to critical and novel situations, most commonly around cardiac arrest.[30] Several studies have shown improvement in both TS and team function using simulation.[31–36]

There have been shifts in the past decade on how to develop mastery learning via simulation, most significantly that of "rapid cycle deliberate practice" (RCDP). It was first published in 2014[37] and since then has gained support for SBME in many scenarios, including cardiac arrest and application of resuscitation algorithms. Learners have reported that they appreciated the interruptions in this technique of simulation, found them beneficial,[38] and recognized that the frequent interruptions helped minimize cognitive load. RCDP has been used to train specific actions within scenarios, such as more quickly initiating chest compression and defibrillation, and this training has correlated to increases in in-hospital arrest survival rates.[39] RCDP was also used to refine the process of basic life support, resulting in a "CPR coach" role, which increased compliance with the American Heart Association's Basic Life Support guidelines during in-hospital cardiac arrest.[36]

Critical care intersects with several specialties at the bedside, and simulation is often used to coordinate workplace education of teams that are not routinely educated together for complex patient care scenarios, specifically in the real clinical environment.[40,41] Practicing in this environment and using in situ resources allows for testing of the system and processes when faced with complex challenges that cross disciplines. In this way, simulation may provide an opportunity to expose system vulnerabilities, identify latent safety threats, and immediately debrief participants, while allowing for learning and maintaining psychological safety. For instance, a pediatric anaphylaxis scenario performed in 28 hospitals identified a high medication error rate, and debriefing revealed a common latent safety threat.[42] Learning opportunities from these system-focused simulations can be maximized by using a specific debriefing framework such as PEARLS,[43] which in turn is based on Systems Engineering Initiative for Patient Safety 2.0, a human-factors model of patient safety and the health-care system.[44] Acute care patient episodes also require strong leadership,[45,46] and leadership is now being studied in both simulated[47] and real[48] acute care patient episodes.

The SARS-CoV-2 pandemic provided another opportunity to use SBME and furthered the use of telesimulation.[49] Teams implemented both low-fidelity and high-fidelity simulations to take care of patients with COVID-19.[50] These simulations were implemented at several levels, focused on individuals as well as processes.[51] For example, Ramanathan and colleagues described using simulation training on a team level in full personal protective equipment during provision of extracorporeal membrane oxygenation services during a pandemic.[52] Dieckmann and colleagues detailed how simulation might be used in the future to prepare for a pandemic response using simulation on several different scales to practice different coordinated responses.[53] These simulations were carried out on team levels with intubations or code events, as well as simulating process changes required to accommodate more patients than usual during a pandemic surge. These simulations allow participants to be stakeholders in implementation of new processes.

Challenges and Future Directions

Both simulation and simulation research are evolving rapidly, and those supporting such research are identifying priorities for future simulation.[54,55] Harwayne-Gidansky and colleagues used a 3-round modified Delphi process to identify critical care topics taught using simulation and developed a list of topics and domains for critical care educators to focus on. The domains included (1) diagnosis and management, (2) procedural skills, (3) teamwork and communication skills, and (4) general knowledge.[54]

Separately, Anton and colleagues also used a 3-round modified Delphi approach to identify research priorities in simulation. Although 10 priorities were identified using this approach, the top 3 research questions identified were (1) understanding the impact of system-level simulation interventions on system efficiency, patient safety, and patient outcomes; (2) understanding the return on investment of simulation for health-care systems; and (3) whether a dose–response relationship exists between simulation training and outcomes.[55]

Specific challenges in health-care simulation include the developing technologies of virtual reality (VR), augmented reality (AR), and artificial intelligence (AI); further understanding teamwork; moving from outcomes toward program evaluation; as well as broader issues of diversity in medical education. We will discuss each of these in turn.

Although simulation is better characterized as a technique for learning rather than a technology itself, newer technologies such as VR, AR, and AI platforms are all being studied with increasing frequency as an adjunct to medical education and simulation for health professional training.[56] The advantage that these digital platforms offer is to allow trainees from multiple disciplines to learn independently and/or asynchronously from other users.

VR is a technology that provides the user with a completely computer-generated environment (such as a three-dimensional [3D] virtual world) through a computer-based device, including through mobile devices, projectors, or head-mounted devices.[57] VR technology use has increased for skills-based surgical simulation training in general surgery, urology, anesthesia, and orthopedic surgery. The use of VR has been reported in other health professions education settings including cadaveric dissection and human anatomy training and across disciplines including nursing skills training.[58–60] In a recent systematic review and meta-analysis, there was evidence to suggest that VR improves skills and knowledge postintervention when compared with traditional methods of education.[57] VR also has been used for NTS simulation including team building and effective communication, although evidence is limited on the effects.[61]

AR is defined as computer-generated technology that enhances the real-life environment perception via different sensory modalities.[62,63] The use of this technology has increased in recent years and has been applied in medical education training for multiple surgical specialties including neurosurgery, orthopedics, oral and maxillofacial surgery, and urology.[64,65] For example, an AR headset was created for placement of a ventricular drain for neurosurgery.[66] There is limited evidence that AR affects the development and outcomes postintervention.[62]

AI is defined as a machine or technological device built with the capacity to learn, reason, and perform other human tasks.[67] This is a rapidly advancing technology that is being applied to different aspects of health professions education including curriculum assessment and adjunctive virtual alternative to simulation for learners; however, data for use in simulation is limited.[67] Alonso-Silverio and colleagues recently published a study describing the development of a laparoscopic box trainer that incorporated AI algorithms and AR for surgical skills simulation.[67,68] These technologies will continue to evolve and may transform the field of medical education and simulation; however, further studies are needed to demonstrate the effectiveness of these platforms.

Several frameworks have informed the study of teamwork in simulation and clinical care thus far,[69] including CRM,[70,71] TeamSTEPPS,[72] and team reflexivity.[73] One stream of research studying teamwork uses a construct of relational coordination (RC). RC theory describes the factors that facilitate optimal work.[74,75] It specifies 3 attributes of relationships within organizations that support coordination: shared goals that transcend specific tasks, shared knowledge that enables team members to understand how their tasks interrelate, and mutual respect that allows members to overcome status barriers and positively regard the work of others. RC is a particularly helpful construct in situations where teams are faced with high levels of task interdependence, uncertainty, and time constraint.[75] Early studies in trauma care are promising and have resulted in interventions targeted at improving the relational foundations of trauma care delivery.[76,77]

For assessing outcomes, Kirkpatrick's model has been widely used[70,71,78,79] as previously discussed. However, its focus on outcomes fails to consider the factors that can affect those outcomes.[80] Level 1 and 2 outcomes are measured more frequently, likely because they are easier to measure.[71,78,81] Level 3 and 4 outcomes are more challenging to evaluate. There is also an assumption that the higher the level, the more important the outcome but this depends on the reason for the evaluation. By focusing on intended outcomes, Kirkpatrick's model neglects unintended impacts.[80]

In contrast to Kirkpatrick's model, program evaluation assumes that educational interventions are complex, and program evaluation is concerned with the design of the program in addition to outcomes.[80,82] Allen and colleagues[80] describe 6 theoretically situated frameworks for program evaluation that were chosen to aid exploration of unintended outcomes, understand factors influencing program implementation, as well and how and why impacts occur.

A final consideration on the future of simulation in critical care is that of diversity. Health professions education scholarship has not yet fully incorporated perspectives of minoritized groups in the development of educational theories and best practices.[83] There has been a sharp increase in studies of diversity in the past 2 years but, by contrast, relatively little research has been done on inclusion, which has important implications for simulation. When considering minoritized trainees and researchers in SBME, further delineation of what an "inclusive" environment is and how to create one is necessary.[84] Equity in SBME is directly related to issues of health-care equity in the broader sense. Further, there may be times when the goals of simulation and those of minoritized communities (eg, as standardized patients) may be at odds, and further research is required to delineate best practices in these situations.[85]

SUMMARY

The use of simulation has greatly expanded since its inception, broadening from simple task trainers to multidisciplinary simulations throughout hospital systems. Simulation is an ideal educational model because of its use of multiple educational theories to underpin its effectiveness, is flexible enough to be used for broad swath of learner topics, configurations, and technologies, and is evolving rapidly. Within critical care, simulation is ideal for focus on procedures, team training, resuscitation, and understanding the larger system of care. It provides a modality by which the objectives of individual learning may converge with broader objectives of improving patient care downstream. Research in critical care simulation continues a trajectory toward better frameworks for understanding teamwork as well as increased diversity. It has tremendous capacity to effect positive change by improving the knowledge base of learners and improving the complex processes in critical care.

CLINICS CARE POINTS

- Simulation is an evidence-based platform for medical education in critical care.
- Multiple learning theories underpin the validity of use of simulation for various objectives, including diagnostics, management, and teamwork.
- Increasing diversity and understanding teamwork are future directions of simulation research.

DISCLOSURE

M.E. McBride is a paid consultant for the American Heart Association.

REFERENCES

1. Ericsson KA. Deliberate practice and the Acquisition and Maintenance of Expert performance in medicine and related domains. Acad Med 2004;79(10):S70–81.
2. Page RL. Brief History of Flight Simulation. Presented at: SimTecT 2000 Proceedings; 2000.
3. Rosen KR. The history of medical simulation. J Crit Care 2008;23(2):157–66.
4. Ballestriero R. Anatomical models and wax Venuses: art masterpieces or scientific craft works? J Anat 2010;216(2):223–34.
5. ACGME Common Program Requirements. Accreditation program for graduate medical education. 2017. Available at: https://www.acgme.org/Portals/0/PFAssets/ProgramRequirements/CPRs_2017-07-01.pdf.
6. Kohn L, Corrigan J, Molla S. To Err is human: building a safer health system. National Academy Press; 1999.
7. Tjomsland N, Baskett P. Åsmund S. Lærdal. Resuscitation 2002;53(2):115–9. https://doi.org/10.1016/s0300-9572(02)00033-3.
8. Denson JS, Abrahamson S. A computer-controlled patient simulator. Jama 1969;208(3):504–8. https://doi.org/10.1001/jama.1969.03160030078009.

9. Gaba DM, DeAnda A. A comprehensive anesthesia simulation environment. Anesthesiology 1988;69(3):387–94. https://doi.org/10.1097/00000542-198809000-00017.

10. Cooper JB, Taqueti VR. A brief history of the development of mannequin simulators for clinical education and training. Qual Saf Heal Care 2004;13(suppl_1): i11–8. https://doi.org/10.1136/qhc.13.suppl_1.i11.

11. Gaba DM. Improving anesthesiologists' performance by simulating reality. Anesthesiology 1992;76(4):491–4. https://doi.org/10.1097/00000542-199204000-00001.

12. Aebersold M. The history of simulation and its impact on the future. Aacn Adv Crit Care 2016;27(1):56–61. https://doi.org/10.4037/aacnacc2016436.

13. Felix H, Simon L. Conceptual frameworks in medical simulation. In: StatPearls. 2022. Available at: https://www-ncbi-nlm-nih-gov.ezproxy.galter.northwestern.edu/books/NBK547741/.

14. McGaghie WC, Harris IB. Learning theory foundations of simulation-based mastery learning. Simul Healthc J Soc Simul Healthc 2018;13(3S):S15–20. https://doi.org/10.1097/sih.0000000000000279.

15. Burke H, Mancuso L. Social cognitive theory, metacognition, and simulation learning in nursing education. J Nurs Educ 2012;51(10):543–8. https://doi.org/10.3928/01484834-20120820-02.

16. Chauvin SW. Applying educational theory to simulation-based training and assessment in surgery. Surg Clin N Am 2015;95(4):695–715. https://doi.org/10.1016/j.suc.2015.04.006.

17. Cheung JJH, Koh J, Brett C, et al. Preparation with Web-based observational practice improves efficiency of simulation-based mastery learning. Simul Healthc J Soc Simul Healthc 2016;11(5):316–22. https://doi.org/10.1097/sih.0000000000000171.

18. Fraser K, Ma I, Teteris E, et al. Emotion, cognitive load and learning outcomes during simulation training. Med Educ 2012;46(11):1055–62. https://doi.org/10.1111/j.1365-2923.2012.04355.x.

19. Fraser KL, Ayres P, Sweller J. Cognitive load theory for the design of medical simulations. Simul Healthc J Soc Simul Healthc 2015;10(5):295–307. https://doi.org/10.1097/sih.0000000000000097.

20. Kirkpatrick D. Evaluating training programs. San Francisco, CA: McGaw-Hill Education; 1975.

21. McGaghie WC. Medical education research as translational science. Sci Trans Med 2010;17(2). https://doi.org/10.1126/scitranslmed.3000679.

22. Dougherty D, Conway PH. The "3T's" Road Map to transform US health care: the "how" of high-quality care. Jama 2008;299(19):2319–21. https://doi.org/10.1001/jama.299.19.2319.

23. Roussin CJ, Weinstock P. SimZones. Acad Med 2017;92(8):1114–20. https://doi.org/10.1097/acm.0000000000001746.

24. Harwayne-Gidansky I, Panesar R, Maa T. Recent Advances in simulation for pediatric critical care medicine. Curr Pediatr Rep 2020;8(4):147–56. https://doi.org/10.1007/s40124-020-00226-5.

25. Henricksen JW, Troy L, Siefkes H. Pediatric critical care medicine fellowship simulation Use survey. Pediatr Crit Care Me 2020;21(10):e908–14. https://doi.org/10.1097/pcc.0000000000002343.

26. Johnson EM, Hamilton MF, Watson RS, et al. An Intensive, simulation-based communication course for pediatric critical care medicine fellows. Pediatr Crit Care Me 2017;18(8):e348–55. https://doi.org/10.1097/pcc.0000000000001241.

27. Fernandez GL, Page DW, Coe NP, et al. Boot camp: educational outcomes after 4 Successive Years of Preparatory simulation-based training at Onset of Internship. J Surg Educ 2012;69(2):242–8. https://doi.org/10.1016/j.jsurg.2011.08.007.

28. Nishisaki A, Hales R, Biagas K, et al. A multi-institutional high-fidelity simulation "boot camp" orientation and training program for first year pediatric critical care fellows. Pediatr Crit Care Me 2009;10(2):157–62. https://doi.org/10.1097/pcc.0b013e3181956d29.

29. Cohen ER, Barsuk JH, Moazed F, et al. Making july safer. Acad Med 2013;88(2): 233–9. https://doi.org/10.1097/acm.0b013e31827bfc0a.

30. Weile J, Nebsbjerg MA, Ovesen SH, et al. Simulation-based team training in time-critical clinical presentations in emergency medicine and critical care: a review of the literature. Adv Simul 2021;6(1):3. https://doi.org/10.1186/s41077-021-00154-4.

31. Cheng A, Brown LL, Duff JP, et al. Improving cardiopulmonary resuscitation with a CPR feedback device and Refresher simulations (CPR CARES study): a random-ized clinical trial. Jama Pediatr 2015;169(2):137–44. https://doi.org/10.1001/jamapediatrics.2014.2616.

32. Cheng A, Duff JP, Kessler D, et al. Optimizing CPR performance with CPR coach-ing for pediatric cardiac arrest: a randomized simulation-based clinical trial. Resuscitation 2018;132:33–40. https://doi.org/10.1016/j.resuscitation.2018.08.021.

33. Cheng A, Kessler D, Lin Y, et al. Influence of cardiopulmonary resuscitation coaching and provider role on perception of cardiopulmonary resuscitation qual-ity during simulated pediatric cardiac arrest. Pediatr Crit Care Me 2019. https://doi.org/10.1097/pcc.0000000000001871.

34. Dewan M, Tegtmeyer K. Let's Get it Right, set it up Again: Achieving high Reli-ability through simulation and debriefing. Pediatr Crit Care Me 2019;20(5): 497–9. https://doi.org/10.1097/pcc.0000000000001908.

35. Cory MJ, Colman N, McCracken CE, et al. Rapid cycle deliberate practice versus reflective debriefing for pediatric Septic Shock training. Pediatr Crit Care Me 2019. https://doi.org/10.1097/pcc.0000000000001891.

36. Hunt EA, Jeffers J, McNamara L, et al. Improved cardiopulmonary resuscitation performance with code ACES2: a resuscitation quality Bundle. J Am Hear Assoc Cardiovasc Cerebrovasc Dis 2018;7(24):e009860. https://doi.org/10.1161/jaha.118.009860.

37. Hunt EA, Duval-Arnould JM, Nelson-McMillan KL, et al. Pediatric resident resus-citation skills improve after "Rapid Cycle Deliberate Practice" training. Resuscita-tion 2014;85(7):945–51. https://doi.org/10.1016/j.resuscitation.2014.02.025.

38. Chancey RJ, Sampayo EM, Lemke DS, et al. Learners' Experiences during rapid cycle deliberate practice simulations. Simul Healthc J Soc Simul Healthc 2019; 14(1):18–28. https://doi.org/10.1097/sih.0000000000000324.

39. Andreatta P, Saxton E, Thompson M, et al. Simulation-based mock codes signif-icantly correlate with improved pediatric patient cardiopulmonary arrest survival rates&ast. Pediatr Crit Care Me 2011;12(1):33–8. https://doi.org/10.1097/pcc.0b013e3181e89270.

40. Sawyer T, Burke C, McMullan DM, et al. Impacts of a pediatric extracorporeal car-diopulmonary resuscitation (ECPR) simulation training program. Acad Pediatr 2019;19(5):566–71. https://doi.org/10.1016/j.acap.2019.01.005.

41. Lind MM, Corridore M, Sheehan C, et al. A multidisciplinary approach to a pedi-atric Difficult airway simulation course. Otolaryngol Head Neck Surg 2018;159(1): 127–35. https://doi.org/10.1177/0194599818758993.

42. Maa T, Scherzer DJ, Harwayne-Gidansky I, et al. Prevalence of errors in anaphylaxis in Kids (PEAK): a Multicenter simulation-based study. J Allergy Clin Immunol Pract 2020;8(4):1239–46. https://doi.org/10.1016/j.jaip.2019.11.013, e3.

43. Dubé MM, Reid J, Kaba A, et al. PEARLS for systems Integration: a modified PEARLS framework for debriefing systems-focused simulations. Simul Healthc J Soc Simul Healthc 2019;14(5):333–42. https://doi.org/10.1097/sih.0000000000000381.

44. Holden RJ, Carayon P, Gurses AP, et al. Seips 2.0: a human factors framework for studying and improving the work of healthcare professionals and patients. Ergonomics 2013;56(11):1669–86. https://doi.org/10.1080/00140139.2013.838643.

45. Hunziker S, Johansson AC, Tschan F, et al. Teamwork and leadership in cardiopulmonary resuscitation. J Am Coll Cardiol 2011;57(24):2381–8. https://doi.org/10.1016/j.jacc.2011.03.017.

46. Grimsley EA, Cochrane NH, Keane RR, et al. A pulse Check on leadership and teamwork. Pediatr Emerg Care 2021;37(12):e1122–7. https://doi.org/10.1097/pec.0000000000001923.

47. Nadkarni LD, Roskind CG, Auerbach MA, et al. The development and Validation of a Concise Instrument for formative assessment of team leader performance during simulated pediatric resuscitations. Simul Healthc J Soc Simul Healthc 2018;13(2):77–82. https://doi.org/10.1097/sih.0000000000000267.

48. Florez AR, Shepard LN, Frey ME, et al. The Concise assessment of leader management tool: evaluation of healthcare provider leadership during real-life pediatric Emergencies. Simul Healthc J Soc Simul Healthc 2022. https://doi.org/10.1097/sih.0000000000000669.

49. Lin E, You AX, Wardi G. Comparison of in-Person and Telesimulation for critical care training during the COVID-19 pandemic. Ats Scholar 2021;2(4):581–94. https://doi.org/10.34197/ats-scholar.2021-0053oc.

50. Huda T, Greig D, Strang T, et al. Preparation for COVID-19: lessons from simulation. Clin Teach 2020;18(1). https://doi.org/10.1111/tct.13262.

51. Mastoras G, Farooki N, Willinsky J, et al. Rapid deployment of a virtual simulation curriculum to prepare for critical care triage during the COVID-19 pandemic. Cjem 2022;1–8. https://doi.org/10.1007/s43678-022-00280-6.

52. Ramanathan K, Antognini D, Combes A, et al. Planning and provision of ECMO services for severe ARDS during the COVID-19 pandemic and other outbreaks of emerging infectious diseases. Lancet Respir Med 2020;8(5):518–26. https://doi.org/10.1016/s2213-2600(20)30121-1.

53. Dieckmann P, Torgeirsen K, Qvindesland SA, et al. The use of simulation to prepare and improve responses to infectious disease outbreaks like COVID-19: practical tips and resources from Norway, Denmark, and the UK. Adv Simul 2020;5(1):3. https://doi.org/10.1186/s41077-020-00121-5.

54. Harwayne-Gidansky I, Zurca A, Maa T, et al. Defining priority Areas for critical care simulation: a modified Delphi consensus Project. Cureus 2021;13(6): e15844. https://doi.org/10.7759/cureus.15844.

55. Anton N, Calhoun AC, Stefanidis D. Current research priorities in healthcare simulation: results of a Delphi survey. Simul Healthc J Soc Simul Healthc 2022;17(1): e1–7. https://doi.org/10.1097/sih.0000000000000564.

56. Walsh C, Lydon S, Byrne D, et al. The 100 most Cited articles on healthcare simulation. Simul Healthc J Soc Simul Healthc 2018;13(3):211–20. https://doi.org/10.1097/sih.0000000000000293.

57. Kyaw BM, Saxena N, Posadzki P, et al. Virtual reality for health professions education: systematic review and meta-analysis by the digital health education Collaboration. J Med Internet Res 2019;21(1). https://doi.org/10.2196/12959.

58. Foronda CL, Fernandez-Burgos M, Nadeau C, et al. Virtual simulation in nursing education: a systematic review Spanning 1996 to 2018. Simul Healthc J Soc Simul Healthc 2020;15(1):46–54. https://doi.org/10.1097/sih.0000000000000411.

59. Ralston BH, Willett RC, Namperumal S, et al. Use of virtual reality for pediatric cardiac critical care simulation. Cureus 2021;13(6):e15856. https://doi.org/10.7759/cureus.15856.

60. Uruthiralingam U, Rea PM. Augmented and virtual reality in anatomical education – a systematic review. Adv Exp Med Biol 2020;89–101. https://doi.org/10.1007/978-3-030-37639-0_5.

61. Bracq MS, Michinov E, Jannin P. Virtual reality simulation in nontechnical skills training for healthcare professionals. Simul Healthc J Soc Simul Healthc 2018. https://doi.org/10.1097/sih.0000000000000347.

62. Barsom EZ, Graafland M, Schijven MP. Systematic review on the effectiveness of augmented reality applications in medical training. Surg Endosc 2016;30(10):4174–83. https://doi.org/10.1007/s00464-016-4800-6.

63. Eckert M, Volmerg JS, Friedrich CM. Augmented reality in medicine: systematic and Bibliographic review. JMIR Mhealth Uhealth 2019;26(7). https://doi.org/10.2196/10967.

64. Yoon JW, Chen RE, Kim EJ, et al. Augmented reality for the surgeon: systematic review. Int J Med Robotics Comput Assisted Surg 2018;14(4):e1914. https://doi.org/10.1002/rcs.1914.

65. Cannizzaro D, Zaed I, Safa A, et al. Augmented reality in neurosurgery, state of art and future Projections. A systematic review. Front Surg 2022;9:864792. https://doi.org/10.3389/fsurg.2022.864792.

66. Schneider M, Kunz C, Pal'a A, et al. Augmented reality–assisted ventriculostomy. Neurosurg Focus 2021;50(1):E16. https://doi.org/10.3171/2020.10.focus20779.

67. Chan KS, Zary N. Applications and challenges of implementing artificial intelligence in medical education: Integrative review. JMIR Med Educ 2019;5(1). https://doi.org/10.2196/13930.

68. Alonso-Silverio GA, Pérez-Escamirosa F, Bruno-Sanchez R, et al. Development of a laparoscopic box trainer based on open Source Hardware and artificial intelligence for objective assessment of surgical Psychomotor skills. Surg Innov 2018;25(4):380–8. https://doi.org/10.1177/1553350618777045.

69. Weaver SJ, Dy SM, Rosen MA. Team-training in healthcare: a narrative synthesis of the literature. Bmj Qual Saf 2014;23(5):359–72. https://doi.org/10.1136/bmjqs-2013-001848.

70. Issenberg SB, Mcgaghie WC, Petrusa ER, et al. Features and uses of high-fidelity medical simulations that lead to effective learning: a BEME systematic review. Med Teach 2009;27(1):10–28. https://doi.org/10.1080/01421590500046924.

71. Steinert Y, Mann K, Anderson B, et al. A systematic review of faculty development initiatives designed to enhance teaching effectiveness: a 10-year update: BEME Guide No. 40. Med Teach 2016;38(8):1–18. https://doi.org/10.1080/0142159x.2016.1181851.

72. TeamSTEPPS 2.0. Agency for healthcare research and quality. 2019. Available at: https://www.ahrq.gov/teamstepps/instructor/onlinecourse.html.

73. Schmutz JB, Lei Z, Eppich WJ. Reflection on the fly: development of the team reflection behavioral observation (TuRBO) system for acute care teams. Acad Med 2021;96(9):1337–45. https://doi.org/10.1097/acm.0000000000004105.

74. Gittell J. High performance healthcare: using the Power of relationships to achieve quality, efficiency and resilience. McGraw-Hill; 2009.

75. Gittell J. Transforming relationships for high performance. Stanford University Press; 2016.

76. Purdy EI, McLean D, Alexander C, et al. Doing our work better, together: a relationship-based approach to defining the quality improvement agenda in trauma care. Bmj Open Qual 2020;9(1):e000749. https://doi.org/10.1136/bmjoq-2019-000749.

77. Purdy E, Alexander C, Shaw R, et al. The team briefing: setting up relational co-ordination for your resuscitation. Clin Exp Emerg Med 2020;7(1):1–4. https://doi.org/10.15441/ceem.19.021.

78. Leslie K, Baker L, Egan-Lee E, et al. Advancing faculty development in medical education. Acad Med 2013;88(7):1038–45. https://doi.org/10.1097/acm.0b013e318294fd29.

79. Onyura B, Baker L, Cameron B, et al. Evidence for curricular and instructional design approaches in undergraduate medical education: an umbrella review. Med Teach 2015;38(2):150–61. https://doi.org/10.3109/0142159x.2015.1009019.

80. Allen LM, Hay M, Palermo C. Evaluation in health professions education—is measuring outcomes enough? Med Educ 2022;56(1):127–36. https://doi.org/10.1111/medu.14654.

81. Yardley S, Dornan T. Kirkpatrick's levels and education 'evidence. Med Educ 2012;46(1):97–106. https://doi.org/10.1111/j.1365-2923.2011.04076.x.

82. Frye AW, Hemmer PA. Program evaluation models and related theories: AMEE Guide No. 67. Med Teach 2012;34(5):e288–99. https://doi.org/10.3109/0142159x.2012.668637.

83. Maduakolam E, Madden B, Kelley T, et al. Beyond diversity: Envisioning inclusion in medical education research and practice. Teach Learn Med 2020;32(5):459–65. https://doi.org/10.1080/10401334.2020.1836462.

84. Fernandez A. Further incorporating diversity, equity, and inclusion into medical education research. Acad Med 2019;94:S5–6. https://doi.org/10.1097/acm.0000000000002916, 11S Association of American Medical Colleges Learn Serve Lead: Proceedings of the 58th Annual Research in Medical Education Sessions).

85. Picketts L, Warren MD, Bohnert C. Diversity and inclusion in simulation: addressing ethical and psychological safety concerns when working with simulated participants. Bmj Simul Technology Enhanc Learn 2021;7(6):590–9. https://doi.org/10.1136/bmjstel-2020-000853.

Translating Guidelines into Practical Practice

Point-of-Care Ultrasound for Pediatric Critical Care Clinicians

Mark D. Weber, RN, CPNP-AC, FCCM[a],*, Joel K.B. Lim, MBBS, MRCPCH[b],
Sarah Ginsburg, MD[c], Thomas Conlon, MD[a],
Akira Nishisaki, MD, MSCE[a]

KEYWORDS

• Pediatric critical care • Ultrasound • POCUS • Guidelines

KEY POINTS

- Point-of-care ultrasound (POCUS) is an emerging technology that can provide immediate answers to clinical questions at the bedside.
- Expert guidelines are now available to direct the application of POCUS for the critical care provider.
- Recognizing the limitations of the current guidelines and formalizing the next steps in POCUS development will further increase the utility of this valuable tool.

INTRODUCTION

During the 1990s, the broad use of point-of-care ultrasound (POCUS) by nonradiologists within the emergency department was met with misgivings.[1] Since that time, clinicians have realized measurable benefits of POCUS, resulting in American College of Emergency Physicians guidelines published in 2001.[2] Adult and pediatric critical care providers now also use POCUS applications for procedural and diagnostic applications frequently encountered in their respective care settings.[3–5] With the rapid growth in critical care POCUS, there is a need for a more structured approach to education, credentialing, and its application at the bedside.

[a] Division of Critical Care Medicine, Department of Anesthesiology and Critical Care Medicine, Children's Hospital of Philadelphia, University of Pennsylvania, Philadelphia, PA 19104, USA; [b] Children's Intensive Care Unit, Department of Pediatric Subspecialties, KK Women's and Children's Hospital, Singapore; [c] Division of Critical Care Medicine, Department of Pediatrics, University of Texas Southwestern Medical Center, Dallas, TX, USA
* Corresponding author. Wood 6025, 3401 Civic Center Boulevard, Philadelphia, PA 19104.
E-mail address: weberm@chop.edu

Crit Care Clin 39 (2023) 385–406
https://doi.org/10.1016/j.ccc.2022.09.012
0749-0704/23/© 2022 Elsevier Inc. All rights reserved.

In 2015 and 2016, the Society of Critical Care Medicine (SCCM) published both procedural and diagnostic evidence-based guidelines for POCUS applications in adult critical care with pediatric considerations included.[6,7] In 2020, the European Society of Pediatric and Neonatal Intensive Care (ESPNIC) published guidelines specific to pediatric and neonatal populations, including 41 statements on the use of POCUS[8] (Supplemental Table 1). Although both SCCM and ESPNIC guidelines provide an important beginning toward incorporating relevant POCUS applications in clinical practice, they are not meant to deliver a comprehensive POCUS education curriculum for pediatric critical care practitioners. The authors review SCCM and ESPNIC guidelines within cores of applications (ie, procedural, cardiac, thoracic, abdominal, and neurologic), discuss strengths and limitations of statements, explore unanswered questions, and suggest important considerations when translating POCUS education to the care of critically ill children.

PROCEDURAL ULTRASOUND

The dawn of ultrasound for vascular access procedures was heralded by the use of doppler to localize the internal jugular vein (IJV) in the late 1970s.[9,10] Several years later, ultrasound was used for direct visualization of the IJV and subclavian veins (SCVs).[11] POCUS to both visualize vessels and guide cannulation became accepted practice for frequently accessed central vessels, including IJVs,[12] femoral veins,[13] and SCVs.[14] With the progression of its adoption for central venous access, there has been a parallel acceptance of the use of POCUS as an adjunct for securing both peripheral venous and arterial access.[15,16]

Both SCCM and ESPNIC guidelines presented strong expert agreement for the use of POCUS for IJV and femoral venous access (**Table 1**). The data demonstrate a decrease in insertion attempts, decrease in arterial punctures, and increased success rates.[17–20] Although the SCCM guidelines cited strong evidence in the adult population, they reported a paucity of data in support of POCUS for IJV placement in children, citing a meta-analysis with equivocal support for POCUS use versus the landmark technique in infants and children.[21] The ESPNIC group subsequently found strong pediatric evidence, grade A, to support the use of POCUS for pediatric IJV line placement. Notably, the meta-analysis cited by SCCM guidelines was in pediatric cardiac populations, and increased benefits of POCUS were noted when POCUS was used by novice providers in the operating room. This may reflect the challenges of training experienced providers new techniques.

POCUS for the use of SCV and axillary vein cannulation had strong agreement in ESPNIC guidelines but conditional agreement in SCCM guidelines.[6–8] Data in the pediatric and adult population demonstrate safe cannulation of the subclavian and brachiocephalic veins using POCUS for guidance.[22–25] These benefits translate even to neonates weighing less than 1500 g.[26]

Arterial access may also benefit from the use of POCUS. The strength of data is not as robust, leading to both ESPNIC and SCCM giving agreement and conditional support, respectively.[6–8] Literature suggests integration of POCUS results in shorter time to arterial cannulation with fewer attempts compared with palpation technique.[15,27,28] These benefits are also found in the neonatal population.[29] Despite growing literature supporting use of POCUS in peripheral vascular access to improve provider performance and patient outcomes in both children and neonates, neither guidelines commented on this important application.

Technically, a short-axis out-of-plane (SA-OOP) approach is most commonly used for POCUS-guided vascular access.[11] The SA-OOP approach is recommended by the

Table 1
Vascular access procedural statements achieving strong agreement in European Society of Pediatric and Neonatal Intensive Care guidelines with corresponding Society of Critical Care Medicine statement

Summary of POCUS Application Statement	ESPNIC Level of Evidence	SCCM Strength of Recommendation	SCCM Pediatric Discussion	SCCM Pediatric-Specific	SCCM Level of Evidence
Internal jugular line placement	A	1	Yes	No	A
Subclavian line placement	B	2	No	No	C
Femoral line placement	B	1	Yes	No	A
Verification of catheter tip position	C	2	No	No	B

Table 1 summarizes the point-of-care ultrasound application within ESPNIC statements with strong agreement among experts. Corresponding level of evidence within the ESPNIC guidelines is defined using GRADE criteria with A as "high," B as "moderate," C as "low," and D as "very low." SCCM guidelines were reviewed to evaluate whether a statement was made corresponding to the ESPNIC statement achieving strong agreement. Strength of recommendation within SCCM guidelines is defined as 1, "strong recommendation"; 2, "weak/conditional recommendation"; and 3, "not reaching agreement." The table also indicates whether pediatric data are included in the discussion of the statement or the statement is pediatric-specific.

SCCM guidelines,[6] as it is an easier skill to acquire over the long-axis in-plane (LA-IP) approach, with early studies showing increased success of SA-OOP over the LA-IP approach.[30–32] Over time, more data have been published on the benefits of an LA-IP approach, with reports of reduced arterial punctures, increased first attempt success, and decreased catheter misplacements.[25,26,33,34] In studies using gel-based phantoms, fewer posterior wall punctures were noted when using the LA-IP approach as opposed to the SA-OOP approach.[35] Although it may be a more challenging technique to master, the above benefits of the LA-IP approach may allow for safer access of the vessel over the SA-OOP approach.

Numerous publications exist regarding the approach to POCUS training for procedural applications. Both manikins and more advanced dynamic haptic trainers provide educational benefits to trainees in IJV placement, including a decrease in procedural time.[36] Another potential training modality includes a real-time 3-dimensional mixed reality simulator. This training approach has led to improved provider confidence with more technically challenging approaches, such as landmark approaches in the supraclavicular subclavian catheter placement.[37] The use of newer needle navigation technology has had mixed reviews with trainees. A study of anesthesia residents within an adult intensive care unit (ICU) revealed that needle navigation technology led to lower satisfaction scores and longer procedure times among experienced providers.[38] On the other hand, a study wherein the technology was implemented with radiology residents found it to be beneficial. It may be that the radiology residents are more comfortable with newer technologies that require complex spatial relations.[39]

In addition, there have been novel approaches to the didactic component of POCUS education. Didactic educational formats have been successfully implemented using an online approach. This online approach could be applied to geographic areas where POCUS educators are limited and is particularly relevant in the era of the SARS-CoV-2 pandemic when large gatherings are avoided. When an online approach is used, follow-up hands-on simulation sessions to solidify a learner's psychomotor skill are essential.[40] As with any education experience, POCUS trainees with the highest level of motivation will benefit most from online training, leading to greater confidence and independence.[41,42]

Following the implementation of hands-on and didactic training, it is imperative to follow the procedural competency of trainees to ensure their skills are progressing as expected. Tools capable of measuring procedural competency are essential to develop and may identify areas of weakness for targeted education.[43–45] Such tools should measure not only psychomotor technique but also essential aspects of preprocedural planning, patient safety considerations, communication skills, and teamwork.[44] Educators can use cumulative sum (CUSUM) analysis charts to track individual skill acquisition over time. CUSUM charts have been used in ultrasound-guided peripheral intravenous cannulation skill acquisition among anesthesiology trainees to determine competency.[45] The investigators noted that with the CUSUM charts it was possible to detect an individual's deterioration in competency before their averages of failed attempts identify issues. With this approach, remediation in training can be implemented early before poor techniques become engrained into practice.

CARDIAC ULTRASOUND

Cardiac ultrasonography has become a valuable tool in assessing critically ill patients, including patients with shock,[46] dyspnea,[47] and cardiac arrest.[48] Although acknowledging the extensive utility of this application, it is important to distinguish the scope of cardiac POCUS compared with traditional echocardiography performed by cardiologists. Singh and colleagues[49] define cardiac POCUS as a tool for intensivists to "answer a defined clinical question" that informs patient management, often in a time-sensitive manner (**Table 2**). These scans can help providers decide on therapies, further evaluation, and when to involve advanced consultants.

Globally, the scope of cardiac POCUS addresses basic questions of qualitative ventricular function, ventricular size relationships, gross estimates of right ventricular (RV) pressure, preload and fluid responsive conditions, and the presence of pericardial effusion. Further training in cardiac POCUS can allow for "semiquantitative" measurements of function and pressure by intensivists at the bedside.[8] However, comprehensive evaluation of cardiac structure and function falls into the realm of formal cardiology-performed echocardiography. As such, the ESPNIC guidelines state with strong agreement that ultrasound should not be used for screening or evaluation of congenital heart disease without advanced cardiology training. The SCCM guidelines support this conclusion, although on lower strength of evidence. Similarly, the guidelines do not support evaluation for acquired defects, such as acquired valvular disease, per SCCM, or endocarditis, per ESPNIC.

One caveat to the statements on structural evaluation involves the assessment of patent ductus arteriosus (PDA) in neonates. Once a formal echocardiogram has excluded ductal-dependent structural heart disease, serial POCUS can be used to assess and trend PDA patency over time or to assess hypotensive patients without congenital heart disease. With advanced training, bedside providers may be able to delineate PDA characteristics, such as diameter, flow direction, velocity, and hemodynamic significance of the shunt.[50,51] ESPNIC supports POCUS PDA assessment with strong agreement, whereas SCCM cites good consensus although low quality of evidence (2C) and indicates that the scans should be performed specifically by providers with advanced training.

The assessment of patients' fluid status and volume responsiveness is an essential part of critical care, yet remains complicated by the lack a gold-standard method for measurement.[52,53] On the topic of fluid status, the ESPNIC guidelines suggest, with strong agreement, POCUS "may be helpful" for determining volume status and preload responsiveness, although cites grade D (very low) evidence. In comparison, SCCM guidelines support similar recommendations for pediatrics with very good consensus and grade 1B evidence. Evaluation of the inferior vena cava (IVC) dimension and respiratory variation is the most easily accessible parameter for assessing preload conditions via POCUS. However, although studies in intubated adults demonstrated an association between IVC distensibility and volume status[54] as well as fluid responsiveness,[55] a similar study of pediatric patients intubated for surgery did not find that IVC respiratory variation accurately predicted fluid responsiveness.[56] In spontaneously breathing patients, an IVC collapsibility index greater than 50% has been considered highly predictive for fluid responsiveness.[57] However, meta-analyses in both adult[58] and pediatric settings[59] failed to show a consistent association between IVC variation and fluid responsiveness. This may be explained by the complex interactions between variables that impact on IVC dimensions, such as volume status, venous capacitance, tricuspid regurgitation (TR), cardiac compliance and function, respiratory effort, and intrathoracic and intra-abdominal pressures. In an attempt to standardize conditions for IVC assessment, adult studies often cite a goal of 8 mL/kg of tidal volume in a sedated patient without spontaneous respiratory effort.

The respiratory variation of both the peak aortic blood flow velocity and the velocity-time integral (VTI) measured across the left ventricular (LV) outflow tract has been

Table 2
Cardiac statements achieving strong agreement in European Society of Pediatric and Neonatal Intensive Care guidelines with corresponding Society of Critical Care Medicine statement

Summary of POCUS Application Statement	Advanced Training Recommended	ESPNIC Level of Evidence	SCCM Strength of Recommendation	SCCM Level of Evidence	SCCM Pediatric-specific
Screening for congenital heart defects	Yes	A	2	C	Yes
Assessment of preload	No	D	1	B	Yes
Assessment of fluid responsiveness	No	D	1	B	Yes
Qualitative assessment of function	No	D	1	C	Yes
Assessment of pulmonary artery pressure	Yes	B	1	B	Yes
Semiquantitative assessment of PAH	No	B	1	B	Yes
Assessment of pericardial effusion	No	B	1	C	No
Guide pericardiocentesis	No	B	1	C	No
Assess patency of ductus arteriosus	Yes	A	2	C	Yes

Table 2 summarizes the POCUS application within ESPNIC statements with strong agreement among experts. Corresponding level of evidence within the ESPNIC guidelines is defined using GRADE criteria with A as "high," B as "moderate," C as "low," and D as "very low." SCCM guidelines were reviewed to evaluate whether a statement was made corresponding to the ESPNIC statement achieving strong agreement. Strength of recommendation within SCCM guidelines is defined as 1, "strong recommendation"; 2, "weak/conditional recommendation"; and 3, "not reaching agreement." The table also indicates whether pediatric data are included in the discussion of the statement or the statement is pediatric-specific.

Abbreviations: N/A, statements were not applicable and without recommendations due to lack of agreement; PAH, pulmonary artery hypertension.

demonstrated to accurately predict fluid responsiveness in both adults and children.[59–65] Using VTI, stroke volume and cardiac output can be calculated and trended over time in critically ill patients. Measuring VTI requires an appropriately oriented apical 5-chamber view and the ability to capture pulse-wave doppler, making it a higher-level skill compared with IVC measurement.

For ventricular function, basic cardiac POCUS uses a qualitative approach to "eyeball" systolic function. Studies have shown such assessments are accurate when compared with formal echocardiographic measurements, particularly for LV systolic function.[66–69] The ESPNIC guidelines state with strong agreement that POCUS "may be helpful" for qualitative assessment, although citing grade D evidence. Quantitative assessments of systolic function, including shortening fraction and ejection fraction for the LV and tricuspid annular plane systolic excursion for the RV, are noted as "helpful" by ESPNIC with grade C evidence. Such calculations require more advanced POCUS skills and should be learned under expert guidance.[70,71]

Cardiac POCUS should be used as a part of holistic clinical hemodynamic assessment of critically ill patients.[46,72,73] As such, the SCCM guidelines do not comment on specific types of functional evaluation but rather applications to shock states. In suspected pediatric cardiogenic shock, the guidelines suggest using cardiac POCUS with an overall recommendation grade of 2C with good consensus. Because of lack of data, the guidelines do not make a recommendation on using cardiac POCUS to evaluate function in pediatric septic shock, although there is growing literature that POCUS can guide resuscitation in pediatric septic shock.[74,75]

Citing similar lack of evidence, the SCCM guidelines do not make a recommendation on the use of cardiac POCUS to specifically evaluate RV function in pediatric patients. In comparison, ESPNIC, with strong agreement, supports the use of cardiac POCUS to evaluate for pulmonary hypertension in neonates and children on grade B evidence (moderate quality evidence). With basic cardiac views, the shape of the interventricular septum in the parasternal short-axis view can indicate RV hypertension when the septum is flattened or bowing. More advanced studies include measurement of the TR velocity, when a TR jet is present, to calculate pulmonary artery systolic pressure using the Bernoulli equation.[71,76] Because of transitional physiology and risk of persistent pulmonary hypertension in neonates, bedside assessment of TR is part of the recommended evaluation for POCUS performed by the neonatologist.[51]

Last, the ESPNIC guidelines recommend that cardiac POCUS is helpful with assessment and drainage of pericardial effusions with strong agreement and grade B evidence. Pericardial effusions can be seen in multiple basic cardiac views, with the subcostal view being the first choice.[77] Evaluation for hemodynamically significant pericardial effusion is an essential part of the ultrasound assessment of an acutely decompensating patient.[78,79] When pericardiocentesis is required for an effusion, the procedure should be done under ultrasound guidance rather than a blind approach.[80,81] Although the SCCM guidelines do not make specific recommendations on pericardial effusion evaluation, they do recommend that cardiac POCUS be used to evaluate for reversible causes of pediatric cardiac arrest and specifically mention evaluation for cardiac tamponade as part of this process with very good consensus (Supplemental Table 3.2).[48]

LUNG ULTRASOUND

Initially, the lung was deemed unsuitable for interrogation via ultrasound. The inability of ultrasound waves to penetrate air and the surrounding thoracic cage was thought to prevent an adequate sonographic assessment.[82] Subsequently, the recognition of ultrasound artifacts generated at the interface between normal and abnormal lung tissues formed the basis for sonographic evaluation of the lung.[83,84] This has been followed by progressive interest and growth in the use of POCUS for the assessment of respiratory failure in the emergency department and ICU, in both adult and pediatric settings.[84–86]

In 2015, guidelines published by SCCM, predominantly focused on applications of POCUS for critically ill adults, included 4 recommendations for the use of lung ultrasound (LUS).[6] In comparison, guidelines from ESPNIC included 11 recommendations for the use of LUS in critically ill neonates and children (**Table 3**).[8] This reflected a rapid expansion of LUS use in emergency departments and ICUs around the world, accompanied by a significant growth of evidence for LUS in neonates and children over several years[83–85,87,88] (Supplemental Table 4.2).

In general, recommendations from the SCCM and ESPNIC guidelines regarding LUS assessment of pleural disorders are well aligned with each other. As the role of LUS in this context is well established, both guidelines have put forth strong recommendations (or strong agreement) in the following: (1) detecting pleural effusions; (2) providing ultrasound guidance for thoracocentesis or drainage of pleural effusions; and (3) detecting a pneumothorax.[83,84,89–91] In addition, the ESPNIC guidelines proposed "strong agreement" that LUS is useful for guiding chest tube insertion or needle aspiration in neonatal tension pneumothorax. Because of limited pediatric evidence, this recommendation is extrapolated from adult studies reporting reduced complications and improved success rates. This was also based on the rationale that LUS may be used to identify margins of the lung, diaphragm, and subdiaphragmatic organs throughout the respiratory cycle so as to safely avoid them during needle or chest tube insertion.[92]

Regarding the assessment of lung parenchyma, the SCCM guidelines make a conditional recommendation that a systematic approach with LUS may be used as a

Table 3
Pulmonary statements achieving strong agreement in European Society of Pediatric and Neonatal Intensive Care guidelines with corresponding Society of Critical Care Medicine statement

Summary of POCUS Application Statement	ESPNIC Level of Evidence	SCCM Strength of Recommendation	SCCM Level of Evidence	SCCM Pediatric-specific
Describe viral bronchiolitis	A	N/A	N/A	N/A
Detect pneumothorax	B	1	A	No
Evacuation of pneumothorax	B	N/A	N/A	N/A
Detect pleural effusions	B	1	A	No
Guided thoracentesis	B	1	B	No

Table 3 summarizes the POCUS application within ESPNIC statements with strong agreement among experts. Corresponding level of evidence within the ESPNIC guidelines is defined using GRADE criteria with A as "high," B as "moderate," C as "low," and D as "very low." SCCM guidelines were reviewed to evaluate whether a statement was made corresponding to the ESPNIC statement achieving strong agreement. Strength of recommendation within SCCM guidelines is defined as 1, "strong recommendation"; 2, "weak/conditional recommendation"; and 3, "not reaching agreement." The table also indicates whether pediatric data are included in the discussion of the statement or the statement is pediatric-specific.
Abbreviation: N/A, not available as a statement within guidelines.

primary diagnostic modality for assessing interstitial and parenchymal lung pathologic condition in critically ill patients with respiratory failure. This recommendation is based on evidence that LUS (complemented by venous analysis where relevant) has a diagnostic accuracy of more than 90% in identifying common causes of acute respiratory failure in adults, including cardiogenic pulmonary edema, pneumonia, decompensated chronic obstructive pulmonary disease, acute asthma, pneumothorax, and pulmonary embolism.[82,93]

In contrast, the ESPNIC guidelines have crafted their recommendations for the role of LUS in assessing interstitial and parenchymal lung disease into 7 separate statements, with several specific to neonates and children. Of the 7 recommendations, the role of LUS in describing features of viral bronchiolitis was the only one assigned "strong agreement." This is supported by reports that LUS is superior to chest radiography in detecting lung abnormalities, with LUS features of bronchiolitis correlating well with clinical severity, facilitating timely identification of patients who may require escalating respiratory support.[94–98] The remaining 6 recommendations were assigned "agreement" and include the utility of LUS in the following: (1) distinguishing between neonatal respiratory distress syndrome and transient tachypnea of the neonate[99–108]; (2) detecting pneumonia in neonates and children[109–112]; (3) recognizing meconium aspiration syndrome[113,114]; (4) evaluating lung edema in neonates and children[115,116]; (5) detecting anesthesia-induced atelectasis in neonates and children[117]; and (6) semi-quantitatively evaluating lung aeration and guiding management of respiratory interventions in acute respiratory distress syndrome (ARDS) in neonates and children.[118,119]

These guidelines are undeniably a welcome step in the evolution of POCUS in the ICU, providing evidence-based recommendations for LUS in critically ill neonates and children. There is little doubt that compared with chest radiography or computed tomography (CT), LUS provides an economical, timely, nonirradiative, and easily repeatable bedside assessment with immediate results, without having to move a critically ill patient. LUS should be used in the appropriate context to answer specific clinical questions, bearing its limitations in mind: (1) LUS is limited in its ability to reliably determine the size of pneumothorax, necessitating clinical considerations or chest radiography to decide between conservative or surgical management; (2) LUS is unable to evaluate the extent of lung hyperinflation; (3) LUS is unable to assess the central areas of the thorax for hilar or mediastinal disorders, such as pneumomediastinum, pneumopericardium, or interstitial emphysema; (4) LUS cannot visualize areas beneath the scapulae, and patients with obesity, subcutaneous emphysema, wounds, or dressings may pose additional challenges with acquiring adequate images; and (5) radiographs are still considered the gold standard for determining the exact position of tubes and lines.

The publication of these recommendations has set the stage for future studies to determine if LUS improves clinical outcomes, particularly for applications related to parenchymal disease. Although it is generally accepted that LUS improves outcomes in the management of pleural disorders, there remains a paucity of evidence for the benefit of LUS in parenchymal disease, such as LUS-guided interventions to mitigate atelectasis via chest physiotherapy or lung recruitment maneuvers and ventilator titration during mechanical ventilation.[120,121] There is a need for consensus on the optimal LUS scoring system that incorporates the spectrum of LUS findings, to accurately reflect the severity of lung parenchymal disease in pediatric ARDS, the impact of clinical interventions, and correlates with outcomes. In the future, such advances in LUS may guide titration of mechanical ventilation at the bedside and lay the foundation for crafting a standardized curriculum for LUS and its applications in the ICU.

ABDOMINAL ULTRASOUND

The Focused Assessment with Sonography in Trauma (FAST) examination arose alongside the development of Emergency Medicine as a distinct clinical practice. Ultrasound now not only found itself in the hands of nonradiology and noncardiology providers, but data suggested POCUS use resulted in better clinical performance and patient outcomes in acute clinical care.[122–126] The historical growth and accumulated evidence are most apparent in abdominal applications of POCUS.

SCCM guidelines recommend the use of ultrasound for paracentesis (1A) and to exclude mechanical causes of renal failure (2C) with no mention of the pediatric population.[6] ESPNIC guidelines (**Table 4**) include the identification of free fluid and paracentesis guidance (strong agreement) as well as solid organ assessment, identifying obstructive uropathy, visualizing bowel peristalsis, and diagnosing necrotizing enterocolitis (agreement).[8] The traditional purpose for abdominal POCUS was to provide definitive, often dichotomous, answers to a focused question. For example, direct ultrasound visualization of "normal versus abnormal" and "present versus absent" (abdominal fluid, renal calyx dilation, peristalsis) provides additional data points for diagnostic considerations. Abdominal POCUS now includes the assessment pathophysiologic evolution resulting in less definitive and more nuanced diagnostic capabilities relevant to care and outcomes. For example, in assessing necrotizing enterocolitis, there are multiple ultrasonographic findings characterizing the varied stages of disease, including the presence of pneumatosis, portal venous air, large/complex ascites, aperistaltic bowel, and an evolution of bowel hyperemia to overt ischemia.[127] Individually these findings may be nonspecific but together improve the accuracy in diagnosis and clearly depict the progression of pathophysiology. Some diagnoses will have pathognomonic image findings (eg, pyloric stenosis), whereas others may require a constellation of findings similar to necrotizing enterocolitis (eg, appendicitis). Guidelines can hardly capture the complex interplay between ultrasound findings and clinical diagnostics specifically in the assessment of abdominal pathophysiologic processes in the pediatric patient.

The "signs and symptoms" traditionally obtained from clinical examination (eg, palpation, percussion) and history now require consideration of real-time ultrasound imaging data. However, the question of *what to do* with the data remains the same,

Table 4
Abdominal statements achieving strong agreement in European Society of Pediatric and Neonatal Intensive Care guidelines with corresponding Society of Critical Care Medicine statement

Summary of POCUS Application Statement	ESPNIC Level of Evidence	SCCM Strength of Recommendation	SCCM Level of Evidence	SCCM Pediatric-specific
Detect intra-abdominal free fluid	C	1	B	No
Guide drainage of peritoneal fluid	D	1	B	No

Table 4 summarizes the POCUS application within ESPNIC statements with strong agreement among experts. Corresponding level of evidence within the ESPNIC guidelines is defined using GRADE criteria with A as "high," B as "moderate," C as "low," and D as "very low." SCCM guidelines were reviewed to evaluate whether a statement was made corresponding to the ESPNIC statement achieving strong agreement. Strength of recommendation within SCCM guidelines is defined as 1, "strong recommendation"; 2, "weak/conditional recommendation"; and 3, "not reaching agreement." The table also indicates whether pediatric data are included in the discussion of the statement or the statement is pediatric-specific.

and one that ultrasound alone cannot answer. Take, for example, the FAST examination in children. Whereas randomized trials demonstrate decreased abdominal CT use, hospital lengths of stay, complications, and hospital charges when ultrasound is used in adult assessment,[128,129] a randomized trial including 925 hemodynamically stable children with blunt abdominal trauma found no outcome differences when FAST was integrated in management decisions.[130] Furthermore, there was only moderate agreement (k = 0.45) between FAST performer and expert reviewer, suggesting needs for improved training and potential risks of misdiagnosis at the bedside.

Although both psychomotor and interpretative skill development is of paramount importance, just because we *can* use ultrasound does not mean we *should* use it when a clinical benefit is in doubt. Thus, as demonstrated by controversies in performing the pediatric FAST examination, we need to move beyond a simple argument related to diagnostic accuracy to better understand how ultrasound is best used within a clinical context. Despite the expert consensus agreement, are longitudinal ultrasound evaluations of abdominal solid organ injuries really in the scope of the acute care provider in a tertiary care institution with radiology services? These are questions that guidelines cannot directly address but should be asked when reaching for a probe.

NEUROLOGIC ULTRASOUND

One of the earliest translations of ultrasound technology to clinical practice was in attempts to identify brain anatomy and pathophysiology as theorized by Dr Karl Dussik[131] in the 1940s. Nonradiology specialty learners in both adult and pediatric clinical practice have only recently explored training in neurosonographic clinical applications. SCCM guidelines did not provide guidance regarding any ultrasound applications related to the evaluation of the nervous system. ESPNIC guidelines did suggest a role for ultrasound use by acute care providers with strong agreement regarding the evaluation of intraventricular hemorrhage in neonates and agreement with its integration in evaluating both changes to and absence of cerebral blood flow in varied clinical settings. Furthermore, ESPNIC guidelines endorsed the evaluation of the optic nerve for assessing elevated intracranial pressure (ICP) (**Table 5**).[8]

Neurosonographic imaging uses both what is seen and what is not seen. Direct visualization of the neonatal brain and an understanding of normal anatomy and corresponding symmetry allow for improved interpretation of gross abnormalities by

Table 5
Neurosonography statements achieving strong agreement in European Society of Pediatric and Neonatal Intensive Care guidelines with corresponding Society of Critical Care Medicine statement

Summary of POCUS Application Statement	ESPNIC Level of Evidence	SCCM Strength of Recommendation	SCCM Level of Evidence	SCCM Pediatric-Specific
Detect intraventricular hemorrhage	A	N/A	N/A	N/A

Table 5 summarizes the POCUS application within ESPNIC statements with strong agreement among experts. Corresponding level of evidence within the ESPNIC guidelines is defined using GRADE criteria with A as "high," B as "moderate," C as "low," and D as "very low." SCCM guidelines were reviewed to evaluate whether a statement was made corresponding to the ESPNIC statement achieving strong agreement. Strength of recommendation within SCCM guidelines is defined as 1, "strong recommendation"; 2, "weak/conditional recommendation"; and 3, "not reaching agreement." The table also indicates whether pediatric data are included in the discussion of the statement or the statement is pediatric-specific.

neonatology providers following brief training.[132] Although ESPNIC guidelines support the evaluation of neonatal intraventricular hemorrhage with grade A level of evidence, there is no cited literature regarding image acquisition and interpretation performed in the clinical setting by neonatology, emergency medicine, or critical care subspecialists.

Direct imaging of the optic nerve sheath diameter (ONSD) may provide important information regarding increased ICP. Meta-analysis of adult data suggests that an increased ONSD measured using ultrasound is accurate for assessing ICP[133–135]; however, a recently published systematic review of pediatric literature suggests ONSD strong sensitivity with only moderate specificity (ie, overdiagnosing increased ICP).[136] Of the 11 studies evaluated for the pediatric systematic review, the investigators found heterogeneity in assessment techniques, including use of different probes for evaluation as well as different standards for measurements. Pediatric caveats, such as the presence of an open fontanelle as well as whether elevated ICP is a chronic or acute clinical change, need to also be considered in ONSD measurements.

Transcranial doppler (TCD) is increasingly used in pediatric acute care settings. TCD provides important information regarding cerebral blood flow in select pediatric populations, most prominently in children with sickle cell disease.[137] A recent Expert Consensus Statement for use of TCD in critically ill children resulted in the development of standardized methods of assessing and reporting TCD findings.[138] TCD can be categorized as imaging and nonimaging. Imaging TCD combines pulsed-wave doppler with 2-dimensional assessment of corresponding anatomy to decipher not only flow patterns but also potential structural abnormalities.[139] Nonimaging TCD is "blind" and uses knowledge of normal anatomy to assess blood flow integrating the spectral display and sound acquired by imaging within a cranial window. ESPNIC guidelines do not specify preferred methods of TCD, and the quality of evidence is C for the limited scope of identified TCD applications.[8] Although TCD is increasingly used in pediatric critical care settings, the vast majority of studies are performed in institutions with dedicated neurocritical care centers, and they are currently interpreted by vascular sonography specialists.[140]

MOVING FORWARD

Considerable time and effort by experts in the POCUS field resulted in SCCM and ESPNIC guidelines providing important guideposts for the integration of ultrasound technology in the pediatric critical care practice setting. Although guidelines are important first steps toward developing curricular platforms, the critical care community must now focus on POCUS clinical practice *guidance*. There appear to be some notable common considerations relevant to translating and expanding all core guidelines in clinical care.

First, we need to understand the educational needs within each core of applications and define implementation strategies that coincide with those educational needs. Common educational domains include knowledge and affective and psychomotor skill development.[141] The authors suggest that an additional domain, interpretative skill, be considered within ultrasound education. This domain necessarily incorporates knowledge and psychomotor skills and also requires contextual understanding of ultrasound data within the scope of the clinical setting. The interpretative domain must teach what ultrasound both *can* and *cannot* tell us at time of performance, as well as during longitudinal incorporation in care. Acquiring mastery skill level within educational domains is vital to the quality of POCUS image acquisition, interpretation, and integration in quality care.

Second, we need to clarify the purpose of each POCUS study and identify whether ultrasound is a simple tool to provide a definitive answer versus an advanced diagnostic tool to provide constellation of findings and/or stage of the disease. The former will have questions that will be easier to answer and therefore easier to master. The latter will require more advanced training with detailed practice parameters. Defining the purpose of POCUS will allow the images gathered to be translated into clinically meaningful outcomes. As more clinical evidence accumulates, we may shift the type of POCUS study from those we *can* perform to those we *should* perform.

Third, it is necessary to tailor the use of POCUS to meet the needs of specific patients, providers, and clinical practice contexts. Should we create practice guidance that meets the needs of both beginner and advanced POCUS providers? Should we account for clinical resources, that is, resource-rich versus resource-limited settings? Local resource availability may likely require tailored curricular design and methods of delivery.

Fourth, education delivery should target measurable clinical competency development by learners. The American College of Graduate Medical Education now emphasizes use of Entrustable Professional Activities to monitor educational growth and ensure competency in clinical practice.[142] Defining thresholds for translation of education to independent bedside performance within cores of applications is an important step to help identify relevant methods of measurement.

Finally, clinical practice guidance may require programmatic support mechanisms. These are present within the current emergency medicine guidelines[143] and suggested within adult critical care literature.[144] These support mechanisms may be difficult to build in pediatric critical care at a unit level and require community support, whether through the institution or external mechanisms.[145] Multicenter database built with common elements can provide longitudinal educational and clinical outcome measures to monitor implementation and translational effectiveness at local, regional, national, and international levels.

SUMMARY

The development of SCCM and ESPNIC guidelines was an important first step to assessing existing evidence and providing support for the use of POCUS in core clinical applications. POCUS is an important adjunct to a systematic clinical assessment in many clinical contexts. Thus, there is a need to develop clinical practice guidance to facilitate the translation of these guidelines into meaningful curriculum that will support the needs of our pediatric critical care community and those it serves.

DISCLOSURE

The authors have nothing to disclose.

CLINICS CARE POINTS

- The use of POCUS for vascular access procedures decreases insertion attempts, time to cannulation and procedural complications.

- Cardiac POCUS can provide rapid answers to defined clinical questions thereby informing management in critically ill children, particularly those with hemodynamic instability.

- Lung US can rapidly diagnose a pneumothorax but cannot accurately quantify its size, requiring clinical considerations or chest radiography to decide between conservative or invasive management.

SUPPLEMENTARY DATA

Supplementary data related to this article can be found online at https://doi.org/10.1016/j.ccc.2022.09.012.

REFERENCES

1. Abbott J. Emergency department ultrasound: is it really time for real time? J Emerg Med 1990;8(4):491–2.
2. American College of Emergency P. American College of Emergency Physicians. ACEP emergency ultrasound guidelines-2001. Ann Emerg Med 2001;38(4): 470–81.
3. Lichtenstein D, Axler O. Intensive use of general ultrasound in the intensive care unit. Prospective study of 150 consecutive patients. Intensive Care Med 1993; 19(6):353–5.
4. Miller LE, Stoller JZ, Fraga MV. Point-of-care ultrasound in the neonatal ICU. Curr Opin Pediatr 2020;32(2):216–27.
5. Conlon TW, Nishisaki A, Singh Y, et al. Moving beyond the stethoscope: diagnostic point-of-care ultrasound in pediatric practice. Pediatrics 2019;144(4): e20191402.
6. Frankel HL, Kirkpatrick AW, Elbarbary M, et al. Guidelines for the appropriate use of bedside general and cardiac ultrasonography in the evaluation of critically ill patients-Part I: general ultrasonography. Crit Care Med 2015;43(11):2479–502.
7. Levitov A, Frankel HL, Blaivas M, et al. Guidelines for the appropriate use of bedside general and cardiac ultrasonography in the evaluation of critically ill patients-Part II: cardiac ultrasonography. Crit Care Med 2016;44(6):1206–27.
8. Singh Y, Tissot C, Fraga MV, et al. International evidence-based guidelines on point of care ultrasound (POCUS) for critically ill neonates and children issued by the POCUS working group of the European society of paediatric and neonatal intensive care (ESPNIC). Crit Care 2020;24(1):65.
9. Ullman JI, Stoelting RK. Internal jugular vein location with the ultrasound Doppler blood flow detector. Anesth Analg 1978;57(1):118.
10. Legler D, Nugent M. Doppler localization of the internal jugular vein facilitates central venous cannulation. Anesthesiology 1984;60(5):481–2.
11. Machi J, Takeda J, Kakegawa T. Safe jugular and subclavian venipuncture under ultrasonographic guidance. Am J Surg 1987;153(3):321–3.
12. Denys BG, Uretsky BF. Anatomical variations of internal jugular vein location: impact on central venous access. Crit Care Med 1991;19(12):1516–9.
13. Kwon TH, Kim YL, Cho DK. Ultrasound-guided cannulation of the femoral vein for acute haemodialysis access. Nephrol Dial Transpl 1997;12(5):1009–12.
14. Skolnick ML. The role of sonography in the placement and management of jugular and subclavian central venous catheters. AJR Am J Roentgenol 1994;163(2):291–5.
15. Kantor DB, Su E, Milliren CE, et al. Ultrasound guidance and other determinants of successful peripheral artery catheterization in critically ill children. Pediatr Crit Care Med 2016;17(12):1124–30.
16. Joing S, Strote S, Caroon L, et al. Ultrasound-guided peripheral IV placement. N Engl J Med 2012;366(25):e38.
17. de Souza TH, Brandao MB, Santos TM, et al. Ultrasound guidance for internal jugular vein cannulation in PICU: a randomised controlled trial. Arch Dis Child 2018;103(10):952–6.

18. Verghese ST, McGill WA, Patel RI, et al. Ultrasound-guided internal jugular venous cannulation in infants: a prospective comparison with the traditional palpation method. Anesthesiology 1999;91(1):71–7.
19. Aouad MT, Kanazi GE, Abdallah FW, et al. Femoral vein cannulation performed by residents: a comparison between ultrasound-guided and landmark technique in infants and children undergoing cardiac surgery. Anesth Analg 2010; 111(3):724–8.
20. Verghese ST, McGill WA, Patel RI, et al. Comparison of three techniques for internal jugular vein cannulation in infants. Paediatr Anaesth 2000;10(5):505–11.
21. Sigaut S, Skhiri A, Stany I, et al. Ultrasound guided internal jugular vein access in children and infant: a meta-analysis of published studies. Paediatr Anaesth 2009;19(12):1199–206.
22. Merchaoui Z, Lausten-Thomsen U, Pierre F, et al. Supraclavicular approach to ultrasound-guided brachiocephalic vein cannulation in children and neonates. Front Pediatr 2017;5:211.
23. Pirotte T, Veyckemans F. Ultrasound-guided subclavian vein cannulation in infants and children: a novel approach. Br J Anaesth 2007;98(4):509–14.
24. Byon HJ, Lee GW, Lee JH, et al. Comparison between ultrasound-guided supraclavicular and infraclavicular approaches for subclavian venous catheterization in children–a randomized trial. Br J Anaesth 2013;111(5):788–92.
25. Kim YJ, Ma S, Yoon HK, et al. Supraclavicular versus infraclavicular approach for ultrasound-guided right subclavian venous catheterisation: a randomised controlled non-inferiority trial. Anaesthesia 2022;77(1):59–65.
26. Lausten-Thomsen U, Merchaoui Z, Dubois C, et al. Ultrasound-guided subclavian vein cannulation in low birth weight neonates. Pediatr Crit Care Med 2017;18(2):172–5.
27. Siddik-Sayyid SM, Aouad MT, Ibrahim MH, et al. Femoral arterial cannulation performed by residents: a comparison between ultrasound-guided and palpation technique in infants and children undergoing cardiac surgery. Paediatr Anaesth 2016;26(8):823–30.
28. Gu WJ, Tie HT, Liu JC, et al. Efficacy of ultrasound-guided radial artery catheterization: a systematic review and meta-analysis of randomized controlled trials. Crit Care 2014;18(3):R93.
29. Liu L, Tan Y, Li S, et al. Modified dynamic needle tip positioning" short-axis, out-of-plane, ultrasound-guided radial artery cannulation in neonates: a randomized controlled trial. Anesth Analg 2019;129(1):178–83.
30. Chittoodan S, Breen D, O'Donnell BD, et al. Long versus short axis ultrasound guided approach for internal jugular vein cannulation: a prospective randomised controlled trial. Med Ultrason 2011;13(1):21–5.
31. Mahler SA, Wang H, Lester C, et al. Short- vs long-axis approach to ultrasound-guided peripheral intravenous access: a prospective randomized study. Am J Emerg Med 2011;29(9):1194–7.
32. Blaivas M, Brannam L, Fernandez E. Short-axis versus long-axis approaches for teaching ultrasound-guided vascular access on a new inanimate model. Acad Emerg Med 2003;10(12):1307–11.
33. Brescia F, Biasucci DG, Fabiani F, et al. A novel ultrasound-guided approach to the axillary vein: oblique-axis view combined with in-plane puncture. J Vasc access 2019;20(6):763–8.
34. Takeshita J, Tachibana K, Nakajima Y, et al. Long-axis in-plane approach versus short-axis out-of-plane approach for ultrasound-guided central venous

catheterization in pediatric patients: a randomized controlled trial. Pediatr Crit Care Med 2020;21(11):e996–1001.

35. Davda D, Schrift D. Posterior wall punctures between long- and short-axis techniques in a phantom intravenous model. J Ultrasound Med 2018;37(12):2891–7.

36. Chen HE, Yovanoff MA, Pepley DF, et al. Evaluating surgical resident needle insertion skill gains in central venous catheterization training. J Surg Res 2019;233:351–9.

37. Sappenfield JW, Smith WB, Cooper LA, et al. Visualization improves supraclavicular access to the subclavian vein in a mixed reality simulator. Anesth Analg 2018;127(1):83–9.

38. Chew SC, Beh ZY, Hakumat Rai VR, et al. Ultrasound-guided central venous vascular access-novel needle navigation technology compared with conventional method: a randomized study. J Vasc access 2020;21(1):26–32.

39. England JR, Fischbeck T, Tchelepi H. The value of needle-guidance technology in ultrasound-guided percutaneous procedures performed by radiology residents: a comparison of freehand, in-plane, fixed-angle, and electromagnetic needle tracking techniques. J Ultrasound Med 2019;38(2):399–405.

40. Chenkin J, Lee S, Huynh T, et al. Procedures can be learned on the Web: a randomized study of ultrasound-guided vascular access training. Acad Emerg Med 2008;15(10):949–54.

41. Calcutt T, Brady R, Liew K. Paediatric ultrasound-guided vascular access: experiences and outcomes from an emergency department educational intervention. J Paediatr Child Health 2021;58(5):830–5.

42. Vusse LV, Shepherd A, Bergam B, et al. Procedure training workshop for internal medicine residents that emphasizes procedural ultrasound: logistics and teaching materials. MedEdPORTAL 2020;16:10897.

43. Hartman N, Wittler M, Askew K, et al. Validation of a performance checklist for ultrasound-guided internal jugular central lines for use in procedural instruction and assessment. Postgrad Med J 2017;93(1096):67–70.

44. Kahr Rasmussen N, Nayahangan LJ, Carlsen J, et al. Evaluation of competence in ultrasound-guided procedures-a generic assessment tool developed through the Delphi method. Eur Radiol 2021;31(6):4203–11.

45. Narayanasamy S, Ding L, Yang F, et al. Feasibility study of cumulative sum (CUSUM) analysis as a competency assessment tool for ultrasound-guided venous access procedures. Can J Anaesth 2022;69(2):256–64.

46. Perera P, Mailhot T, Riley D, et al. The RUSH exam: rapid Ultrasound in SHock in the evaluation of the critically Ill. Emerg Med Clin North Am 2010;28(1): 29–56, vii.

47. Gartlehner G, Wagner G, Affengruber L, et al. Point-of-Care ultrasonography in patients with acute dyspnea: an evidence report for a clinical practice guideline by the American College of Physicians. Ann Intern Med 2021;174(7):967–76.

48. Avila-Reyes D, Acevedo-Cardona AO, Gomez-Gonzalez JF, et al. Point-of-care ultrasound in cardiorespiratory arrest (POCUS-CA): narrative review article. Ultrasound J 2021;13(1):46.

49. Singh Y, Bhombal S, Katheria A, et al. The evolution of cardiac point of care ultrasound for the neonatologist. Eur J Pediatr 2021;180(12):3565–75.

50. van Laere D, van Overmeire B, Gupta S, et al. Application of NPE in the assessment of a patent ductus arteriosus. Pediatr Res 2018;84(Suppl 1):46–56.

51. de Boode WP, Kluckow M, McNamara PJ, et al. Role of neonatologist-performed echocardiography in the assessment and management of patent ductus arteriosus physiology in the newborn. Semin Fetal Neonatal Med 2018;23(4):292–7.

52. Megri M, Fridenmaker E, Disselkamp M. Where are we heading with fluid responsiveness and septic shock? Cureus 2022;14(4).

53. Vignon P, Repesse X, Begot E, et al. Comparison of echocardiographic indices used to predict fluid responsiveness in ventilated patients. Am J Respir Crit Care Med 2017;195(8):1022–32.

54. Schefold JC, Storm C, Bercker S, et al. Inferior vena cava diameter correlates with invasive hemodynamic measures in mechanically ventilated intensive care unit patients with sepsis. J Emerg Med 2010;38(5):632–7.

55. Feissel M, Michard F, Faller J-P, et al. The respiratory variation in inferior vena cava diameter as a guide to fluid therapy. Intensive Care Med 2004;30(9): 1834–7.

56. Byon HJ, Lim CW, Lee JH, et al. Prediction of fluid responsiveness in mechanically ventilated children undergoing neurosurgery. Br J Anaesth 2013;110(4): 586–91.

57. Preau S, Bortolotti P, Colling D, et al. Diagnostic accuracy of the inferior vena cava collapsibility to predict fluid responsiveness in spontaneously breathing patients with sepsis and acute circulatory failure. Crit Care Med 2017;45(3): e290–7.

58. Orso D, Paoli I, Piani T, et al. Accuracy of ultrasonographic measurements of inferior vena cava to determine fluid responsiveness: a systematic review and meta-analysis. J Intensive Care Med 2020;35(4):354–63.

59. Gan H, Cannesson M, Chandler JR, et al. Predicting fluid responsiveness in children: a systematic review. Anesth Analg 2013;117(6):1380–92.

60. Pereira de Souza Neto E, Grousson S, Duflo F, et al. Predicting fluid responsiveness in mechanically ventilated children under general anaesthesia using dynamic parameters and transthoracic echocardiography. Br J Anaesth 2011; 106(6):856–64.

61. Desgranges FP, Desebbe O, Pereira de Souza Neto E, et al. Respiratory variation in aortic blood flow peak velocity to predict fluid responsiveness in mechanically ventilated children: a systematic review and meta-analysis. Paediatr Anaesth 2016;26(1):37–47.

62. Wang J, Zhou D, Gao Y, et al. Effect of VTILVOT variation rate on the assessment of fluid responsiveness in septic shock patients. Medicine (Baltimore) 2020; 99(47):e22702.

63. Wang X, Jiang L, Liu S, et al. Value of respiratory variation of aortic peak velocity in predicting children receiving mechanical ventilation: a systematic review and meta-analysis. Crit Care 2019;23(1):372.

64. Blanco P. Rationale for using the velocity–time integral and the minute distance for assessing the stroke volume and cardiac output in point-of-care settings. Ultrasound J 2020;12(1):1–9.

65. Feissel M, Mangin I, Ruyer O, et al. Respiratory changes in aortic blood velocity as an indicator of fluid responsiveness in ventilated patients with septic shock. Chest 2001;119(3):867–73.

66. Hope MD, de la Pena E, Yang PC, et al. A visual approach for the accurate determination of echocardiographic left ventricular ejection fraction by medical students. J Am Soc Echocardiogr 2003;16(8):824–31.

67. Pershad J, Myers S, Plouman C, et al. Bedside limited echocardiography by the emergency physician is accurate during evaluation of the critically ill patient. Pediatrics 2004;114(6):e667–71.

68. Vignon P, Mucke F, Bellec F, et al. Basic critical care echocardiography: validation of a curriculum dedicated to noncardiologist residents. Crit Care Med 2011; 39(4):636–42.

69. Spurney CF, Sable CA, Berger JT, et al. Use of a hand-carried ultrasound device by critical care physicians for the diagnosis of pericardial effusions, decreased cardiac function, and left ventricular enlargement in pediatric patients. J Am Soc Echocardiogr 2005;18(4):313–9.

70. Klugman D, Berger JT. Echocardiography and focused cardiac ultrasound. Pediatr Crit Care Med 2016;17(8 Suppl 1):S222–4.

71. Singh Y. Echocardiographic evaluation of hemodynamics in neonates and children. Front Pediatr 2017;5:201.

72. Nikravan S, Song P, Bughrara N, et al. Focused ultrasonography for septic shock resuscitation. Curr Opin Crit Care 2020;26(3):296–302.

73. Sweeney DA, Wiley BM. Integrated multiorgan bedside ultrasound for the diagnosis and management of sepsis and septic shock. Semin Respir Crit Care Med 2021;42(5):641–9.

74. Ranjit S, Aram G, Kissoon N, et al. Multimodal monitoring for hemodynamic categorization and management of pediatric septic shock: a pilot observational study. Pediatr Crit Care Med 2014;15(1):e17–26.

75. Arnoldi S, Glau CL, Walker SB, et al. Integrating focused cardiac ultrasound into pediatric septic shock assessment. Pediatr Crit Care Med 2021;22(3):262–74.

76. Jone PN, Ivy DD. Echocardiography in pediatric pulmonary hypertension. Front Pediatr 2014;2:124.

77. Pérez-Casares A, Cesar S, Brunet-Garcia L, et al. Echocardiographic evaluation of pericardial effusion and cardiac tamponade. Front Pediatr 2017;5:79.

78. Yousef N, Singh Y, De Luca D. Playing it SAFE in the NICU" SAFE-R: a targeted diagnostic ultrasound protocol for the suddenly decompensating infant in the NICU. Eur J Pediatr 2022;181(1):393–8.

79. Hardwick JA, Griksaitis MJ. Fifteen-minute consultation: point of care ultrasound in the management of paediatric shock. Arch Dis Childhood-Education Pract 2021;106(3):136–41.

80. Tsang TS, Freeman WK, Sinak LJ, et al. Echocardiographically guided pericardiocentesis: evolution and state-of-the-art technique. Mayo Clin Proc 1998; 73(7):647–52.

81. Luis SA, Kane GC, Luis CR, et al. Overview of optimal techniques for pericardiocentesis in contemporary practice. Curr Cardiol Rep 2020;22(8):1–10.

82. Lichtenstein DA, Meziere GA. Relevance of lung ultrasound in the diagnosis of acute respiratory failure: the BLUE protocol. Chest 2008;134(1):117–25.

83. Ammirabile A, Buonsenso D, Di Mauro A. Lung ultrasound in pediatrics and neonatology: an update. Healthcare (Basel) 2021;9(8).

84. Musolino AM, Toma P, De Rose C, et al. Ten years of pediatric lung ultrasound: a narrative review. Front Physiol 2021;12:721951.

85. Potter SK, Griksaitis MJ. The role of point-of-care ultrasound in pediatric acute respiratory distress syndrome: emerging evidence for its use. Ann Transl Med 2019;7(19):507.

86. Pietersen PI, Madsen KR, Graumann O, et al. Lung ultrasound training: a systematic review of published literature in clinical lung ultrasound training. Crit Ultrasound J 2018;10(1):23.

87. Cantinotti M, Marchese P, Giordano R, et al. Overview of lung ultrasound in pediatric cardiology. Diagnostics (Basel) 2022;12(3).

88. Kharasch S, Duggan NM, Cohen AR, et al. Lung ultrasound in children with respiratory tract infections: viral, bacterial or COVID-19? A narrative review. Open Access Emerg Med 2020;12:275–85.

89. Raimondi F, Rodriguez Fanjul J, Aversa S, et al. Lung ultrasound in the crashing infant (LUCI) protocol study group. Lung Ultrasound Diagnosing Pneumothorax Critically Ill Neonate J Pediatr 2016;175:74–8.

90. Cattarossi L, Copetti R, Brusa G, et al. Lung ultrasound diagnostic accuracy in neonatal pneumothorax. Can Respir J 2016;2016:6515069.

91. Dahmarde H, Parooie F, Salarzaei M. Accuracy of ultrasound in diagnosis of pneumothorax: a comparison between neonates and adults-a systematic review and meta-analysis. Can Respir J 2019;2019:5271982.

92. Dancel R, Schnobrich D, Puri N, et al. Recommendations on the use of ultrasound guidance for adult thoracentesis: a position statement of the society of hospital medicine. J Hosp Med 2018;13(2):126–35.

93. Lichtenstein D. Lung ultrasound in acute respiratory failure an introduction to the BLUE-protocol. Minerva Anestesiol 2009;75(5):313–7.

94. Caiulo VA, Gargani L, Caiulo S, et al. Lung ultrasound in bronchiolitis: comparison with chest X-ray. Eur J Pediatr 2011;170(11):1427–33.

95. Tsung JW, Kessler DO, Shah VP. Prospective application of clinician-performed lung ultrasonography during the 2009 H1N1 influenza A pandemic: distinguishing viral from bacterial pneumonia. Crit Ultrasound J 2012;4(1):16.

96. Basile V, Di Mauro A, Scalini E, et al. Lung ultrasound: a useful tool in diagnosis and management of bronchiolitis. BMC Pediatr 2015;15:63.

97. Varshney T, Mok E, Shapiro AJ, et al. Point-of-care lung ultrasound in young children with respiratory tract infections and wheeze. Emerg Med J 2016;33(9):603–10.

98. La Regina DP, Bloise S, Pepino D, et al. Lung ultrasound in bronchiolitis. Pediatr Pulmonol 2021;56(1):234–9.

99. Liu J, Wang Y, Fu W, et al. Diagnosis of neonatal transient tachypnea and its differentiation from respiratory distress syndrome using lung ultrasound. Medicine (Baltimore) 2014;93(27):e197.

100. Liu J, Chen XX, Li XW, et al. Lung ultrasonography to diagnose transient tachypnea of the newborn. Chest 2016;149(5):1269–75.

101. Chen SW, Fu W, Liu J, et al. Routine application of lung ultrasonography in the neonatal intensive care unit. Medicine (Baltimore) 2017;96(2):e5826.

102. Sawires HK, Ghany EAA, Hussein NF, et al. Use of lung ultrasound in detection of complications of respiratory distress syndrome. Ultrasound Med Biol 2015;41(9):2319–25.

103. Copetti R, Cattarossi L, Macagno F, et al. Lung ultrasound in respiratory distress syndrome: a useful tool for early diagnosis. Neonatology 2008;94(1):52–9.

104. Vergine M, Copetti R, Brusa G, et al. Lung ultrasound accuracy in respiratory distress syndrome and transient tachypnea of the newborn. Neonatology 2014;106(2):87–93.

105. Raimondi F, Yousef N, Rodriguez Fanjul J, et al. A multicenter lung ultrasound study on transient tachypnea of the neonate. Neonatology 2019;115(3):263–8.

106. Razak A, Faden M. Neonatal lung ultrasonography to evaluate need for surfactant or mechanical ventilation: a systematic review and meta-analysis. Arch Dis Child Fetal Neonatal Ed 2020;105(2):164–71.

107. De Martino L, Yousef N, Ben-Ammar R, et al. Lung ultrasound score predicts surfactant need in extremely preterm neonates. Pediatrics 2018;142(3).

108. Raschetti R, Yousef N, Vigo G, et al. Echography-guided surfactant therapy to improve timeliness of surfactant replacement: a quality improvement project. J Pediatr 2019;212:137–143 e131.

109. Pereda MA, Chavez MA, Hooper-Miele CC, et al. Lung ultrasound for the diagnosis of pneumonia in children: a meta-analysis. Pediatrics 2015;135(4):714–22.

110. Tsou PY, Chen KP, Wang YH, et al. Diagnostic accuracy of lung ultrasound performed by novice versus advanced sonographers for pneumonia in children: a systematic review and meta-analysis. Acad Emerg Med 2019;26(9):1074–88.

111. Yan JH, Yu N, Wang YH, et al. Lung ultrasound vs chest radiography in the diagnosis of children pneumonia: systematic evidence. Medicine (Baltimore) 2020; 99(50):e23671.

112. Lu X, Jin Y, Li Y, et al. Diagnostic accuracy of lung ultrasonography in childhood pneumonia: a meta-analysis. Eur J Emerg Med 2022;29(2):105–17.

113. Liu J, Cao HY, Fu W. Lung ultrasonography to diagnose meconium aspiration syndrome of the newborn. J Int Med Res 2016;44(6):1534–42.

114. Piastra M, Yousef N, Brat R, et al. Lung ultrasound findings in meconium aspiration syndrome. Early Hum Dev 2014;90(Suppl 2):S41–3.

115. Kaskinen AK, Martelius L, Kirjavainen T, et al. Assessment of extravascular lung water by ultrasound after congenital cardiac surgery. Pediatr Pulmonol 2017; 52(3):345–52.

116. Volpicelli G, Skurzak S, Boero E, et al. Lung ultrasound predicts well extravascular lung water but is of limited usefulness in the prediction of wedge pressure. Anesthesiology 2014;121(2):320–7.

117. Acosta CM, Maidana GA, Jacovitti D, et al. Accuracy of transthoracic lung ultrasound for diagnosing anesthesia-induced atelectasis in children. Anesthesiology 2014;120(6):1370–9.

118. Brat R, Yousef N, Klifa R, et al. Lung ultrasonography score to evaluate oxygenation and surfactant need in neonates treated with continuous positive airway pressure. JAMA Pediatr 2015;169(8):e151797.

119. Bouhemad B, Brisson H, Le-Guen M, et al. Bedside ultrasound assessment of positive end-expiratory pressure-induced lung recruitment. Am J Respir Crit Care Med 2011;183(3):341–7.

120. Song IK, Kim EH, Lee JH, et al. Utility of perioperative lung ultrasound in pediatric cardiac surgery: a randomized controlled trial. Anesthesiology 2018; 128(4):718–27.

121. Elayashy M, Madkour MA, Mahmoud AAA, et al. Effect of ultrafiltration on extravascular lung water assessed by lung ultrasound in children undergoing cardiac surgery: a randomized prospective study. BMC Anesthesiol 2019;19(1):93.

122. Ma OJ, Mateer JR, Ogata M, et al. Prospective analysis of a rapid trauma ultrasound examination performed by emergency physicians. J Trauma 1995;38(6):879–85.

123. McKenney MG, Martin L, Lentz K, et al. 1,000 consecutive ultrasounds for blunt abdominal trauma. J Trauma 1996;40(4):607–10 [discussion: 611-602].

124. Jarowenko DG, Hess RM, Herr MS, et al. Use of ultrasonography in the evaluation of blunt abdominal trauma. J Trauma Acute Care Surg 1989;29(7):1031.

125. Gruessner R, Mentges B, Duber C, et al. Sonography versus peritoneal lavage in blunt abdominal trauma. J Trauma 1989;29(2):242–4.

126. Hoffmann R, Nerlich M, Muggia-Sullam M, et al. Blunt abdominal trauma in cases of multiple trauma evaluated by ultrasonography: a prospective analysis of 291 patients. J Trauma 1992;32(4):452–8.

127. Epelman M, Daneman A, Navarro OM, et al. Necrotizing enterocolitis: review of state-of-the-art imaging findings with pathologic correlation. Radiographics 2007;27(2):285–305.

128. Melniker LA, Leibner E, McKenney MG, et al. Randomized controlled clinical trial of point-of-care, limited ultrasonography for trauma in the emergency department: the first sonography outcomes assessment program trial. Ann Emerg Med 2006;48(3):227–35.

129. Rose JS, Levitt MA, Porter J, et al. Does the presence of ultrasound really affect computed tomographic scan use? A prospective randomized trial of ultrasound in trauma. J Trauma Acute Care Surg 2001;51(3):545–50.

130. Holmes JF, Kelley KM, Wootton-Gorges SL, et al. Effect of abdominal ultrasound on clinical care, outcomes, and resource use among children with blunt torso trauma: a randomized clinical trial. JAMA 2017;317(22):2290–6.

131. Dussik K. On the possibility of using ultrasound waves as a diagnostic aid. Neurol Psychiatr 1942;174:153–68.

132. Ben Fadel N, McAleer S. Impact of a web-based module on trainees' ability to interpret neonatal cranial ultrasound. BMC Med Educ 2020;20(1):489.

133. Ohle R, McIsaac SM, Woo MY, et al. Sonography of the optic nerve sheath diameter for detection of raised intracranial pressure compared to computed tomography: a systematic review and meta-analysis. J Ultrasound Med 2015;34(7):1285–94.

134. Robba C, Santori G, Czosnyka M, et al. Optic nerve sheath diameter measured sonographically as non-invasive estimator of intracranial pressure: a systematic review and meta-analysis. Intensive Care Med 2018;44(8):1284–94.

135. Koziarz A, Sne N, Kegel F, et al. Bedside optic nerve ultrasonography for diagnosing increased intracranial pressure: a systematic review and meta-analysis. Ann Intern Med 2019;171(12):896–905.

136. Bhargava V, Tawfik D, Tan YJ, et al. Ultrasonographic optic nerve sheath diameter measurement to detect intracranial hypertension in children with neurological injury: a systematic review. Pediatr Crit Care Med 2020;21(9):e858–68.

137. Adams RJ, McKie VC, Hsu L, et al. Prevention of a first stroke by transfusions in children with sickle cell anemia and abnormal results on transcranial Doppler ultrasonography. N Engl J Med 1998;339(1):5–11.

138. O'Brien NF, Reuter-Rice K, Wainwright MS, et al. Practice recommendations for transcranial Doppler ultrasonography in critically ill children in the pediatric intensive care unit: a multidisciplinary expert consensus statement. J Pediatr Intensive Care 2021;10(2):133–42.

139. Blanco P, Abdo-Cuza A. Transcranial Doppler ultrasound in neurocritical care. J Ultrasound 2018;21(1):1–16.

140. LaRovere KL, Tasker RC, Wainwright M, et al. Transcranial Doppler ultrasound during critical illness in children: survey of practices in pediatric neurocritical care centers. Pediatr Crit Care Med 2020;21(1):67–74.

141. Sousa DA. How the brain learns. Thousand Oaks, CA: Corwin Press; 2016.

142. Ten Cate O. Nuts and bolts of entrustable professional activities. J graduate Med Educ 2013;5(1):157–8.

143. Physicians ACoE. Ultrasound guidelines: emergency, point-of-care and clinical ultrasound guidelines in medicine. Ann Emerg Med 2017;69(5):e27–54.

144. Pustavoitau A, Blaivas M, Brown SM, et al. Recommendations for achieving and maintaining competence and credentialing in critical care ultrasound with focused cardiac ultrasound and advanced critical care echocardiography. Documents/Critical% 20care% 20Ultrasound pdf> Accessed Oct 27, 2016.
145. Conlon TW, Kantor DB, Su ER, et al. Diagnostic bedside ultrasound program development in pediatric critical care medicine: results of a national survey. Pediatr Crit Care Med 2018;19(11):e561–8.

Pediatric Critical Care in the Twenty-first Century and Beyond

Mary Dahmer, PhD[a], Aimee Jennings, CPNP-AC/PC, FCCM[b],
Margaret Parker, MD, MCCM[c], Lazaro N. Sanchez-Pinto, MD, MBI[d],
Ann Thompson, MD, MCCM[e], Chani Traube, MD[f],
Jerry J. Zimmerman, MD, PhD, FCCM[g,h,*]

KEYWORDS

- Children • Critical illness/injury • Omics • Learning health-care system
- Data science • Humanism • Wearable sensors • Clinical decision support tools

Continued

INTRODUCTION

As multidisciplinary pediatric critical care providers, we deliver increasingly complex therapies to increasingly complex patients within increasingly complex environments. Dynamics of change within our profession are nearly palpable. Contemplating how all of this will evolve is at once exciting, inspiring, and perhaps frightening. Using a case presentation format, basing our expectations on the exponential trajectory of medical technology (which we are likely to underestimate), and projecting an enduring necessity for bedside humanism, we provide one vision of pediatric intensive care in the near future. This preview focuses on facilitated diagnostics, continuous advancement of care, the learning health-care environment, and the continuum of critical care beyond the walls of the intensive care unit and hospital.

[a] Division of Critical Care, Department of Pediatrics, University of Michigan, 1500 East Medical Center Drive, F6790/5243, Ann Arbor, MI, USA; [b] Division of Critical Care Medicine, Advanced Practice, FA.2.112, Seattle Children's Hospital, 4800 Sandpoint Way Northeast, Seattle, WA 98105, USA; [c] Department of Pediatrics, Stony Brook University, 7762 Bloomfield Road, Easton, MD 21601, USA; [d] Department of Pediatrics, Ann and Robert H Lurie Children's Hospital of Chicago, Northwestern University Feinberg School of Medicine, 225 East Chicago Avenue, Box 73, Chicago, IL 60611-2605, USA; [e] Department of Critical Care Medicine, University of Pittsburgh, 3550 Terrace Street, Pittsburgh, PA 15261, USA; [f] Department of Pediatrics, Weill Cornell Medicine, 525 East 68th Street, Box 225, New York, NY 10065, USA; [g] Department of Pediatrics, FA.2.300B Seattle Children's Hospital, 4800 Sandpoint Way Northeast, Seattle, WA 98105, USA; [h] Pediatric Critical Care Medicine, Seattle Children's Hospital, Harborview Medical Center, University of Washington, School of Medicine, FA.2.300B, Seattle Children's Hospital, 4800 Sand Point Way Northeast, Seattle, WA 98105, USA
* Corresponding author.
E-mail address: jerry.zimmerman@seattlechildrens.org

Crit Care Clin 39 (2023) 407–425
https://doi.org/10.1016/j.ccc.2022.09.013
0749-0704/23/© 2022 Elsevier Inc. All rights reserved.

criticalcare.theclinics.com

Continued

KEY POINTS

- Data science is increasingly adding sensitivity and specificity to all aspects of critical care and will need to be included in future critical care training curricula.
- A pediatric intensive care unit (PICU) learning health-care environment promotes best clinical practice, clinical research and rigorous quality improvement, and a shared education model.
- Computerized decision support tools, including closed-loop titration algorithms, will drive continuous advancement of care in the PICU.
- Critical care providers will assume responsibility for postintensive care syndrome (prevention, intervention) to insure the continuum of quality pediatric critical care.
- Although technology will increasingly advance the cause of personalized medicine, humanism, practiced at the bedside, will always define the essence of pediatric critical care.

Julian's Story

It was one of those busy mornings in the house: getting the kids ready for school, packing lunch boxes, answering work emails from the phone. Mia was about to start brushing her teeth when she received the phone call that would upend her life for the next two months.

"Hi, Ms. Spencer, this Yolanda, one of the nurses in the remote patient monitoring program at the children's hospital. I'm calling to ask about Julian; how is he feeling this morning?"

Julian was Mia's 15-year-old son, a tall, kind, smart teenager who loved his sisters, basketball, and the family's labradoodle, Leo. He also had leukemia and was undergoing chemotherapy at the children's hospital. Because genetic variants, identified when his DNA was sequenced shortly after birth indicated he had an increased risk of infection, and because he had been diagnosed with leukemia, Julian had been outfitted with a smart watch that monitored his heart rate, blood hemoglobin oxygen saturation and temperature so that any infection could be identified early.

"He says he feels okay now, but he was complaining of some belly ache when he woke up and he barely touched his breakfast," said Mia. "He is in his room now getting dressed for school."

"I see. We detected some abnormal trends in the vital signs from his smartwatch that are a little concerning. We would like Julian to come in for an evaluation."

The next few hours were a whirlwind for Mia and Julian. The nurse had suggested taking Julian to the local emergency department (ED) where providers had a direct connection to the children's hospital and Julian's doctors would be able to see all the results of the tests they performed in real-time. By the time they arrived at the ED, things had worsened. Julian's abdominal pain was more intense, he looked pale, and was breathing faster. He was triaged to a "high-risk sepsis pathway"; two intravenous catheters were inserted; blood was drawn for a variety of laboratory tests; fluid closely resembling plasma and antibiotics were administered, all within 30 minutes of arrival.

A short time later, the ED doctor shared the results of the laboratory tests: "We performed something called a 'sepsis biomarker panel' that identifies the infection in Julian's blood as well as his body's response to the infection. Based on those results, we are almost certain that he has a bloodstream infection with a very aggressive type of bacteria that usually resides in the intestine. Even more concerning is that Julian exhibits many characteristics of patients who develop a type of lung inflammation called *acute respiratory distress syndrome. We are going to start some treatments, but I think he is likely going to get worse before he gets better. Because he requires close monitoring, we are going to transfer him to the pediatric intensive care unit (PICU) at the children's hospital. They are already expecting him."*

TeleICU was initiated in the ED to monitor Julian closely and continuously. Rapid data synthesis and validation with the ED nurse aided the advanced practice provider to identify onset of hypotension, make a best practice recommendation to the ED for the initiation of vasoactive-inotropic support, and prepare the ICU team receiving Julian.

Informing parents that their child has, or is at high risk of developing, serious or life-threatening illness requires communication skills essential to all members of the PICU team. Almost certainly, these skills will be just as essential in the future as they are now, and unlikely to be replaced by advanced science or technology. Human understanding is an equal partner to technical knowledge for optimum medical care of the critically ill child.[1]

It is critical to assess the child's and parent's understanding of the underlying and developing condition and adjust one's explanation of the clinical situation to their level of prior experience and understanding. Recognizing that they are likely to experience very strong emotions in response to this information, including tremendous anxiety, guilt, grief, or anger, allows clinicians to support them appropriately. The amount of information they can absorb is significantly affected by these feelings. Making sure that we seek to understand what they are feeling and acknowledge their emotions as important and normal represents a crucial step in establishing trust between clinicians and the family. Assuring that intensive communication skill training is part of every critical care practitioner's education will remain essential in the future.

FACILITATED DIAGNOSTICS

Effective provision of acute and critical care is often defined by one parameter above all others: time. Time to recognize the onset of an illness, time to access expert care, time to make the correct diagnosis, and time to initiate the correct therapy. Historically, waiting has represented the biggest waste in medicine.[2] However, critical care professionals are increasingly thinking beyond the geographic and time boundaries of the PICU and embracing the continuum of care that starts and ends at patients' homes.[3] Although still relatively immature, the field of remote patient monitoring is evolving at a fast pace, particularly as technological advancements allow for less invasive and more efficient physiologic monitoring.[4] Within the next decade, patients at high risk for physiologic derangement will be routinely equipped with novel sensors and monitored remotely with the aid of machine learning algorithms, enabling early recognition and diagnosis of impending deterioration.[5] Today's sensors are increasingly capable of recording cardiorespiratory signals, temperature, and motion with materials that are flexible and unobtrusive.[6,7] The next decade will likely see the development of sensors capable of analyzing sweat for biomarkers, while harvesting energy from the user's body to prolong battery life.[8,9] Evolution of remote patient monitoring will also parallel the advancement of teleICU (ie, telemedicine in critical care) that will enable supply-limited providers outside of tertiary care centers to coordinate care, make earlier diagnoses, and provide advanced treatments globally at earlier time points in the critical illness continuum.[10,11]

Other advancements in diagnostic technology will enable better, more accurate, and earlier diagnoses (**Fig. 1**). For example, the fields of neonatal and pediatric critical care are poised to begin using whole genome sequencing (WGS) as a clinical test,[12–14]

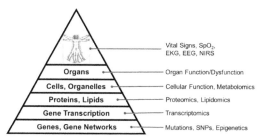

Fig. 1. Facilitated diagnostics. The history of critical care has witnessed insight of the person, then the organ, then the cell, then biochemistry and cellular biology, and most recently genetics. Real-time multimodal monitoring of each of these domains will greatly facilitate critical illness diagnosis and treatment. EEG, electroencephalogram; EKG, electrocardiogram; NIRS, near infrared spectroscopy; SNPs, single nucleotide polymorphisms; SpO$_2$, pulse oximetry hemoglobin oxygen saturation.

and professional organizations have made recommendations related to laboratory standards for sequencing and analyzing genomic data that will enable this.[15,16] Recent studies have demonstrated the feasibility of WGS as a first-line clinical test for children with critical illness, particularly in young children with undiagnosed disease suggestive of a genetic disorder.[14,17–22] Within the next decade, the cost of WGS will decrease enough that it will become feasible and cost-effective to perform on infants to better understand the risk for acute and chronic diseases throughout their lifetime. Assuming associated significant ethical and legal dilemmas can be equitably addressed, the relevant information could be made both portable and accessible while insuring confidentiality.

Other molecular and multiomics technologies are also advancing at a fast pace. Metagenomics to evaluate the microbiome and identify pathogens at earlier time points are already a reality.[23] Similarly, advancement in transcriptomics, metabolomics, proteomics, and clinical data science can be leveraged to detect disease subtypes that have both prognostic and therapeutic implications.[24] Evidence suggests the failure of treatments tested in randomized control trials in patients with critical illness such as sepsis or acute respiratory distress syndrome (ARDS) is due, at least in part, to patient heterogeneity.[25,26] Detection of disease subtypes will enable both prognostic enrichment (ie, identifying patients more likely to suffer an event) and predictive enrichments (ie, identifying a group of patients more likely to respond to a treatment) and transform the way we conduct clinical trials and treat critically ill patients.[27,28] Examples of prognostic and predictive enrichment are emerging in pediatric ARDS, sepsis, and other critical illnesses.[29]

A recent study using latent class analysis (LCA) of demographic, clinical and plasma biomarker variables revealed hypoinflammatory and hyperinflammatory subphenotypes in pediatric ARDS,[30] similar to the LCA subphenotypes previously reported in adults with ARDS that were associated with heterogeneity of treatment effects.[31,32] Sepsis phenotypes and endotypes in children have also been identified using several approaches including clinical characteristics,[33] plasma biomarkers,[34] and transcriptomics.[35,36] It is likely this field of research will continue to advance rapidly with more sophisticated diagnostics and digital technology that will enable the implementation and use of enrichment strategies in real-time.[36] In the future, it will be essential that when we apply demographic information, we are using biological, not social, descriptions, to avoid building our current biases into these novel analyses.[37]

Recent studies examining single cell RNA sequencing (scRNAseq) have reported substantial monocyte heterogeneity in sepsis and identified an early monocyte gene signature in ARDS.[38,39] In addition, metabolomics, proteomics, and methylomics are now being used in studies of critically ill patients. Several recent studies of adult COVID-19 patients have used a multiomics approach. Using longitudinal blood and plasma biomarker measurements, flow cytometry, methylomics, and bulk and scRNA-seq, investigators demonstrated complex changes in immune cells over time, as well as a link between megakaryocytes and erythroid cells and clinical outcomes.[40] Another study using integrative analysis of genomic, transcriptomic, proteomic, metabolomic, and lipidomic profiles found that neutrophil overactivation, arginine depletion, and accumulation of tryptophan metabolites correlated with T cell dysfunction in critically ill COVID-19 patients.[41] To date only a few studies using metabolomics or proteomics have included critically ill children.[42–44] However, the field is starting to flourish with promising studies underway that will facilitate future critical diagnostics.[45]

Preventing progression of illness severity requires recognition of the patient's risks, monitoring and early detection of signs of deterioration, and interventions to address the abnormalities detected. Technology will be invaluable in monitoring and early detection of patient changes[46] but clinical evaluation and treatment by a trained multidisciplinary critical care team is equally important in identifying and preventing patient deterioration.

As the ED physician had predicted, Julian's condition continued to worsen in the PICU. Based on the identified bacteria and Julian's individual immune response to the infection, he was enrolled in an adaptive platform trial for sepsis. Julian would be randomized to receive several novel therapies at different time points in his clinical course. As foreseen, he developed ARDS and required mechanical ventilation and several medication infusions for vasoactive-inotropic support and sedation. The bedside nurse explained to Mia that the medications were being titrated automatically by a best-practice, evidence-based algorithm monitoring Julian's blood pressure, his brain electrical activity, and other vital signs. "That way he receives only the minimum drug necessary, allowing us to wean these medications as soon as possible," the nurse explained. "We are also changing his antibiotic class and dose to ensure killing of the bacteria causing sepsis while preserving Julian's 'healthy bacteria.' Some bacteria can be difficult to treat, especially as Julian's body changes the way he processes the antibiotics, based on his genetics and his organ dysfunction."

Serial blood samples for the multiomic analyses were obtained to follow Julian's response to therapy. Once intubated, tracheal aspirates were also obtained to examine the lung microbiome. Eventually all the data related to biomarkers and the multiomic analyses would be deidentified and added to a federated data repository to facilitate sepsis research in children, particularly identification of novel therapies.

A wave of activity and lots of new information evolved during the next several days. Mia worked in the marketing industry, so she was not very well versed on medicine before this but since Julian's cancer diagnosis, and especially since he was admitted to the PICU with sepsis and ARDS, she had been absorbing information like a sponge. She wanted to understand everything that was happening, and a lot was happening.

LEARNING HEALTH-CARE ENVIRONMENT

Elements of a learning health-care system include provision of best-available, evidence-based care, participation in translational/clinical research and rigorous continuous quality improvement, and engagement in a shared education model (**Fig. 2**).

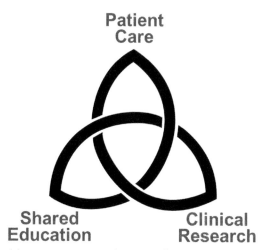

Patient
Care

Shared
Education

Clinical
Research

Fig. 2. Learning health-care system. Key elements of a learning health-care system include best-evidence clinical care, clinical research and rigorous quality improvement, and a shared education model. In addition, awareness of implementation science and need for humanism are both essential in a successful learning health-care environment.

Ideally, these elements are so integrated that each benefits from and informs the others.[47,48]

Implementation of science infrastructure is a frequently underappreciated additional essential component of a learning health-care system.[49] Advancement of pediatric critical care will not only depend on the development of novel diagnostics and therapeutics, but also depend on how we test and implement those technologies in an effective, efficient, and equitable manner. Many experts advocate for the design and implementation of multicenter, adaptive, platform trials in critical care to facilitate this process.[50,51] Characteristics of such trials include (1) embedding into routine care and leveraging the electronic health record (EHR) to complete large portions of the protocols and reduce costs, (2) engaging multifactorial statistical approaches that facilitate comparison of multiple interventions across subgroups of patients with unique characteristics, (3) using adaptive randomization with preferential assignment to those interventions that seem most favorable while maintaining robust causal inference, and 4) using a platform design that allows for continuous (and potentially perpetual) enrollment of patients after the first sets of interventional trials are completed.[50] One such trial, Randomized Embedded Multifactorial Platform for Community Acquired Pneumonia, was leveraged during the COVID-19 pandemic to rapidly test and determine the effectiveness of various immunomodulatory and anticoagulation strategies.[52–55]

Equally important in the future of our field will be the standardization of best available care using protocols and bundles to increase the value and reduce the harm associated with PICU care. Adequately explicit (eventually closed-loop) computer protocols (informed by evidence, experience, EHR data, and individual patient status) that result in consistent clinician actions will reduce unwarranted variation, increase quality of critical care and research, and enable a learning health-care system.[56] Approaches such as the ABCDEF bundle to liberate patients from the PICU more rapidly and protocols to prevent iatrogenic harm such as hospital-acquired infections will be consistently implemented and supported by EHR-based clinical decision support tools (CDST).[57–59] Increased value of critical care will be further proactively promoted by avoiding tests and interventions (interactive EHR interface) that provide no benefit to the patient but increase waste.[60,61] Personalized care provided to high-risk patients will be seamlessly integrated with standardized care for all patients to provide maximal benefit and minimize harm.

PICU providers must be aware of important differences in the ways families respond to a child's illness and the people caring for them, as well as their own responses to diverse family experiences, values, and styles, and work to address biases they may have that interfere with fully appreciating a family's needs and creating trust. Establishing confidence is difficult with families whose earlier health-care or life experiences warrant suspicion that the health-care team cannot be trusted to have their or their loved one's best interest at heart. This is currently the case for many families from racial, ethnic, or other minority groups, who need only review medical history and often their own experiences to have reason for mistrust. Until meaningful progress is made overcoming persistent health-care disparities, such suspicion is likely to persist well into the future. Acknowledging the truth of past atrocities and establishing processes that effectively reverse inequities in our patients' family experiences is critical to regaining trust.[62] Certainly, a dramatic increase in the diversity within our health profession will be essential for enhancing trust. Even as the PICU team becomes much more diverse, the need for every team member to demonstrate cultural humility and excellent communication skills will continue.[63] This expertise will need to be taught with the same conviction as PICU procedural skills.[64]

Essential skills include providing information in language that is understandable to families, using skilled translators when necessary, and then listening carefully to their responses and valuing what they say, acknowledging their emotions, and soliciting questions, repeatedly, as needed. Communication training helps practitioners speak clearly and empathically, ask open-ended questions to be sure family concerns are fully addressed, and respond more appropriately to cues from family members. PICU conversations are commonly difficult and charged with emotion. Training and experience facilitate team members to manage their own feelings while remaining open and available to families.[65] These same communications skills are also essential for good team functioning, helping assure that with all the technology at our fingertips, we trust and value the contributions of all members of the team and avoid communicating conflicting information to families.[66,67] Good communication includes the ability to provide and respond to constructive feedback from colleagues and families so that the care we provide can steadily improve.

Ongoing and just-in-time education of critical care providers will be central to maintaining the highest quality critical care. Highly trained and certified staff will apply evidence-based care and adapt to novel approaches to patient care as new evidence is generated.[68] Voice recognition/translation programs will ensure that quality pediatric critical care education is available to providers anywhere.

Importantly, the PICU of the future will learn from the past. We cannot effectively care for others without also caring for ourselves. As the SARS-CoV-2 pandemic demonstrated, overstretched and stressed providers represent not just a danger to their own well-being but also to the patients for whom they care.[69] Recognizing the importance of staff wellness to avoid burnout is, and will continue to be, critical. Wellness programs and novel approaches to self-care for all PICU staff must become a routine part of critical care shared education.[70] Grief support for health-care workers will also need to be a part of the institutional culture.[71] Ongoing, judgment-free, value-added services will be continuously available for the health-care providers, including therapeutic breaks, scheduled exercise, planned daily transitions, encouraged creativity, and surround support.[72] These programs may be informed by high-quality

RCTs that compare different interventions but will also be part of "continuous quality improvement" in the PICU.[73]

Julian's course in the PICU continued with a steady and reassuring trajectory toward recovery. The PICU team changed his feeding formula and added additional fiber and nutrients after a stool study demonstrated low levels of some types of healthy bacteria. His antibiotics were stopped after only 6 days once all traces of infection disappeared from the bloodstream and the risk for antibiotic resistance became concerning. His central catheter was also removed because a machine learning algorithm indicated a very high risk for catheter-related bloodstream infection. Julian started physical therapy shortly after admission to the PICU and continued in earnest after his ARDS improved and he was extubated. The hospital provided informative and user-friendly modules in the patient's portal that were tailored to Julian's case. Mia watched and read everything she could on sepsis, ARDS, and mechanical ventilation. Delirium, which she had not previously encountered, became the epicenter of their lives for several days.

CONTINUOUS ADVANCEMENT OF CARE

Biomedical "big data," data science, and clinical informatics will likely have a major influence on continuously advancing PICU care in the coming decade (**Fig. 3**). The widespread implementation of EHRs in the last 15 years has established a digital infrastructure to support the future of health care.[74] Few places are as data-intensive and are as likely to benefit from data-driven technologies as the PICU. Multicenter data collaborative projects that leverage interoperable EHR technologies will enable more rapid development, validation, dissemination, and implementation of machine learning algorithms and CDST.[75–77] Algorithms based in the EHR that facilitate proactive weaning of titratable PICU therapies (mechanical ventilation, vasoactive-inotropic support, analgesia/anxiolytic infusions) when it is safe to do so, will add value to critical care.[56] Future mechanical ventilators will be sophisticated enough to sense changes in patient lung compliance and work of breathing. Using a data algorithm feedback loop, such ventilators will be programmed to automatically adjust/respond and titrate ventilator support in real time. Intravenous pumps with medication infusions will integrate patient data and sense physiologic changes to automatically titrate analgesia/

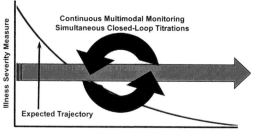

Fig. 3. Continuous advancement of care. Critical care includes treatment of the primary illness/injury as well as avoiding iatrogenic injury associated with treatment. In the future, patients' trajectories will be anticipated with precision. Off-course from anticipated trajectory, based on multimodal monitoring (see **Fig. 1**), will generate alarms indicating need for closer clinical scrutiny. Infusions will be continuously titrated using closed loop systems again linked to multimodal monitoring. This will facilitate escalation as well as weaning, to create a pull system (red horizontal *arrow*) to decrease the duration of organ support and PICU stay.

anxiolysis and vasoactive-inotropic medications in a closed loop fashion using evidenced-based metrics for optimal recovery and management. Capturing and analyzing high-frequency physiologic data from bedside monitors will also likely lead to a whole host of novel algorithms for high-risk patients, as demonstrated by recent studies in PICU patients with the use of so-called physiomarkers.[78,79] Some of these algorithms using physiologic data may be able to be extended beyond the walls of the PICU to both pre-PICU and post-PICU settings to predict deterioration and monitor recovery.[80,81]

As we develop and refine CDST and other data-driven systems enabled by machine learning algorithms, special attention will need to be paid to the human factors involved in the implementation and evaluation of these technologies.[82] Prediction models powering bedside CDST systems must first and foremost position human users at the center of their design that must be interpretable, informative, and actionable.[83] These tools need to be seamlessly integrated into clinical workflows, making it easy to do the right thing and provide the right care for the right patient at the right time, which is to continuously advance care.[84] Furthermore, advancements in monitoring technology and integration with routine care practices may finally liberate clinicians from some of the menial documentation tasks of today and allow them to focus on the needs of their patients and their families.[85] Clinical data science and computational biology will also help us answer questions about the complex systems involved in critical illness that for years have eluded us and cannot be answered with reductionist approaches.[86] This includes better understanding the role of the microbiome in critical illness.[87]

Whole metagenome sequencing of human microbiota has been used to examine the composition of the microbiome and to identify pathogenic microbes in critically ill children and adults.[20,88,89] Dysbiosis, or an imbalance in the composition of the commensal microbial communities, often characterized by a decrease in diversity in the gut and lung microbiota, influences host immunity and disease, including critical illness.[90,91] Therapeutic interventions targeting the gut are now being explored as an additional approach to treating critically ill patients and reestablishing a normal microbiota after critical illness.[90] Getting patients back to, "you are what you eat," will represent another aspect of continuous advancement of critical care.

Not every aspect of continuous advancement of care will require cutting-edge technology to make a big impact. With increasing integration of technology, automated protocols, and enhanced clinical decision support, one might assume that the future of pediatric critical care would be an automated one, with less need for skilled leadership and empathetic human caregivers. This could not be further from the truth.[92] By leveraging technology, we may be able to improve outcomes but only if we do not lose sight of the humanism that is essential in pediatric critical care.

As a case in point, in 2017, delirium occurred in approximately 25% of critically ill children.[93] A subset of delirium is probably a function of sedation and polypharmacy and can be minimized with the use of CDST as previously described.[94] However, this likely accounts for less than half of pediatric delirium cases. The mainstay of delirium prevention and treatment is, in fact, human interaction. Studies have shown that the presence of a familiar caregiver, frequent orientation, cognitive stimulation, and physical exercise are all effective ways to decrease delirium prevalence.[95–97] A personalized approach, taking the child's developmental stage into consideration, and incorporating family customs, is essential. Intelligent, thoughtful use of technology, rather than replacing the need for medical providers at the bedside, should allow more time for provider-to-patient interactions.

Family presence has long been recognized as a critical aspect of the continuous advancement of PICU care.[98] Technological advancements may allow us to assist families in being part of the care team with reliable and pertinent information and communication at any time of day. For example, a pilot study in Taiwan demonstrated the feasibility of a self-service, self-directed information portal to deepen understanding of elements of critical care by family members.[99] Virtual visiting through video conferencing can reduce feelings of isolation and psychological stress, while maintaining morale and feelings of connectedness even when access to the hospital by family members and friends is limited.[100] Therapeutic PICU environments and patient rooms can also promote healing using evidence-based design, inclusion of elements of nature, views of outdoors, and peaceful spaces.[101,102]

One of the most exciting—and low hanging—arenas for improvement in the care we provide regards language services. Limited English proficiency has been recently identified as a risk factor for poor pediatric outcomes.[103] By 2030, population predictions for the United States indicate that the number of ethnic minority children will exceed the number of non-Latino white children.[104] The PICU of the future will leverage technology to provide real-time, language concordant services to enable effective provider–parent and provider–patient communication. The cumbersome systems currently in place in many large centers will be replaced by smooth and efficient user-friendly services.[105] Of course, language alone will not be enough; cultural humility is necessary as well.[106] Advancing workforce diversity to mirror the populations we serve should allow us to appreciate one another's humanity both in the learning as well as working environment ultimately facilitating improved care for patients of all backgrounds.

The make-up of the future PICU team will continue to be multidisciplinary.[10,107] Ongoing shortages of adequately trained critical care team members remains problematic—this is true for physicians, nurses, respiratory therapists, pharmacists, and other team members.[108–111] One health-care role that is likely to expand is that of the advanced practice provider (APP), a nurse practitioner or physician assistant. Both APP professions are growing but with rising demand for PICU services, workforce demand continues to outpace supply. As previously noted, teleICU will expand individual provider reach to more patients at any given time. There will be advances in the methods for deploying additional medical provider staffing on a regional or national scale.[112] If the future of pediatric critical care includes more personal interactions and less pharmacology, there will likely be a need for bedside sitters or surrogate patient "aunties" to enhance human interactions particularly when family members cannot be present.[113,114]

An ongoing practical challenge is how to implement effective data modeling to improve PICU care delivery.[115] In the PICU of the future, sophisticated, integrated predictive modeling will be applied to correctly size the health care team make-up. Patients' illness/recovery trajectories will be collated and analyzed to assist healthcare leaders in adjusting workforce staffing needs. In the current state, staffing adjustments for front line providers such as rgistered nurses (RNs), respiratory therapists (RTs), and ancillary staff occurs shift-to-shift and day-to-day. In an ideal future state, patient trajectory modeling will facilitate avoidance of overstaffing and understaffing. The PICU of the future will have an expandable ICU staffing pool with a full range of multidisciplinary team members using regional and national strategies to deploy health-care providers who have critical care training in response to surges, pandemics, or national disasters.[116]

After 3 weeks in the hospital, Julian went home and continued an intense rehabilitation program. His school developed a study plan for him, and his pediatrician worked with the hospital team to design a care plan that included several follow-up blood tests, cognitive examinations, and physical activity challenges. The hospital also put Julian in touch with a group of teenagers who had also experienced sepsis, and he started texting with some of them. The stress and trauma of Julian's hospitalization and acute illness resulted in residual negative psychological effects on Julian's parents and siblings. The household was strained by acute-on-chronic worry and uncertainty. Julian's parents and siblings participated in hospital-based workshops and programs to help them channel and manage anxiety and distress. They were also connected with a support group focused on stress management for caregivers and family members. As a monitoring tool and for peace of mind, Julian continued to wear his smartwatch. It was upgraded with additional functionality to monitor pharmacokinetic processes in the body as well as early warning signs of stress and depression.

CONTINUUM OF PEDIATRIC CRITICAL CARE

Surviving critical illness is of course the priority but survival is only the beginning; as mortality associated with pediatric critical illness is decreasing, long-term morbidity is increasingly recognized as another crucial outcome[117–121] (**Fig. 4**). We are learning to identify risks for morbidity among PICU survivors and developing strategies in the PICU to minimize long-term harm from critical illness/injury and its treatments. In the future, critical care providers will own postintensive care syndrome. Participation in PICU follow-up clinics is gaining momentum and can provide value not only to patients but also to critical care practitioners.[122] By participating in critical care follow-up clinics, PICU providers can learn more about their patients and their families and have the benefit of continuing relationships with them, especially following a long and complicated course in the PICU. Effects of pediatric critical illness on the

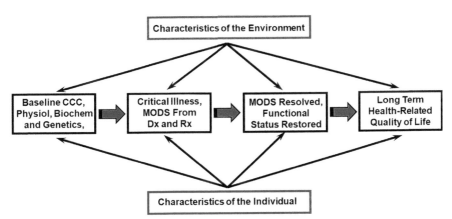

Fig. 4. Continuum of pediatric critical care. Each critically ill child presents with a unique baseline. Critical care largely focuses on preventing, diagnosing, and treating organ dysfunction but also includes iatrogenic injury related to critical care. With resolution of organ dysfunction, significant functional status abnormalities are frequently restored and the PICU Team may celebrate a "great save." However, children and their families surviving critical illness typically face a long-term burden of impaired health-related quality of life in relation to baseline status. Trajectory of recovery toward baseline is affected by characteristics of the patient and the environment in which the patient resides. biochem, biochemistry; CCC, chronic comorbid conditions; Dx, primary diagnosis; MODS, multiple organ dysfunction syndrome; physiol, physiology; Rx, treatment-related injury. (*Original concept from* Wilson IB, Cleary PD. Linking clinical variables with health-related quality of life. A conceptual model of patient outcomes. JAMA 1995; 273: 59-65.)

family members do not end on discharge from the PICU. For many families, this is only the beginning of the journey.[123] More than 20% of parents have symptomatic levels of posttraumatic stress disorder months after their child who survives critical illness is discharged home.[124] Parents' mental health is inextricably bound with that of the child's well-being. Parental posttraumatic stress disorder has been shown to be associated with impaired family functioning and decreased parenting efficacy, with downstream effects on the health and well-being of the child survivor.[125] Future pediatric critical care will be exceptionally aware of this. This will require responsibility not just for the child's well-being but also the larger family unit. The recent emergence of post-PICU clinics will continue to grow, and provide an opportunity to identify families who are struggling.[122] However, rather than waiting until after discharge, providers will begin to intervene earlier while the parents and children are still in the PICU. Randomized clinical trials will have taught us which interventions work during the PICU stay to decrease the long-term effects of pediatric critical illness. All families will be automatically screened before discharge for psychological symptomatology and psychosocial risk assessment to identify those at highest risk.

The PICU team can play an important role in assuring that care provided before, during, and after a patient's critical care needs are resolved is entirely equitable. The quality of treatment before PICU admission has been shown to be an important factor in severity of illness and outcome, and minority groups are disproportionately likely to be treated in lower quality care institutions.[126,127] Critical care providers have a window on social and environmental factors that increase the risk of life-threatening illness or injury, suboptimal access to primary, preventive care, and inequitable access to needed rehabilitation services. Although the primary focus will probably remain assuring excellent, equitable PICU care for all children, PICU providers will be in an excellent position to educate families, policy makers, and the larger health-care system about the need to optimize prevention, assure that adequate resources are available for primary care physicians to receive expert advice, and assure that excellent support is available to all families, regardless of their ancestry, zip code, or socioeconomic status.[63,128,129]

SUMMARY

After 2 months, Julian was able to join his regular class schedule in school and started training with the basketball team again. Moreover, the best news: Julian's leukemia was in remission and all the surveillance tests were coming back negative. Just this morning, he had asked Mia permission to learn how to play the drums. His friends from the sepsis group wanted to form a rock band called, "The Resistant Biomes." A few months ago, the idea of drums in the house would have been a hard "no," but today Mia hugged her son and decided she would just need to buy earplugs.

DISCLOSURES

All authors disclose that they have no real or perceived conflicts of interest related to composition of this article.

REFERENCES

1. Todres ID. Communication between physician, patient, and family in the pediatric intensive care unit. Crit Care Med 1993;21(9 Suppl):S383–6.

2. Bagheri Lankarani K, Ghahramani S, Roozitalab M, et al. What do hospital doctors and nurses think wastes their time? SAGE Open Med 2019;7. 2050312118813680.
3. Cabrini L, Landoni G, Antonelli M, et al. Critical care in the near future: patient-centered, beyond space and time boundaries. Minerva Anestesiol 2016;82(5): 599–604.
4. Vegesna A, Tran M, Angelaccio M, et al. Remote patient monitoring via non-invasive digital technologies: a systematic review. Telemed J E Health 2017; 23(1):3–17.
5. Xu S, Jayaraman A, Rogers JA. Skin sensors are the future of health care. Nature 2019;571(7765):319–21.
6. Lee SP, Ha G, Wright DE, et al. Highly flexible, wearable, and disposable cardiac biosensors for remote and ambulatory monitoring. NPJ Digit Med 2018;1:2.
7. Tavakoli Golpaygani A, Mehdizadeh AR. Future of wearable health devices: smartwatches VS smart headphones. J Biomed Phys Eng 2021;11(5):561–2.
8. Heikenfeld J, Jajack A, Feldman B, et al. Accessing analytes in biofluids for peripheral biochemical monitoring. Nat Biotechnol 2019;37(4):407–19.
9. Wu W, Zhang Y, Ding D, et al. A high-performing direct carbon fuel cell with a 3D architectured anode Operated below 600 degrees C. Adv Mater 2018;30(4).
10. Welsh C, Rincon T, Berman I, et al. TeleICU interdisciplinary care teams. Crit Care Nurs Clin North Am 2021;33(4):459–70.
11. Dayal P, Hojman NM, Kissee JL, et al. Impact of telemedicine on severity of illness and outcomes among children transferred from referring emergency departments to a children's hospital PICU. Pediatr Crit Care Med 2016;17(6): 516–21.
12. Marshall CR, Bick D, Belmont JW, et al. The Medical Genome Initiative: moving whole-genome sequencing for rare disease diagnosis to the clinic. Genome Med 2020;12(1):48.
13. Dahmer MK. Whole genome sequencing as a first-line clinical test: almost ready for prime time. Crit Care Med 2021;49(10):1815–7.
14. Australian Genomics Health Alliance Acute Care F, Lunke S, Eggers S, et al. Feasibility of Ultra-rapid exome sequencing in critically ill infants and children with suspected Monogenic conditions in the Australian public health care system. JAMA 2020;323(24):2503–11.
15. Aziz N, Zhao Q, Bry L, et al. College of American Pathologists' laboratory standards for next-generation sequencing clinical tests. Arch Pathol Lab Med 2015; 139(4):481–93.
16. Roy S, Coldren C, Karunamurthy A, et al. Standards and Guidelines for validating next-generation sequencing Bioinformatics pipelines: a Joint recommendation of the association for molecular pathology and the college of American pathologists. J Mol Diagn 2018;20(1):4–27.
17. Willig LK, Petrikin JE, Smith LD, et al. Whole-genome sequencing for identification of Mendelian disorders in critically ill infants: a retrospective analysis of diagnostic and clinical findings. Lancet Respir Med 2015;3(5):377–87.
18. French CE, Delon I, Dolling H, et al. Whole genome sequencing reveals that genetic conditions are frequent in intensively ill children. Intensive Care Med 2019; 45(5):627–36.
19. Sanford EF, Clark MM, Farnaes L, et al. Rapid whole genome sequencing has clinical utility in children in the PICU. Pediatr Crit Care Med 2019;20(11): 1007–20.

20. Wu B, Kang W, Wang Y, et al. Application of full-spectrum rapid clinical genome sequencing improves diagnostic rate and clinical outcomes in critically ill infants in the China neonatal genomes project. Crit Care Med 2021;49(10):1674–83.

21. Gubbels CS, VanNoy GE, Madden JA, et al. Prospective, phenotype-driven selection of critically ill neonates for rapid exome sequencing is associated with high diagnostic yield. Genet Med 2020;22(4):736–44.

22. Dimmock DP, Clark MM, Gaughran M, et al. An RCT of rapid genomic sequencing among seriously ill infants results in high clinical utility, changes in management, and low perceived harm. Am J Hum Genet 2020;107(5): 942–52.

23. Pendleton KM, Erb-Downward JR, Bao Y, et al. Rapid pathogen identification in bacterial pneumonia using real-time Metagenomics. Am J Respir Crit Care Med 2017;196(12):1610–2.

24. Wong HR. Personalized medicine, endotypes, and intensive care medicine. Intensive Care Med 2015;41(6):1138–40.

25. Iwashyna TJ, Burke JF, Sussman JB, et al. Implications of heterogeneity of treatment effect for reporting and analysis of randomized trials in critical care. Am J Respir Crit Care Med 2015;192(9):1045–51.

26. Seymour CW, Kennedy JN, Wang S, et al. Derivation, validation, and potential treatment implications of novel clinical phenotypes for sepsis. JAMA 2019; 321(20):2003–17.

27. Prescott HC, Calfee CS, Thompson BT, et al. Toward smarter Lumping and smarter splitting: rethinking strategies for sepsis and acute respiratory distress syndrome clinical trial design. Am J Respir Crit Care Med 2016;194(2):147–55.

28. Stanski NL, Wong HR. Prognostic and predictive enrichment in sepsis. Nat Rev Nephrol 2020;16(1):20–31.

29. Sanchez-Pinto LN, Stroup EK, Pendergrast T, et al. Derivation and validation of novel phenotypes of multiple organ dysfunction syndrome in critically ill children. JAMA Netw Open 2020;3(8). e209271.

30. Dahmer MK, Yang G, Zhang M, et al. Identification of phenotypes in paediatric patients with acute respiratory distress syndrome: a latent class analysis. Lancet Respir Med 2022;10(3):289–97.

31. Calfee CS, Delucchi K, Parsons PE, et al. Subphenotypes in acute respiratory distress syndrome: latent class analysis of data from two randomised controlled trials. Lancet Respir Med 2014;2(8):611–20.

32. Famous KR, Delucchi K, Ware LB, et al. Acute respiratory distress syndrome subphenotypes respond differently to randomized fluid management strategy. Am J Respir Crit Care Med 2017;195(3):331–8.

33. Carcillo JA, Berg RA, Wessel D, et al. A multicenter Network assessment of three inflammation phenotypes in pediatric sepsis-induced multiple organ failure. Pediatr Crit Care Med 2019;20(12):1137–46.

34. Wong HR, Salisbury S, Xiao Q, et al. The pediatric sepsis biomarker risk model. Crit Care 2012;16(5):R174.

35. Wong HR, Cvijanovich N, Lin R, et al. Identification of pediatric septic shock subclasses based on genome-wide expression profiling. BMC Med 2009;7: 34 1.

36. Wong HR, Cvijanovich NZ, Anas N, et al. Developing a clinically feasible personalized medicine approach to pediatric septic shock. Am J Respir Crit Care Med 2015;191(3):309–15.

37. Zurca AD, Suttle ML, October TW. An antiracism approach to conducting, reporting, and evaluating pediatric critical care research. Pediatr Crit Care Med 2022;23(2):129–32.

38. Wen M, Cai G, Ye J, et al. Single-cell transcriptomics reveals the alteration of peripheral blood mononuclear cells driven by sepsis. Ann Transl Med 2020; 8(4):125.

39. Jiang Y, Rosborough BR, Chen J, et al. Single cell RNA sequencing identifies an early monocyte gene signature in acute respiratory distress syndrome. JCI Insight 2020;5(13).

40. Bernardes JP, Mishra N, Tran F, et al. Longitudinal multi-omics analyses identify responses of megakaryocytes, erythroid cells, and plasmablasts as hallmarks of severe COVID-19. Immunity 2020;53(6):1296–12314 e9.

41. Wu P, Chen D, Ding W, et al. The trans-omics landscape of COVID-19. Nat Commun 2021;12(1):4543.

42. Grunwell JR, Rad MG, Stephenson ST, et al. Cluster analysis and profiling of airway fluid metabolites in pediatric acute hypoxemic respiratory failure. Sci Rep 2021;11(1):23019.

43. Yehya N, Fazelinia H, Lawrence GG, et al. Plasma Nucleosomes are associated with mortality in pediatric acute respiratory distress syndrome. Crit Care Med 2021;49(7):1149–58.

44. Yehya N, Fazelinia H, Taylor DM, et al. Differentiating children with sepsis with and without acute respiratory distress syndrome using proteomics. Am J Physiol Lung Cell Mol Physiol 2022;322(3):L365–72.

45. Feinstein Y, Walker JC, Peters MJ, et al. Cohort profile of the Biomarkers of Acute Serious Illness in Children (BASIC) study: a prospective multicentre cohort study in critically ill children. BMJ Open 2018;8(11). e024729.

46. Joshi R, Kommers D, Oosterwijk L, et al. Predicting neonatal sepsis using features of heart rate variability, respiratory characteristics, and ECG-derived Estimates of infant motion. IEEE J Biomed Health Inform 2020;24(3):681–92.

47. Institute of Medicine. The learning healthcare system: Workshop summary. Washington, DC: National Academies Press; 2007.

48. Bakken S. Progress toward a science of learning systems for healthcare. J Am Med Inform Assoc 2021;28(6):1063–4.

49. Barr J, Paulson SS, Kamdar B, et al. The coming of age of implementation science and research in critical care medicine. Crit Care Med 2021;49(8):1254–75.

50. Angus DC, Berry S, Lewis RJ, et al. The REMAP-CAP (randomized embedded multifactorial adaptive platform for community-acquired pneumonia) study. Rationale and design. Ann Am Thorac Soc 2020;17(7):879–91.

51. Noor NM, Pett SL, Esmail H, et al. Adaptive platform trials using multi-arm, multi-stage protocols: getting fast answers in pandemic settings. F1000Res 2020;9: 1109.

52. Investigators R-C, Gordon AC, Mouncey PR, et al. Interleukin-6 receptor antagonists in critically ill patients with covid-19. N Engl J Med 2021;384(16): 1491–502.

53. Angus DC, Derde L, Al-Beidh F, et al. Effect of hydrocortisone on mortality and organ support in patients with severe COVID-19: the REMAP-CAP COVID-19 corticosteroid domain randomized clinical trial. JAMA 2020;324(13):1317–29.

54. Remap-Cap Writing Committee for the REMAP-CAP Investigators, Bradbury CA, Lawler PR, et al. Effect of antiplatelet therapy on survival and organ support-free days in critically ill patients with COVID-19: a randomized clinical trial. JAMA 2022;327(13):1247–59.

55. The REMAP-CAP, ACTIV-4a, and ATTACC Investigators. Therapeutic anticoagulation with heparin in critically ill patients with covid-19. N Engl J Med 2021; 385(9):777–89.

56. Morris AH, Stagg B, Lanspa M, et al. Enabling a learning healthcare system with automated computer protocols that produce replicable and personalized clinician actions. J Am Med Inform Assoc 2021;28(6):1330–44.

57. Barnes-Daly MA, Phillips G, Ely EW. Improving hospital survival and reducing brain dysfunction at seven California community hospitals: implementing PAD Guidelines via the ABCDEF bundle in 6,064 patients. Crit Care Med 2017; 45(2):171–8.

58. Pun BT, Balas MC, Barnes-Daly MA, et al. Caring for critically ill patients with the ABCDEF bundle: results of the ICU liberation collaborative in over 15,000 adults. Crit Care Med 2019;47(1):3–14.

59. Geva A, Albert BD, Hamilton S, et al. eSIMPLER: a dynamic, electronic health record-integrated checklist for clinical decision support during PICU daily rounds. Pediatr Crit Care Med 2021;22(10):898–905.

60. Halpern SD, Becker D, Curtis JR, et al. The choosing Wisely(R) top 5 list in critical care medicine. Am J Respir Crit Care Med 2014;190(7):818–26.

61. Zimmerman JJ, Harmon LA, Smithburger PL, et al. Choosing Wisely for critical care: the next five. Crit Care Med 2021;49(3):472–81.

62. Suttle M, Hall MW, Pollack MM, et al. Therapeutic alliance between Bereaved parents and physicians in the PICU. Pediatr Crit Care Med 2021;22(4):e243–52.

63. Metzl JM, Hansen H. Structural competency: theorizing a new medical engagement with stigma and inequality. Soc Sci Med 2014;103:126–33.

64. Fryer-Edwards K, Arnold RM, Baile W, et al. Reflective teaching practices: an approach to teaching communication skills in a small-group setting. Acad Med 2006;81(7):638–44.

65. Meert KL, Eggly S, Pollack M, et al. Parents' perspectives on physician-parent communication near the time of a child's death in the pediatric intensive care unit. Pediatr Crit Care Med 2008;9(1):2–7.

66. October TW, Dizon ZB, Hamilton MF, et al. Communication training for interspecialty clinicians. Clin Teach 2019;16(3):242–7.

67. Michalsen A, Long AC, DeKeyser Ganz F, et al. Interprofessional shared decision-making in the ICU: a systematic review and recommendations from an expert panel. Crit Care Med 2019;47(9):1258–66.

68. Hickey PA, Gauvreau K, Porter C, et al. The impact of critical care nursing certification on pediatric patient outcomes. Pediatr Crit Care Med 2018;19(8): 718–24.

69. Restauri N, Sheridan AD. Burnout and posttraumatic stress disorder in the coronavirus disease 2019 (COVID-19) pandemic: intersection, impact, and interventions. J Am Coll Radiol 2020;17(7):921–6.

70. National academy of medicine. National plan for health workforce well being. 2022. https://nap.nationalacademies.org/catalog/26744/national-plan-for-health-workforce-well-being. [Accessed 13 October 2022].

71. Rabow MW, Huang CS, White-Hammond GE, et al. Witnesses and victims both: healthcare workers and grief in the time of COVID-19. J Pain Symptom Manage 2021;62(3):647–56.

72. Haupt A. What burnout really means, and what bosses and employees can do about it15. Washington, DC: Washington Post; 2021. p. 2021.

73. Hysong SJ, Best RG, Pugh JA. Audit and feedback and clinical practice guideline adherence: making feedback actionable. Implement Sci 2006;1:9.

74. Sanchez-Pinto LN, Luo Y, Churpek MM. Big data and data science in critical care. Chest 2018;154(5):1239–48.

75. Bennett TD, Russell S, Albers DJ. Neural Networks for mortality prediction: ready for prime time? Pediatr Crit Care Med 2021;22(6):578–81.

76. Brant EB, Kennedy JN, King AJ, et al. Developing a shared sepsis data infrastructure: a systematic review and concept map to FHIR. NPJ Digit Med 2022;5(1):44.

77. Sanchez-Pinto LN, Dziorny AC. From bedside to Bytes and back: data quality and standardization for research, quality improvement, and clinical decision support in the Era of electronic health records. Pediatr Crit Care Med 2020; 21(8):780–1.

78. Kamaleswaran R, Akbilgic O, Hallman MA, et al. Applying artificial intelligence to identify physiomarkers predicting severe sepsis in the PICU. Pediatr Crit Care Med 2018;19(10):e495–503.

79. Badke CM, Marsillio LE, Carroll MS, et al. Development of a heart rate variability risk score to predict organ dysfunction and death in critically ill children. Pediatr Crit Care Med 2021;22(8):e437–47.

80. Mayampurath A, Volchenboum SL, Sanchez-Pinto LN. Using photoplethysmography data to estimate heart rate variability and its association with organ dysfunction in pediatric oncology patients. NPJ Digit Med 2018;1:29.

81. Badke CM, Swigart L, Carroll MS, et al. Autonomic Nervous system dysfunction is associated with Re-hospitalization in pediatric septic shock survivors. Front Pediatr 2021;9:745844.

82. Shortliffe EH, Sepulveda MJ. Clinical decision support in the Era of artificial intelligence. JAMA 2018;320(21):2199–200.

83. Sanchez-Pinto LN, Bennett TD. Evaluation of machine learning models for clinical prediction problems. Pediatr Crit Care Med 2022;23(5):405–8.

84. Meissen H, Gong MN, Wong AI, et al. The future of critical care: Optimizing technologies and a learning healthcare system to potentiate a more humanistic approach to critical care. Crit Care Explor 2022;4(3):e0659.

85. Poncette AS, Mosch L, Spies C, et al. Improvements in patient monitoring in the intensive care Unit: survey study. J Med Internet Res 2020;22(6):e19091.

86. Seymour CW, Gomez H, Chang CH, et al. Precision medicine for all? Challenges and opportunities for a precision medicine approach to critical illness. Crit Care 2017;21(1):257.

87. Mittal R, Coopersmith CM. Redefining the gut as the motor of critical illness. Trends Mol Med 2014;20(4):214–23.

88. Langelier C, Kalantar KL, Moazed F, et al. Integrating host response and unbiased microbe detection for lower respiratory tract infection diagnosis in critically ill adults. Proc Natl Acad Sci U S A 2018;115(52):E12353–62.

89. Zinter MS, Dvorak CC, Mayday MY, et al. Pulmonary metagenomic sequencing suggests Missed infections in immunocompromised children. Clin Infect Dis 2019;68(11):1847–55.

90. Martin-Loeches I, Dickson R, Torres A, et al. The importance of airway and lung microbiome in the critically ill. Crit Care 2020;24(1):537.

91. Petersen C, Round JL. Defining dysbiosis and its influence on host immunity and disease. Cell Microbiol 2014;16(7):1024–33.

92. Kissoon N. Bench-to-bedside review: humanism in pediatric critical care medicine - a leadership challenge. Crit Care 2005;9(4):371–5.

93. Traube C, Silver G, Reeder RW, et al. Delirium in critically ill children: an international point prevalence study. Crit Care Med 2017;45(4):584–90.

94. Patel SB, Poston JT, Pohlman A, et al. Rapidly reversible, sedation-related delirium versus persistent delirium in the intensive care unit. Am J Respir Crit Care Med 2014;189(6):658–65.

95. Inouye SK, Bogardus ST Jr, Charpentier PA, et al. A multicomponent intervention to prevent delirium in hospitalized older patients. N Engl J Med 1999;340(9): 669–76.

96. Simone S, Edwards S, Lardieri A, et al. Implementation of an ICU bundle: an interprofessional quality improvement project to enhance delirium management and monitor delirium prevalence in a single PICU. Pediatr Crit Care Med 2017; 18(6):531–40.

97. Smith HAB, Besunder JB, Betters KA, et al. 2022 society of critical care medicine clinical practice Guidelines on prevention and management of pain, agitation, Neuromuscular Blockade, and delirium in critically ill pediatric patients with consideration of the ICU environment and early Mobility. Pediatr Crit Care Med 2022;23(2):e74–110.

98. Aronson PL, Yau J, Helfaer MA, et al. Impact of family presence during pediatric intensive care unit rounds on the family and medical team. Pediatrics 2009; 124(4):1119–25.

99. Chang IC, Hou YH, Lu LJ, et al. Self-service system for the family members of ICU patients: a pilot study. Healthcare (Basel) 2022;10(3).

100. Rose L, Yu L, Casey J, et al. Communication and virtual visiting for families of patients in intensive care during the COVID-19 pandemic: a UK national survey. Ann Am Thorac Soc 2021;18(10):1685–92.

101. Sundberg F, Fridh I, Lindahl B, et al. Visitor's experiences of an evidence-based designed healthcare environment in an intensive care Unit. HERD 2021;14(2): 178–91.

102. Verderber S, Gray S, Suresh-Kumar S, et al. Intensive care Unit Built environments: a comprehensive Literature review (2005-2020). HERD 2021;14(4): 368–415.

103. Flores G, Rabke-Verani J, Pine W, et al. The importance of cultural and linguistic issues in the emergency care of children. Pediatr Emerg Care 2002;18(4): 271–84.

104. United States census Bureaqu. Population projections of the United States by age, sex, race, and hispanic Origin: 1995-2050. 1995 (revised 2021). https://www.census.gov/library/publications/1996/demo/p25-1130.html. [Accessed 13 October 2022].

105. Regenstein M, Huang J, West C, et al. Hospital language services: quality improvement and performance Measures. Rockville (MD): Agency for Healthcare Research and Quality; 2008.

106. Greene-Moton E, Minkler M. Cultural competence or cultural humility? Moving beyond the debate. Health Promot Pract 2020;21(1):142–5.

107. Brilli RJ, Spevetz A, Branson RD, et al, for the American College of Critical Care Medicine Task Force on Models of Critical Care Delivery. Critical care delivery in the intensive care unit: defining clinical roles and the best practice model. Crit Care Med 2001;29(10):2007–19.

108. Bourgault AM. The nursing shortage and work expectations are in critical condition: is anyone listening? Crit Care Nurse 2022;42(2):8–11.

109. Vera San Juan N, Clark SE, Camilleri M, et al. Training and redeployment of healthcare workers to intensive care units (ICUs) during the COVID-19 pandemic: a systematic review. BMJ Open 2022;12(1):e050038.

110. Halpern NA, Pastores SM, Oropello JM, et al. Critical care medicine in the United States: addressing the intensivist shortage and image of the specialty. Crit Care Med 2013;41(12):2754–61.
111. Association of. American medical colleges. The complexities of physician supply and demand: projections from 2018 to 2033. 2020. https://www.aamc.org/system/files/2020-06/stratcomm-aamc-physician-workforce-projections-june-2020.pdf. [Accessed 13 October 2022].
112. Lustbader D, Fein A. Emerging trends in ICU management and staffing. Crit Care Clin 2000;16(4):735–48.
113. Carr FM. The role of sitters in delirium: an update. Can Geriatr J 2013;16(1): 22–36.
114. Greeley AM, Tanner EP, Mak S, et al. Sitters as a patient safety strategy to reduce hospital falls: a systematic review. Ann Intern Med 2020;172(5):317–24.
115. Carra G, Salluh JIF, da Silva Ramos FJ, et al. Data-driven ICU management: using Big Data and algorithms to improve outcomes. J Crit Care 2020;60:300–4.
116. Arabi YM, Azoulay E, Al-Dorzi HM, et al. How the COVID-19 pandemic will change the future of critical care. Intensive Care Med 2021;47(3):282–91.
117. Pollack MM, Banks R, Holubkov R, et al. And the Eunice Kennedy shriver national institute of child H, human development collaborative pediatric critical care research N. Long-term outcome of PICU patients discharged with new, functional status morbidity. Pediatr Crit Care Med 2021;22(1):27–39.
118. Fink EL, Maddux AB, Pinto N, et al. A core outcome set for pediatric critical care. Crit Care Med 2020;48(12):1819–28.
119. Killien EY, Farris RWD, Watson RS, et al. Health-related quality of life among survivors of pediatric sepsis. Pediatr Crit Care Med 2019;20(6):501–9.
120. Maddux AB, Pinto N, Fink EL, et al. Postdischarge outcome domains in pediatric critical care and the instruments used to evaluate them: a scoping review. Crit Care Med 2020;48(12):e1313–21.
121. Zimmerman JJ, Banks R, Berg RA, et al. Trajectory of mortality and health-related quality of life morbidity following community-acquired pediatric septic shock. Crit Care Med 2020;48(3):329–37.
122. Ducharme-Crevier L, La KA, Francois T, et al. PICU follow-up clinic: patient and family outcomes 2 Months after discharge. Pediatr Crit Care Med 2021;22(11): 935–43.
123. Ely W. Every Deep-drawn Breath. New York: Scribner; 2021.
124. Ko MSM, Poh PF, Heng KYC, et al. Assessment of long-term psychological outcomes after pediatric intensive care Unit admission: a systematic review and Meta-analysis. JAMA Pediatr 2022;176(3):e215767.
125. Christie H, Hamilton-Giachritsis C, Alves-Costa F, et al. The impact of parental posttraumatic stress disorder on parenting: a systematic review. Eur J Psychotraumatol 2019;10(1):1550345.
126. McGowan SK, Sarigiannis KA, Fox SC, et al. Racial disparities in ICU outcomes: a systematic review. Crit Care Med 2022;50(1):1–20.
127. Sample M, Acharya A, O'Hearn K, et al. The relationship between remoteness and outcomes in critically ill children. Pediatr Crit Care Med 2017;18(11): e514–20.
128. Cooke CR, Kahn JM. Deconstructing racial and ethnic disparities in critical care. Crit Care Med 2010;38(3):978–80.
129. Mayr FB, Yende S, D'Angelo G, et al. Do hospitals provide lower quality of care to black patients for pneumonia? Crit Care Med 2010;38(3):759–65.

9780323938754